Fatigue in Cancer

Fatigue in Cancer
A Multidimensional Approach

Maryl L. Winningham

and

Margaret Barton-Burke

Jones and Bartlett Publishers
Sudbury, Massachusetts
BOSTON • TORONTO • LONDON • SINGAPORE

World Headquarters
Jones and Bartlett Publishers
40 Tall Pine Drive
Sudbury, MA 01776
978-443-5000
info@jbpub.com
www.jbpub.com

Jones and Bartlett Publishers Canada
2100 Bloor Street West
Suite 6-272
Toronto, ON M6S 5A5
CANADA

Jones and Bartlett Publishers International
Barb House, Barb Mews
London W6 7PA
UK

PRODUCTION CREDITS
Senior Acquisitions Editor: Greg Vis
Production Editor: Linda S. DeBruyn
Manufacturing Director: Therese Bräuer
Editorial and Production Service: Bookwrights
Cover Design: Dick Hannus
Text Design: Anne Spencer
Printing and Binding: Malloy Lithographing

Library of Congress Cataloging-in-Publication Data
Fatigue in cancer / [edited by] Maryl L. Winningham, Margaret Barton-Burke
    p. cm.
  Includes bibliographical references and index.
  ISBN 0-7637-0630-2
  1. Cancer–Complications. 2. Fatigue. I. Winningham, Maryl Lynn, 1947– .
II. Barton-Burke, Margaret.
  [DNLM: 1. Neoplasms–complications. 2. Fatigue. 3. Rehabilitation QZ 200 F253 2000]
RC262.F   2000
616.99'4–dc21
DNLM/DLC
for Library of Congress   98-43133
                                      CIP

Printed in the United States of America
03 02 01 00 99   10 9 8 7 6 5 4 3 2 1

Dedication

*To the many who suffered
from confusion and devastating fatigue
for so long,
who were mocked
or accused of malingering,
or ignored,
or whose suffering was treated as insignificant:
This is your Vindication!*

Las Phantasmas De Tiral

I come gentle to this place,
Not wanting to disturb the spirits
Fleeting through this
fractured landscape.

I am an intruder from another time,
I have no business here.

I come gentle to this place,
Not wishing to disrupt
The ancient rhythms of the stories
Swirling through these crumbled ruins,
The dancing embers
of the ghosts.

I am an intruder from another space,
I have no business here.

I come gentle to this place,
Pleading with the jungle gods
To hide me in their world
Just long enough for me to glimpse
The silent moon procession
of these souls.

Please, may I be a guest?
I have no time or space.
So you see, I do have business here.

I come hopeful to this place,
Searching for the peace of mind
So violently wrenched from me.
I am not callous to the
healing magic here.

I will not overstay my time
I know it cannot last
It's just that I'm so very tired
I simply need to rest.

Tricia C. Corbett. Oaxaca Mexico, March 1998

Contents

Preface

We hope this book is different from anything you have read before. First, the study of fatigue as a major focus in cancer clinical practice and research is a relatively new phenomenon. Second, the style of this book is different from that of most books. It is a series of essays and interviews representing the perspectives of many creative, insightful, clinically oriented people who keep an active communication network with patients, families, and other professionals. We encouraged the contributors to go beyond research in the cancer-related fatigue syndrome (CRFS) to their clinical observations and to other associated phenomena. We especially encouraged them to be free in sharing their opinions. Because of the diverse backgrounds represented by our contributors, we hope the readers come to see the CRFS from the point of view of many disciplines and develop fresh insights as a basis for research. Several of our contributors have experienced some aspects of the CRFS, or fatigue related to other chronic health conditions, so the topic is not merely academic. Third, this book is not meant to be a rehash of information that can be obtained easily through a review of the recent literature. Those who are looking for a literature review will be disappointed. They would be better served by going to a library or by conducting an on-line search in a computerized database. Since the CRFS is such a rapidly developing area, a-literature-review book would be out-of-date by the time of publication. Further, good researchers not referenced in such a book would not get the credit they deserve. Hopefully, this book will encourage readers to go to the research databases on a regular basis for reports on the most recent work and to pursue new ideas for research and clinical practice.

It is common for articles on the CRFS to repeat the same line (with some variation): "Very little is known about cancer fatigue." This is not entirely true. We know a good deal about fatigue in humans in general. There is no reason why much of this information cannot be extrapolated to understanding fatigue in people with cancer. People with cancer may have more problems than healthy humans, but they are not less than human. Indeed, people experiencing CRFS phenomena often say, "This is different from anything I've ever experienced before." How are we to understand CRFS if we don't tease out the sources of fatigue in general?

There is nearly a century of physiological and psychological fatigue-oriented research that can be applied to understanding fatigue as experienced by people with cancer. The scientific roots go back even farther by several centuries. In fact, the origins can be found in the quotes of Hippocrates. Conceptually, we could view this problem in the form of a mathematical equation:

Overall experience of fatigue phenomena in cancer
− Known experience of fatigue (in healthy individuals)
_____
= Cancer-specific fatigue phenomena

Although we know a great deal about fatigue in general, little of that knowledge has been applied to the CRFS. We need to start by identifying what we know. This means learning from a broad variety of disciplines, each able to lend insight into this issue. Then we need to prevent that which is known to be preventable. In addition, we need to develop an understanding, a comprehension of conceptual relationships, particularly those that bridge disciplines. Lacking knowledge of historical developments and research in various other disciplines, we have difficulty synthesizing useful information, filtering out the issues specific to and useful in understanding the CRFS.

As long as people have had cancer, there has been the CRFS. While treatment developments have given life, they have introduced harsh side effects and frequently leave residual effects that result in lasting exhaustibility and functional impairments. Why have we just now started to notice it? As anyone who has experienced it will tell you, the word fatigue is grossly inadequate. This book most appropriately can be used as an adjunct to ongoing research and more traditional reviews. We hope it invigorates with fresh ideas and new insights, and encourages a broader understanding of what it is like to live with fatigue in the setting of cancer. Perhaps we will begin to get a feel for why it is so devastating for so many.

It is expected that the full spectrum of health care providers may be interested in this book. In addition, this book is intended for a broad variety of lay readers. Patients and families may find affirmations or solutions in its pages. We hope this book will find its way onto the shelves of cancer survivors' resource libraries and onto clinic shelves, and be used by individuals struggling to obtain recognition and treatment of pathologies influencing their fatigue by insurance companies and the disability system.

You will find a great deal of controversy in this book. We believe that is good. Many who have or who had cancer prefer to call themselves "cancer survivors." This is the term preferred by many of the cancer support and activist organizations including the Wellness Community and the National Coalition for Cancer Survivorship. Some of our contributors use this term. On the other hand, there are those, including those who had cancer, who prefer to use "cancer patient." We elected to let the contributors exercise their own choice and hope that readers are generous with respect to personal preference. After all, regardless of the term, we need to remember that each one is a person, a human being with cancer, never just a medical label or the name *du jour*.

You will find some information overlap from chapter to chapter. Some chapters can be read independently or out of sequence. In some places, you will find contradictions between the opinions of the contributors. Since we asked each contributor to be creative and share from their clinical experience, we decided to restrain the editorial pen and let the readers draw their own conclusions. Where there are contradictions, they may indicate the need for more focused research or an appreciation of various points of view.

There has been an academic trend toward discouraging "outdated references" (sometimes as little as five years!). This is good when it discourages undergraduates from doing "quick and lazy" literature reviews out of reference books. However, as a general rule, it represents poor scientific training. Interest in some phenomena goes back as much as two millennia; their study is as relevant today as it was then. Interest in life and vitality (words often used synonymously with *energetic* today) had roots in the writings of Aristotle and gave rise to an influential philosophy called *vitalism*. Florence Nightingale and medical experts of her day wrote about a deficit of "vital force" or "vital powers" because they observed what we today would term *fatigue* in a variety of patients. *Vitality* and *energy* are words still associated with life, health, and well-being. It is crucial that graduate students and neophyte researchers be able to trace the origins of concepts and constructs in theory and the foundations of their research despite alterations in terminology. Slavish worship of "political correctness" is the death of scientific progress and is the worst form of mind control. It brings about stagnation and stifles creativity. It also contributes to the Woozle effect as suffered by Winnie the Pooh and his research assistant, Piglet. If you remember, Pooh and Piglet found themselves going around in circles, following tracks (artifacts) of their own making, while ascribing them to a very fearsome Hostile Animal called a Woozle. Readers are encouraged to challenge and explore, to resist the tendency to fall victim to the Woozle effect as they search for answers.

Since this book is a composite of ideas from many sources, we cannot begin to acknowledge them all. Further, it is likely there will be many gaps revealed in our knowledge–this is a rapidly growing area of research and clinical practice. Where we have omitted some important things, we ask your forgiveness and ask that you bring them to our attention for the next edition (we may even ask you to write something for the next edition). If we have omitted reference to the accomplishments of many fine researchers and clinicians, it is not from lack of respect. We believe their work speaks for itself. The purpose of this book is to supplement their contributions with a variety of different or new perspectives.

We have tried to encourage an examination of the interdisciplinary nature of fatigue as well as the art of living with it, by asking many of our contributors to write about objective as well as subjective reports and clinical observations. Finally, we encouraged contributors to suggest areas that may provide fruit for research in the hopes that the future of the study of fatigue might be rich and deep in knowledge and clinical solutions.

The original title of this book was supposed to be "Fatigue in Cancer: The Art and the Science," but for awhile we could not locate sufficient art describing the fatigue phenomenon to justify the title. It was only after we changed the title that we received many choice examples of art, brief reports, and poetry reflecting personal experiences. Throughout the book, we have displayed the creative communications survivors and their families shared from their experiences–illustrations, insights, and vignettes–in the hope that we might all grow in insight and sensitivity and be inspired in our search for answers.

Maryl L. Winningham
Margaret Barton-Burke

Repression

Dedicated to Eric, who survived Dachau but died of cancer.

Who guards my mind
from treachery
in slumber?
Who saves my soul
from terror
in the night?
How could I live
if Sentinel were not
so vigilant to shield
and to defend?
How could I stand
my stern betrayer's might?

Throughout the day
my life is filled
with busyness.
With iron will
I govern fear
and dread.
But when, each night
I'm forced to yield
to torpid helplessness at last
Then Sentinel stands watch
lest fears break forth
from memories long dead.

So on I live
in slumber unmolested.
No nightmare dares
betray this solemn sleep.
So deep the fear
of horrors from my past
has been repressed
I sell my life, my soul,
my sanity,
To Sentinel to keep.

Now I yield my soul to sleep
Repression serves my mind to keep
If I should dream before I wake
I pray the Lord my soul will take.
Amen

To Florence Nightingale (1820–1910)

Statistician, public health visionary, leader in the development of health care models, and founder of modern nursing, and her book Notes on Nursing: What It Is and What It Is Not, *published 1859 in London. Many of her insightful observations are scattered throughout this book. She understood what we need to learn if we are to understand those suffering from the effects of illnesses such as the cancer-related fatigue syndrome. Those who have to live with it have been trying to tell us all along . . . but are we listening? Perhaps now, after nearly a century and a half, we are ready for her wisdom.*

Acknowledgments

We gratefully acknowledge the many individuals who contributed to this book. Without them, it would never have come to fruition. These individuals have been most generous in sharing and giving of themselves. So that we don't jeopardize any confidentialities, the names are listed without any reference to the content of their contribution. Some contributed but asked not to be identified; we have honored their requests. For individuals who gave permission to include personally identifying comments with their contributions, we have included those identifiers in context. When all is said and done, the credit goes to them. We will take the blame for any deficiencies and errors.

We especially thank the editorial staff at Jones and Bartlett: Greg Vis, Senior Acquisitions Editor, who saw us through to completion by his positive reinforcement and encouraging words; Amy Austin, Associate Editor, who looked after the details and gave us frequent reality checks; Linda DeBruyn, Production Editor; John Danielowich and Christine Tridente, Editorial Assistants; and the layout, editorial, and production staff at Bookwrights who brought order out of chaos.

We are greatly indebted to those who contributed to the creative content and helped us understand the personal side of cancer-related fatigue: Frederick P. and Susan Kesler, Diana Dean, Linda S. Jimison, Karen Rabus, Daniel and Debra Witman, Sherri Taylor, Lennett F. Radke, Barbara and Todd Richardson, Jessica Flores, Keith Grace, and Brenda Heil and her husband, Robert.

Last but not least, we thank the following for their expertise and professional advice: Barbara F. Piper, RN, PhD; Lori Precht Lindsey, RNC, FNO, OCN; and Barbara A. Preusser, PhD, FNPc, who helped with content review and critique.

Most of all, our thanks go to the many hundreds of cancer survivors and their families who have taught us, out of their struggle, what fatigue means to them in their lives and how they have found meaning in the midst of it. They have challenged us to do what we can to alleviate this source of suffering and discouragement.

Contributors

Margaret Barton-Burke, PhD (candidate), RN, AOCN; *Principal,* Oncology Consulting Services, Boston, MA; *Doctoral Student,* University of Rhode Island, Kingston, RI

Marilyn Bookbinder, PhD, RN; *Director of Nursing Education and Quality Improvement,* Pain Medicine and Palliative Care, Beth Israel Medical Center, New York, NY

Patricia C. Buchsel, RN, MSN; *Oncology Nurse Educator/Clinical Instructor,* University of Washington School of Nursing, Seattle, WA

Kathryn Ann Caudell, PhD, RN; *Assistant Professor,* College of Nursing, University of New Mexico, Edgewood, NM

Tricia C. Corbett, MSPH; *President,* Corbett Consulting, Inc., Issaquah, WA

Eileen S. Donovan, PT, M.ED; *Assistant Director,* Rehabilitation Services and Rehabilitation Services Team, University of Texas M. D. Anderson Cancer Center, Houston, TX

Renata J. M. Engler, MD, FACAAI, FAAAAI; *Colonel,* U.S. Army; *Chief,* Allergy and Immunology Department; Walter Reed Army Medical Center, Washington, DC

Theresa A. Gillis, MD; *Assistant Professor and Chief,* Section of Physical Medicine and Rehabilitation, Department of Pain and Symptom Management, University of Texas MD Anderson Cancer Center, Houston, TX

Marcia Grant, RN, DNSC, FAAN; *Director and Research Scientist,* Nursing Research and Education, City of Hope National Medical Center, Duarte, CA

Wendy S. Harpham, MD, FACP, *Internal Medicine Physician,* Dallas, TX

Pamela S. Hinds, PhD, RN, CS; *Coordinator of Nursing Research* and *Associate Director of Research for Behavioral Medicine,* St. Jude Children's Research Hospital, Memphis, TN

Marilyn Hockenberry-Eaton, PhD, RN, CS, PNP, FAAN; *Associate Professor,* Department of Pediatric, Pediatric Hematology-Oncology Division, Baylor College of Medicine, Houston, TX

Gerald Kelly, M. DIV; *Director,* Supportive Care, The Don and Sybil Harrington Cancer Center, Amarillo, TX

Theodore P. McDade, MD, SM (Engineering); *Resident in General Surgery,* Massachusetts General Medical Center, Boston, MA

Lisa N. Meadows, R.PH; *Oncology Pharmacy Specialist,* Dana Farber Cancer Center, Boston, MA

Christina A. Meyers, PhD, ABPP; *Associate Professor of Neuropsychology,* Department of Neuro-Oncology, University of Texas, M. D. Anderson Cancer Center, Houston, TX

Henry Olders, MD, P. Eng., FRCPC; Sir Mortimer B. Davis–Jewish General Hospital, Montreal, Quebec

Brian T. Pruitt, MD; *Chief,* Division of Oncology, Texas Tech University Health Sciences Center, School of Medicine and School of Pharmacy; *Associate Medical Director for Clinical Trials,* The Don and Sybil Harrington Cancer Center, Amarillo, TX

Marjorie H. Royle, PhD; *Consulting Psychologist,* Lincoln Park, NJ

Sandra J. Smeeding, MS, FNPC, CSC; *General Surgery Nurse Practitioner,* Veterans Administration Medical Center, Salt Lake City, UT

Claudette G. Varricchio, DSN, RN, FAAN; *Program Director / Nurse Consultant,* Division of Cancer Prevention, National Cancer Institute, Rockville, MD

Maryl L. Winningham, APRN, PhD, FACSM; *Executive Director and Senior Research Associate,* Institute for the Advancement of Health Care Engineering, Salt Lake City, UT

Introduction

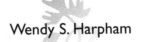

Wendy S. Harpham

Fatigue presents a unique challenge to cancer survivors and those who care for them. Defined as a feeling of weariness during or following exertion, fatigue is a near-universal symptom during treatment. For many, it persists long after remission is achieved. Its effect on individual survivors is often not appreciated or addressed. Even when fatigue is acknowledged as a problem by patients, caretakers, and the health care teams, a sense of helplessness may follow: "What can we do?" The diagnosis and treatment of fatigue are especially difficult. Invisible and without an objective unit of measure, fatigue nevertheless affects and is affected by patients' medical, intellectual, emotional, spiritual, social, and financial conditions.

Fatigue is expressed in relation to effort: It has a volitional component and is impossible to separate from patients' personality, mood, and sense of hope. Our current vocabulary does little to differentiate survivors' fatigue from the tiredness that healthy people feel at the end of a long day, even though patients describe it as different and more distressing. This problem led me, in 1995, to coin the term, postcancer fatigue (PCF) to represent the distinctive fatigue that persists after completion of treatment when remission is achieved and all known causes of fatigue have resolved or been ruled out. Grateful patients' letters and calls followed, sharing how the label helped them open useful dialogue with their physicians and family. But naming a problem is only one step. Research into the causes of fatigue in cancer patients during and after treatment is still in its infancy.

The psychosocial impact and consequences of fatigue are just now being addressed in professional and survivor forums. An important obstacle to dealing with fatigue seems to be a combination of neglect and denial. Understandably, hospitalized patients' immediate (often life-threatening) medical concerns eclipse the constitutional complaint of fatigue. As for the majority of survivors who are treated as outpatients, illness is experienced in the setting of the well world. Consequently, patients' responses to their invisible wounds of fatigue are colored by the surrounding culture that values productivity. The mystique of the cancer warrior encourages survivors to downplay their fatigue, or bite the bullet and push on in the face of discomfort or disability. Every day, tired survivors interact with family and friends who simply do not understand what is wrong.

As a doctor of internal medicine and a long-term survivor of non-Hodgkin's lymphoma, I have experienced the challenges of fatigue from both sides of the stethoscope. Over the years, I have developed a philosophy of survivorship based on three steps: obtaining sound knowledge, nourishing genuine hope, and acting effectively. Knowledge, hope, and action allow patients to affect the course of their lives in positive directions, and deal in healthy ways with any residual pain, debility, and loss. When applied to the problem of cancer-related fatigue, this approach allows patients to minimize the physiological causes of fatigue and adjust to energy limitations that remain. *Fatigue in Cancer: A Multidimensional Approach* is indeed an innovative exploration that offers sound information, explores creative ways for looking at fatigue, investigates ways to minimize patients' experience of fatigue as well as their associated distress, and provides some suggestions for the future. By bringing both the science and the art of healing from many disciplines and dimensions to the challenge of fatigue, we can begin to transform survivors' experience of fatigue from a pernicious toxin on quality of life to a manageable concern. For some, the changes precipitated by cancer-related fatigue can lead to insights about themselves and their world, and can lead them to a "new normal" life that is, in fact, a better one.

Resources

Harpham, W. S. (1998). *Diagnosis: Cancer. Your Guide Through the First Few Months.* Revised and updated. New York: W. W. Norton.

Harpham, W. S. (1995). *After Cancer: A Guide to Your New Life.* New York: HarperCollins.

Harpham, W. S. (1995). *When a Parent Has Cancer: A Guide to Caring for Your Children.* With a companion children's book, *Becky and the Worry Cup.* New York: HarperCollins.

About the Contributor

In addition to being an internal medicine physician, a long-term cancer survivor, a best-selling author, mother of several children, and an articulate spokesperson for cancer survivors, Wendy S. Harpham is a warm, delightful, insightful, thoughtful human being. Her books (listed at the end of this introduction) have been a source of encouragement to many. She has made numerous radio and television appearances including CBS's This Morning, ABC's Good Morning America, NBC's Today Show, *and NBC's* Nightly News. *Articles about her experiences and work have appeared in the* New York Times, Boston Globe, American Medical News, Dallas Morning News, *and local papers around the country. She was the first to propose the term postcancer fatigue (PCF) to describe the long-term fatigue that affects so many with cancer.*

A few weeks ago, when a cancer survivor and his wife wrote and said, "We wish there were a book to warn you about what life will be like after cancer." I could tell them, "There is! After Cancer: A Guide to Your New Life.*"*

I first met Wendy when we were both speakers at a conference. I knew right away she should be a part of this book. From the section on "postcancer fatigue" in After Cancer, *it is clear that she brings special insight to this subject through her intimate knowledge of medicine and her experience as a cancer survivor.*

M.L.W.

PART
I

Background

When you go through chemo (more so with my bone marrow transplant) you just feel like a pile of wet noodles. There is absolutely _NO_ energy (not even enough to wiggle your toes).

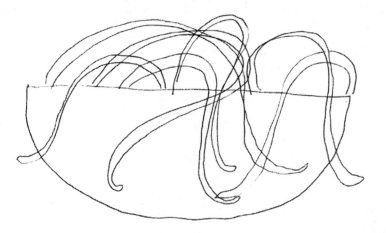

Brenda Heil, 33 years old, 9-year survivor

The Puzzle of Fatigue: How Do You Nail Pudding to the Wall?

Maryl L. Winningham

What cruel mistakes are sometimes made by benevolent men and women in matters of business about which they can know nothing and think they know a great deal.

Florence Nightingale, *Notes on Nursing*

Background

The old fairy tale "Rumpelstiltskin" tells about a Queen whose only child was being extorted from her as the result of a bad debt. When she begged for mercy, her tormentor finally hinted, "If you can guess my name, you will have power over me. I will have to do what you ask." This seemed impossible because the name was so unusual there was no way she could guess it. It was only by accident (and a bit of stealth) that the Queen was able to discover his name and keep her child. The moral of the story is known to all who read it: If you can name something, you gain power over it.

That is how we seem to be treating fatigue with reference to cancer—like a word with incantational powers. Unlike Rumpelstiltskin, we are not quite sure what *fatigue* means or what to do with it. In the recent cancer literature, one frequently reads the statement, "There is no clear definition for *fatigue*." Given the contextual history of the word *fatigue*, that should come as no surprise. The real question is whether it is necessary or desirable to define *fatigue*. The word *definition* implies a precise meaning, clarification, or distinction of a word or condition. It includes determining the outline and limitations. This book will clearly demonstrate that given the diverse phenomena and implications of the fatigue experience, associating the word *fatigue* with *definition* is an oxymoron.

From a more creative perspective, Barton-Burke (1998) posited that fatigue should be explored rather than defined. Those looking to this book to provide a definition for fatigue will be disappointed. As the philosopher Wittgenstein pointed out, the limits of possible experience cannot be drawn because to do so, we would have to stand outside experience to see on both sides (Kaplan, 1964, p. 34). Those interested in an exploration of the phenomena associated with cancer fatigue will find great challenges. This is the beginning of an exploration of fatigue in cancer.

Communication Chasms in Understanding and Investigating Fatigue

One of the biggest hindrances to exploring the knowledge base about the cancer fatigue phenomenon is communication. There are not just barriers to communication; there are chasms to overcome. This communication deficit is at all levels: People with cancer have trouble recognizing the many manifestations of cancer fatigue. It is even more difficult to verbalize about their experience to themselves. It is unlike anything most have ever experienced.[1] It is even more difficult to communicate what cancer fatigue is like to others who have never experienced it. Finally, the problem is compounded because the "experts" do not agree!

Prior to continuing, it is essential to acknowledge my bias: That those who have experienced the fatigue of chronic illness (there are other illnesses with parallel manifestations) are the real experts. Healthy clinicians and researchers can never be experiential experts unless they have lived through something similar. For them, the study of fatigue presents a metaphysical impossibility. With them, one can only try to communicate using imprecise metaphors. Albert Schweitzer understood this when he wrote of "The Fellowship of Those Who Bear the Mark of Pain"[2] (see page 11). That probably is one of the most critical reasons why cancer fatigue has only recently been "discovered." This is not to disparage the

About the Editor

Maryl L. Winningham has been interested in the problem of fatigability in people suffering from chronic illness for more than 20 years. Her first bachelor's and master's degrees were in psychology, music, exercise physiology, and history and philosophy of higher education. She has worked in Canada, Switzerland, and Germany, and has enjoyed living among people from over 20 different cultural origins. Her commitment to studying fatigue is personal as well as professional: While living in Europe, she experienced a serious illness that resulted in several weeks' of bed rest. Afterward, she was confronted by the problem of how to regain her strength and endurance. She started walking every day–slowly and cautiously. After a year or two, someone gave her Dr. Ken Cooper's book The Aerobics Way. *As she tells it, it took her two more years to work up to the lowest, beginning level in his book. She says, "If I only knew then what I tell people now."*

Later, while doing graduate work in the United States, Maryl started working in a hospital as a nursing assistant where she saw health care "from the bottom up." She observed: "I was shocked by how illogical and unscientific many hospital policies and procedures were. Worse, I saw how patients were left unnecessarily exhausted and threatened by what was supposed to make them better." Studies in biochemistry, physiology, nutrition, and physics had convinced her there was only one way to put energy in the body: There is no magic–the body has to make its own. Her doctoral work in exercise science at Ohio State University included studies in physiology, human anatomy, preventive medicine, and nutritional

role of clinicians and researchers who are playing a critical role in facilitating communication, elucidating mechanisms of fatigue, and developing effective interventions. If we truly acknowledge that fatigue, like pain, is what the patient says it is, we will find more effective ways to listen, whether to verbal reports or by using various means of nonverbal or artistic expression.

Teamwork is essential if we are to attack the problem of fatigue in a meaningful way. Clinicians and researchers often do not understand each other's perspectives and disciplinary philosophies. Researchers from different disciplines have difficulty communicating with one another because they have strayed from the essentials of science and have focused on technology and a narrowed disciplinary focus. A historical understanding of the process of scientific thought is necessary to provide a common basis for communication. Only then will there be sufficient interdisciplinary respect and recognition of our common origins for them to work together.

The word *fatigue* is not commonly used in everyday English. The use of the word has come largely from science, from physiology and engineering. During wartime, in particular, a large amount of funding went into fatigue research focused on alertness and performance in pilots flying bombers, in workers manufacturing, and in technicians monitoring instruments. During peacetime, industrialists focused on similar issues but for a different reason, as they sought ways to analyze and optimize efficiency of workers' performance. These

biochemistry. For her dissertation, she developed an exercise program for breast cancer patients, the first of its kind, designed to promote the biochemical resources of all three of the body's energy systems without inducing fatigue or injury. Since there was no set precedent, it was necessary to start from scratch: A questionnaire to monitor symptoms and clinical status, detailed clinical screening, and eligibility criteria were developed. In addition, an exercise testing protocol consistent with international standards, safety guidelines for exercise, and an exercise training protocol to stimulate all three cellular energy systems had to be designed. Data showed improvement in physiological indicators of functional capacity, functional status, body composition, and feelings of control in the exercising group while they were on chemotherapy! Patients in the exercise group also reported reduced symptoms and improved energy for everyday living. This work was completed in 1983–and it was just the beginning. After completing doctoral and postdoctoral work, she earned bachelor's and master's degrees in nursing.

Maryl has written numerous chapters and articles, has proposed theoretical models to explain fatigue-activity–related phenomena, has published guidelines for the conduct of safe exercise in cancer patients, and has been a leader in the field of the cancer-related fatigue syndrome. She enjoys using metaphors and visual aids to demonstrate the principles of biochemistry and physics of energetics and fatigue to professional as well as lay audiences. Her favorite activities include graphic arts and poetry. She is currently at work on a futuristic novel about medical ethics.

studies were all on normal subjects, limited to objective measures of performance. Although some of this work focused on physiological manifestations of fatigue, cognitive factors such as motivation and boredom were also significant foci. On the other hand, physiologically based research largely examined neuromuscular and endocrine aspects of fatigue. This area of science also has included sports medicine and athletic performance. Since World War II, the U.S. National Aeronautics and Space Agency (NASA), as well as the aeronautics and space administrations in Asia and Europe, picked up the trail of fatigue-related research because of its relationship to performance and well-being in astronauts. Graphic records kept by the Soviet cosmonauts of Salyut 6 starkly portrayed the effects of space flight (microgravity) on blunted cognition as well as physical abilities (Tufte, 1997). Comparisons of human responses to NASA bed rest studies versus the effects of space flight provided evidence of obtunded cognitive ability as well as physical weakness. More recent work has focused on elucidating the influence of neurohumoral immunological factors, such as cytokines. All this work has significance for understanding fatigue in cancer.

> *Those who have experienced cancer fatigue are the experts. We must, before anything else, listen and learn from them. Healthy clinicians and researchers can never be experiential experts unless they have gone through something similar.*

Although the phenomena associated with cancer-related fatigue have long been observed, it is only recently that they have become an acknowledged focus of clinical inquiry. Interestingly, we still hang on to the single word *fatigue,* although it is clear that the fatigue experienced by someone with cancer and that of a baseball player or a radar technician are very different. The experiences of people with different types of cancer and undergoing different types of treatment also differ. And now comes the real question: If the fatigue we are currently hearing so much about in cancer practice is such a serious and distressing part of the cancer experience, why has it taken so long for us to recognize the significance and magnitude of the problem?

Over a period of several years, in the process of gathering material for this book, it became obvious that there was no consensus on what the word *fatigue* meant. People with cancer knew they were experiencing something, but the word *fatigue* seemed to be grossly inadequate if not confusing. They were trying to figure out how to name a strange, debilitating condition that health care professionals could not understand. When they tried to explain, they often met with a response like, "What do you expect? You've got cancer!" There was a communication chasm, but what kind? When asked about this general phenomenon, people were inclined to use many words or metaphors, but the word *fatigue* was rarely their first choice. In fact, reducing their suffering to a single word seemed to trivialize it. Further, despite the devastation fatigue caused in the lives of those who experienced it, it was rarely considered dramatic enough to be considered a cause of suffering.

To conceptualize a sense of the problem of communicating something like cancer fatigue with words, Figure 1-1 and Table 1-1 demonstrate the origins of the English word *fatigue* and associated words. Many of these words currently are used in fatigue scales to measure quality of life. (See Chapter 3 for Varricchio's comments on this problem.) From

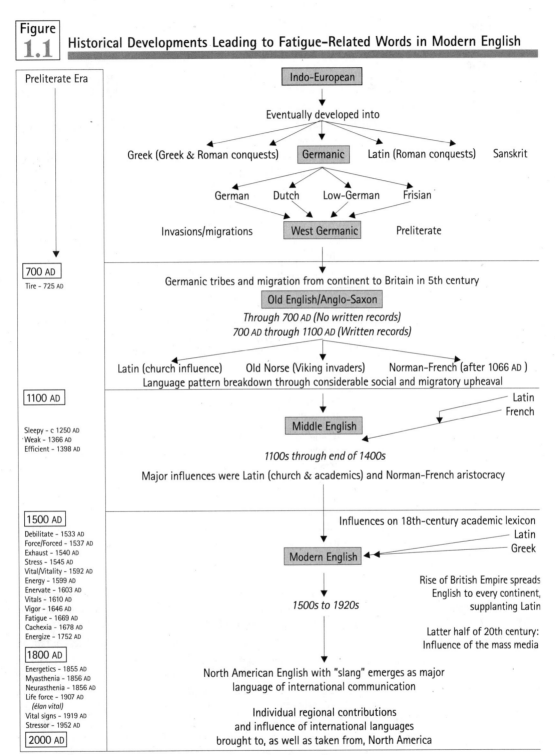

Preliterate Era

Indo-European

↓

Eventually developed into

Greek (Greek & Roman conquests)   Germanic   Latin (Roman conquests)   Sanskrit

German   Dutch   Low-German   Frisian

Invasions/migrations   West Germanic   Preliterate

700 AD
Tire - 725 AD

Germanic tribes and migration from continent to Britain in 5th century

Old English/Anglo-Saxon

Through 700 AD (No written records)
700 AD through 1100 AD (Written records)

Latin (church influence)   Old Norse (Viking invaders)   Norman-French (after 1066 AD)
Language pattern breakdown through considerable social and migratory upheaval

1100 AD

Sleepy - c 1250 AD
Weak - 1366 AD
Efficient - 1398 AD

Latin
French

Middle English

1100s through end of 1400s

Major influences were Latin (church & academics) and Norman-French aristocracy

1500 AD
Debilitate - 1533 AD
Force/Forced - 1537 AD
Exhaust - 1540 AD
Stress - 1545 AD
Vital/Vitality - 1592 AD
Energy - 1599 AD
Enervate - 1603 AD
Vitals - 1610 AD
Vigor - 1646 AD
Fatigue - 1669 AD
Cachexia - 1678 AD
Energize - 1752 AD

Influences on 18th-century academic lexicon

Latin
Greek

Modern English

1500s to 1920s

Rise of British Empire spreads
English to every continent,
supplanting Latin

Latter half of 20th century:
Influence of the mass media

1800 AD
Energetics - 1855 AD
Myasthenia - 1856 AD
Neurasthenia - 1856 AD
Life force - 1907 AD
   (élan vital)
Vital signs - 1919 AD
Stressor - 1952 AD

2000 AD

North American English with "slang" emerges as major
language of international communication

Individual regional contributions
and influence of international languages
brought to, as well as taken from, North America

Table 1.1 The Etymology of Select Life- and Fatigue-Related English Words

Word(s)	Origin(s)	Meaning
Aesthenia	Greek fi New Latin	Weakness and debility as loss of bodily strength; diminution of vital force (medical)
Cachexia	Greek fi New Latin	Wasting and loss of body tissue, especially muscle, which is associated with malnutrition and often with chronic illness
Debilitate	Latin	Enfeebled, weak, and impairment and loss of energy and/or strength
Efficient	Latin fi Middle French fi Middle English	The relationship between effective or useful output (usually money, energy, work, or time) and the total input in any system; in physics or physiology, expressed in terms of a percentage or ratio; focus on production without waste
Energetic/ energetics/ energize	Greek	Exerting or showing energy; relating to energy
Energy	Greek fi Latin fi French	Internal or inherent power; capacity for acting, operating, or producing an effect; strength of expression; force of utterance; work; vigorous exertion of power; capacity for work or power; vitality
Enervate	Latin	To lessen the viability and strength of; lacking physical, mental, or moral vigor
Exhaust	Latin	To wear out completely; to drain of resources; to use up completely; to draw out the contents of something
Fatigue	Latin fi Old French fi Middle French	Weariness (physical or mental) resulting from exertion or activity; a weakening or failure of a person or a material as a result of prolonged stress; the decreased ability of an organism or organ part to function as a result of excessive stimulation and prolonged exertion
Force	Latin fi Vulgate Latin fi Middle French fi Middle English	Strength; vigor; energy of body or mind; capacity for exercising or producing an effect, muscular force, or energy; metabolic force; the influence that controls the metabolism of the body; vital force, which acts toward organization, which is the cause of life in the body
Invigorate	Old English fi Middle English	Enliven; make alert; energetic, sharpen
Life force (*élan vital*)	Modern French (1907)	Term used by French philosopher Henri Bergson as the source of organized causation and evolution in nature; A twentieth-century extension of Aristotle's philosophy of vitalism
Myasthenia	New Latin	Mid-1800s term used to describe unusual muscular weakness or fatigue
Neur- asthenia	New Latin	Mid-1800s term used to describe psychic and emotional disorder as evidenced by easy fatigability; apparent lack of motivation; weakness; loss of memory; generalized aches and pains; formerly thought to result from exhaustion of the nervous system
Sleep/sleepy	Old English fi Middle English	The natural condition of periodic and temporary suspension of consciousness that results in the renewal of the powers of the body and mind; characterized by an absence of alertness

Word(s)	Origin(s)	Meaning
Stress/ stressed/ distressed	Latin fi Old French fi Middle English	Pressure, strain, with implication of urgency or significance; the negative condition of too little as well as too much stress emphasized by early English writers; force or forces that produce strain or tension
Stressor	Modern English (1952)	Term used by Selye to apply the physics and engineering concept of tension or stress to human beings
Tire	Anglo-Saxon fi Old English fi Middle English	Showing weariness, fatigue, failure of strength, usually as a result of toil; labor or excessive strain.
Vigor/ vigorous	Latin fi Old French fi Old English	Active capacity for strength, exertion, force, or energy; applies to body, mind, or moral capability
Vital/ vitality	Latin fi Old French fi Middle English	Used in nineteenth century as vital force, vital powers: characteristic of life, life sustaining, essential to continued existence, full of life, distinguishing the living from nonliving; physical and mental vigor
Vital signs	English (1919)	Signs of life as part of physical observation in medicine—usually includes pulse, temperature, respiration, and blood pressure (not commonly used in first decades of this century)
Weak	Latin fi Old High Gothic fi Gothic fi Anglo-Saxon and Old Norse fi Old English	Lacking physical strength, infirm, debilitated, unable to sustain great strain, frail; also used to refer to moral or intellectual deficiencies of character

Sources: Crabb, 1879; March and March, 1902; Scott, 1952; *The American Heritage Dictionary of the English Language, Third Edition,* 1992; *The Compact Edition of the Oxford English Dictionary,* 1971; Wyld, 1939.

the etymology of these words, it is clear they have a broad variety of linguistic origins. It is doubtful whether most individuals tested by current cancer fatigue scales could give an adequate or accurate description or definition of many of the words on those scales. The middle-class, northeastern U.S. vernacular may differ from, for instance, that of an African-American rapper in Florida to such an extent that it sounds as if they are speaking different languages. English spoken in the United Kingdom, particularly by recent immigrants, is considerably different from that spoken by many North Americans. Consider that people often use slang and metaphors in talking about their cancer fatigue experience. When we force unusual or uncustomary words upon patients and demand that they speak our specialized language, we lose the basis for effective communication. To further the problem, written language often has different nuances from spoken language. We depend on language for communication, and a relatively new field of study, sociolinguistics, examines how essential symbolic language usage contributes insight into social behaviors and interactions.

A concise definition of *fatigue* has escaped elucidation in the study of healthy people, under a broad variety of conditions and circumstances, because the mechanisms appear to be so complex and interactive. In 1921, an exasperated Italian researcher, Muscio, suggested we completely abandon the concept of fatigue. He argued there was no possible way to devise an acceptable test of fatigue because there were no observable criteria. That is, there was no "gold standard" for comparison except any given test against itself (Muscio, 1921). Despite the logic and vehemence of his argument, researchers continued to forge forward in a search for objective indicators. Diverse performance instruments and measures have been developed and tested, but none are in agreement.

Even the most objective, physiologically based gold standard measures of fatigue, such as the maximal force exerted by a muscle group contraction or maximal oxygen uptake under laboratory conditions, can be altered in an instant by increased motivation, fear, boredom, excitement, or enthusiasm. The same variables, in addition to socioeconomic, cultural, and mood factors, can confound well-constructed psychosocial instruments. Early in this century (1915), the eminent medical physiologist Walter B. Cannon (1929) pointed out that physiologically fatigued muscle could instantly be restored to full strength by "adrenin" or adrenaline.[3] Despite the continued inconsistency among the many instrumentation and measurement techniques, methodologies tested and developed by various disciplines have guided changes in the military, business, industrial production, airline and aerospace industries, athletics, and medicine.

Why do we continue to pursue this thing called fatigue? It appears to be, as in the metaphor, like "trying to nail pudding to the wall." The reason is, we know something is there; we feel the effects, we see its influence on performance, and we are becoming increasingly aware of its profound effect on cancer patients' everyday lives. In general, fatigue has long been known to be responsible for life-threatening accidents, errors in judgment, and inattention to details that affect productivity throughout society. It is not only a distressing problem but also a devastating and expensive problem that affects all aspects of life. So why are we just now becoming focused on fatigue in oncology patients?

Fatigue-related phenomena have been the object of extensive research. For more than a century, the multicausality and complexity of fatigue have been acknowledged. We need to consider whether retaining the word *fatigue* in the oncology setting contributes to more confusion and obfuscation rather than less.

In recent study (Fatigue Coalition, 1998), researchers examined some of the economical and emotional aspects of fatigue. Widespread recognition of fatigue by health care professionals as a significant problem in people with cancer is only a few years old. While an increasing number of oncology professionals recognize it to be a major functional and quality of life issue in their patients, they are less certain what to do about it.

Sources of Knowledge

Traditionally, health care professionals are taught that there are two kinds of clinical information to gather in the process of making a differential diagnosis: subjective data and objective data. Subjective data are obtained from a patient or a competent representative. Particular focus is placed on the chief complaint (CC) and descriptions of the symptom or symptoms that prompted the person to initiate contact with the health care system. The CC should be recorded in the patient's own words. An example of a fatigue-related CC could be, "I've been feeling run-down lately." Unfortunately, fatigue, in any clinical condition, is one of the most difficult complaints to analyze. What does *run-down* mean? How long is *lately?* Additional questions (gathering subjective data) are asked to obtain a clinical picture or impression to guide the clinician in further investigation. A good clinician can often spare expensive diagnostic tests by first asking the right questions.

Objective data are obtained from a physical examination and diagnostic procedures. For instance, if the patient's CC corresponds to physical findings of poor circulation, a fever, an infection, wheezing in the lungs, or a laboratory value indicating low hemoglobin, it may be reasonably easy to analyze. Further, if the word *lately* refers to a period of 7 days in someone with cancer, the person received chemotherapy 14 days ago, and the hemoglobin level is 9 milligrams per deciliter (mg/dL), the problem may be anemia. If a person has a hemoglobin of 15 mg/dL, is not receiving any kind of therapy that affects laboratory levels, but has wheezing in the lungs and a slight fever, one of the first additional diagnostic studies ordered may be an x-ray to see if the person has pneumonitis.

Fatigue Is Not a Symptom

As we examine cancer-related fatigue, we must come to a conclusion: Fatigue is not a symptom. Generally speaking, it is a phenomenon. Medically speaking, it is a syndrome. To continue to call it a symptom is misleading and contributes to mischaracterization. A *syndrome* is broadly defined as a group or complex of symptoms that indicates or distinguishes the existence of an undesirable or abnormal condition or quality. The word *fatigue* has proved to be grossly inadequate; in fact, the continuing tendency to lump all the related phenomena under this one word may be our biggest hindrance to understanding it. Hence, fatigue as part of the cancer experience more accurately should be called a syndrome or, specifically, the cancer-related fatigue syndrome (CRFS). Viewing fatigue as a symptom continues to obstruct meaningful communication between clinicians, researchers, and patients, functioning as a barrier to problem solving. If we view it as a syndrome, the widespread, multidimensional nature of fatigue becomes much more logical and promotes

> *The Fellowship of those who bear the Mark of Pain. . . . Who are the members of this fellowship? Those who have learned by experience what physical pain and bodily anguish mean, belong together the world over; they are united by a secret bond. One and all they know the horrors of suffering to which man can be exposed, and one and all they know the longing to be free from pain. He who has been delivered . . . must not think he is now free again to take up life just as it was before, entirely forgetful of the past. He is now a `man whose eyes are open.' . . . And he must bring to others the deliverance which he has himself enjoyed. . . . Such is the Fellowship of those who bear the Mark of Pain.*
>
> Albert Schweitzer
> *Out of My Life and Thought:*
> *An Autobiography*

meaningful exploration. Wittgenstein's proposal of a "family of meanings" applies here (Kaplan, 1964, p. 48). In a family of meanings, it is not a matter of definitive features being common to all the members of the family, but the sharing of some features that show the resemblance by some members of the family with one another. The CRFS is very much a family of meanings.

Cella et al (1998) drafted cancer-related fatigue diagnostic criteria to accompany the ICD-10 (*International Classification of Diseases*) code (World Health Organization, 1998). In their proposal, they list four diagnostic criteria for this code (Cella et al, 1998):

There are many causes and manifestations involved in what we call fatigue. In order to avoid confusion, we should more properly consider this phenomenon (since there are many manifestations) as a syndrome, hence, the cancer-related fatigue syndrome (CRFS).

1. Six or more of 11 criteria are present daily or nearly every day for the same two-week period during the past month of which at least one symptom is significant fatigue.
2. The symptoms contribute to clinically significant distress or impairment in social, occupational, or other important areas of functioning.
3. There are historical, physical, or laboratory findings indicating the symptoms are sequelae of cancer or cancer therapy.
4. The symptoms are not primarily a consequence of comorbid psychiatric conditions such as major depression, somatization disorder, or delirium.

The 11 symptoms associated with item 1 (above) are as follows (Cella et al, 1998):

a. significant fatigue, diminished energy, and increased need for rest that are disproportional to any change in level of exertion;
b. complaints of generalized weakness or limb heaviness;
c. diminished concentration or attention;
d. decreased motivation or willingness to engage in usual activities;
e. insomnia or hypersomnia;
f. experience of sleep as unfreshing or nonrestorative;
g. perceived need to struggle to overcome inactivity;
h. marked emotional reactivity (e.g., sadness, frustration, or irritability) to feeling fatigued;
i. difficulty completing daily tasks attributable to feeling fatigued;
j. perceived problems with short-term memory;
k. postexertional malaise lasting several hours.

These authors also proposed a single-page, cancer-related fatigue diagnostic interview guide to establish a standardized means for the identification of research subjects. Although they emphasized this was a draft, it acknowledges the many manifestations and dimensions of fatigue that should be acceptable to most researchers. Breitbart (personal communication, March 10, 1999), one of the proponents of these documents, even suggested we may be looking at fatigue syndromes (plural) rather than a single syndrome.

The CRFS is particularly important in clinical populations because it influences, and is influenced by, a variety of clinical outcomes ranging from emotional states to social interaction and functional performance in everyday living. The economic implications–from the cost of medications to the cost of assisted care, caregiver exhaustion, and the draining of community resources–are staggering.

The experience of the CRFS has always been a part of the clinical presentation in the various types and diverse stages of cancer. In the "old days," people got cancer (or under whatever label it was or was not diagnosed), they went to bed, and they died. Fatigue was accepted as part of the illness, part of the dying process. It was not questioned. In addition, treatments have multiple effects that reasonably contribute to the fatigue phenomenon. Finally, long-term survival after cancer treatments has brought about issues of cancer as a chronic condition.

> *How do you expect a man who is warm to understand a man who is cold?*
>
> Aleksandr Isayevich Solzhenitsyn, cancer survivor, *One Day in the Life of Ivan Denisovich*

Sources of Error in Understanding the Cancer-Related Fatigue Syndrome

In the past 50 years, aggressive therapies have resulted in improved survival rates for many types of cancer. These therapies have been characterized by many complicated and life-threatening clinical problems and impaired quality of life. Unfortunately, some survivors continue to suffer from disease and treatment-related impairments long after termination of their treatments. Persistent, often unresolved fatigability is one of the most debilitating after-cancer conditions. Associated decrements in functioning inevitably affect every aspect of life and significantly influence quality of life.

Pain and nausea have been the focus of considerable intervention research. The treatment of cancer pain is well codified, with many alternatives. How is it that we have missed fatigue, the most distressing symptom of all? It has been half a century since Karnofsky and Burchenal (1949) proposed outcome measures for chemotherapy that included functional status. Their suggestion was based on the observation that patients may show improved clinical status, yet experience decreased functional status. (The link between functional status and quality of life appeared to be so inviolate that for decades, performance scales were the singular research indicators of patient's well-being in clinical trials.) They saw the need to monitor multidimensional indicators of treatment outcomes. Research has shown that we consistently underestimate how fatigue influences patients' lives. Why? Perhaps part of the reason can be attributed to the arrogance and ignorance of presuming we can understand how other people live and feel on the basis of a five-minute, hurried, clinical observation that usually focuses on a disease process. Further, clinical observations can lead to grossly inaccurate conclusions because they take place in such artificial settings. This cannot be the whole reason: Some very fine and observant clinicians have been fooled by fatigue and the patient's appearance.

In her classic book *Notes on Nursing* (1859, p. 30), Florence Nightingale warned about the likelihood of misjudging the functional well-being of patients based on superficial observation. She observed the effect of excitement on patient behavior. She stated, "It is the highest folly to judge of the sick, as is so often done, when you see them merely during a period of excitement." Perceptive nurses have long remarked about how patients who can barely walk into the clinic will look, talk, and walk miraculously well when the "white coat" walks through the door. Patients themselves are often confused by this apparent enigma.

If observations, or objective data, are the source of error, how is a clinician to know the true state of the patient? Nightingale (1859) advised, "Come back and look at your patient after he has had an hour's animated conversation with you. It is the best test of his real state we know. But never pronounce upon him from merely seeing what he does, or how he looks, during such a conversation. Learn also carefully and exactly, if you can, how he passed the night after it. . . . Almost every effect of over-exertion appears after, not during such exertion." Until recently, we have been assessing patients' functioning based on observations, usually by the Karnofsky Scale or some similar means (Eastern Cooperative Oncology Group, World Health Organization, or Zubrod scales are variants) during a period of excitement. It then becomes clear: We have been grossly overestimating patients' ability to function and underestimating their fatigability for a long time because we did not understand the artifact introduced by the very ones doing the assessment!

> *If the "fatigue" in cancer we are hearing so much about is such a serious and distressing part of the cancer experience, why has it taken so long for us to recognize it?*

The lack of regard for the "classics" in graduate science and medicine today has also contributed to our dilemma. How can we teach that which we do not know? Most faculty, who have been trained in narrow disciplines, are not aware of the tradition of learning that could provide universality in learning. We have ignored or forgotten the very references that could teach us the insights of a science long past. In Chapter 2, the physiological basis of Florence Nightingale's insightful comments will become clear as they are linked to significant, physiologically based work by Harvard's Walter B. Cannon and associates (1929).

Observation is the key to good medicine, taught Lord Lister, establishing one of the most sacred foundations of modern medicine. Indeed, observation has been considered the "objective" key to good medical diagnosis. The objective observations of the professional have been treated as inviolate in comparison with the "subjective" reports of the patient. This is even reflected in our patronizing clinical documentation language: "patient alleges," "patient states," "patient claims." The suspicion is transmitted that the patient is not to be completely believed or trusted.[4]

One frequently heard definition of fatigue is, "Fatigue is what the patient says it is," or, like Muscio (1921) lamented, "The Test = The Test" (no wonder he was frustrated!). This definition tells us nothing more useful than that we finally acknowledge that the patient may be experiencing something real, even if we cannot see it. This may be vaguely sufficient for patient descriptors in the clinical setting, but far more is needed for any kind of meaningful communication to take place. First, we must ask ourselves whether fatigue as we understand it is fatigue as patients are trying to communicate it. Second, vague or forced definitions are likely to result in minimally useful clinical interventions and bad science. There is no doubt that we must find better ways to explore, understand, and communicate about the CRFS in a meaningful way if we are to accomplish anything useful. "Fatigue is what the patient says it is" precludes communicating an individual's experience in a way that can be associated with such specific objective markers as anemia, neurotransmitter activity, cytokines, and other measures that may provide the basis for exciting intervention breakthroughs. It provides no basis for investigating mechanisms or linking those mechanisms to interventions. Finally, to understand "what the patient says it is," we have to learn more effective ways of listening.

As already discussed, many definitions for *fatigue* have been suggested. Most of them represent a conceptual narrowness that reflects the researcher's particular area of expertise. Herein lies the problem: There are three sources of communication chasms relevant to the CRFS (see next section). Each of these types of communication constitutes more of a barrier than we are aware. Because we tend to assume that others think like we do, we frequently fail to be aware of the enormity of the barriers. In fact, it is because healthy health care workers cannot think like someone experiencing the CRFS that we have a problem! To oversimplify this complex phenomenon is to obscure, obliterate, or ignore good information that could lead to effective solutions. Certainly in the area of cancer-related fatigue, the best hope for understanding will be in formulating clear and meaningful bridges to communication in all three of these areas. Without effective communications, we will continue building our conceptual, clinical, and research "Tower of Babel."

Rather than continuing to struggle for a universal definition of fatigue (which is likely to prove futile and counterproductive, for numerous reasons), we can use other approaches to help us understand this phenomenon and develop effective interventions. A two-front attack would yield the most effective results in understanding and developing effective interventions for the CRFS:

1. Focus on differentiating the various types and conditions of fatigue manifestations, as well as linguistic, gender, age, and cultural variations in reported perception. This involves more than qualitative interview research techniques. It involves employing as many communication techniques as creativity can appreciate and allowing people a choice in how they wish to convey that information.
2. Undertake parallel studies in the mechanisms of fatigue and how the different mechanisms (for they are surely legion) influence perception.

Chapter 2 addresses the biophysiological approach to understanding the body's experience of fatigue phenomena. The rest of this chapter addresses communication hindrances to understanding and solving the riddle of the CRFS.

Three Areas of Communication Breakdown

Three sources of communication breakdown hinder understanding and intervention development with respect to the CRFS. On a grander scale, these problems are associated with investigating the age-old questions, What is life?, What is man?, and What is his place in the universe? There are many levels at which answers can be sought.

1. *Definitionally.* Measurement is the time-honored means by which we establish "truth" and define the parameters of scientific investigation. There are two fundamental branches of the sciences, each with very different philosophies and methods of measurement.

   a. The *biophysical* sciences place great emphasis on precision and reproducibility of measurement. They attempt to identify a gold standard and then measure other things by comparing them to this standard. Much of this work takes place under controlled laboratory conditions.

   b. *Psychosocial* research tends to focus on behavioral phenomena. Researchers are concerned with reliability and validity. Since the thoughts or feelings behind the behaviors are not visible, it is necessary to resort to asking questions, or making observations about behavioral patterns. Their instruments, rather than microscopes, barometers, and goniometers, often consist of questionnaires, interviews, and behavioral observation techniques.

   There tends to be a good deal of suspicion between the two groups. The biophysical scientists tend to think their science is purer and of a higher level than that of the psychosocial scientists (perhaps because it usually is much more expensive). Objectivity is the means by which they guard their research from the "sin" of personal bias. Psychosocial scientists also tend to carry a bias. They often think of biophysical scientists as cold, uncaring, and impractical. Van Doren (1991, p. 188) flatly stated ". . . science deals almost exclusively with things, not ideas or feelings, . . . inner states and their working."

   Whereas medicine has tended to emphasize the biophysical tradition of objectivity, most nurse researchers have been trained in various psychosocial traditions. Hence, it is not unexpected that nurses lead the way in pioneering the study of the cancer-related fatigue phenomenon and in exploring interventions. In fact, the first reference to fatigue in cancer was published by Haylock and Hart in 1979—20 years ago! More recently, researchers have bridged the gap between the two philosophies and methodologies by borrowing from both. It is this approach that shows the greatest promise in the CRFS since both approaches and areas of expertise are needed.

2. *Conceptually.* Hypotheses and theoretical frameworks are used to provide direction and focus to scientific inquiry. Without them, we have to wonder whether, despite

efforts to obtain very impressive precise and repeatable measurements, we are measuring the right things, whether those measurement have any meaning, or whether we are doing anything useful at all!

3. *Experientially*. Humans have devised many ways by which they explore and communicate about their experience. Science is but one of these means. Art, music, and dance are among the many ways feelings, experiences, and perceptions are explored. Creativity sometimes leaps across the chasm that science alone cannot breech.

How the human experience of life is perceived can vary greatly, depending on how information is communicated. For instance, using the language of biomedical statistics, we might write, "According to the American Cancer Society, there will be 1,228,600 new cases of cancer this year." There is little human connectivity here, little useful information, but impressive numbers. Now from a psychosocial perspective, it might be written, "Of the 1,228,600 new cases of cancer this year, Native Americans and African Americans have a lesser chance for survival. This is often because of inadequate screening resources. Our research is investigating methods for increasing awareness of screening resources among these populations." But on another level, we may read this poem by a young black woman who was recently diagnosed with advanced ovarian cancer at the age of 15 and has a poor prognosis for survival:

Suddenly I feel alone in my darkness.
Someone pulled the bridge of life out from under me.
All I wanted was to cross over and be with my friends.
Now I don't see anyone on either side and I am falling.

We respond quite differently to this. There is an insight shared in the experience of the one that was not there in describing the experience of the many.

Finally, if we hear, "Your tests have come back. The news is mixed. You have a rare type of cancer. The prognosis is poor, but we're trying some new experimental treatments . . . ," we probably will not hear more before going into emotional shock. No matter how objective and scientific we are, at some level, the human response is still overwhelming and frightening. At this level, we cross a threshold of understanding that is impossible to breech any other way.

The human response to the CRFS is greatly understudied. This is where we most need to learn communication techniques. Without it, our assumptions will continue to lead us into chaos and disorder. Perhaps conceptualizing the CRFS as "plaid" may help. In weaving, there is the woof and the warp. No two threads cross each other at the same place. Similarly, no two experiences are alike, and the resulting colors and the patterns may be quite different.

Studies that fail to involve an interdisciplinary team are more likely to fall into at least one of five sources of error:

1. "discoveries" that are not useful because they are not sufficiently generalizable
2. discoveries that were already published years ago in other disciplinary journals, perhaps expressed under different terms
3. the failure to recognize, discriminate, or distinguish significant phenomena and thus close doors to potential areas of significant discovery
4. claims to have discovered something special when, indeed, there is nothing but artifact (the Woozle effect)
5. the development of clinical interventions, based on ignorance, that may accomplish nothing or may actually lead to harm in patients

It is essential that research projects and committees include patient or consumer representatives, insightful, articulate individuals who have lived through the experience. This helps provide a means whereby researchers can protect themselves from making well-intended, erroneous assumptions and patients or families can be shielded from needlessly burdensome expectations and demands on their time and energy.

Additional Barriers to Communication

Following are three additional barriers to communicating about the CFRS that we need to bridge if we are to accomplish anything meaningful.

1. We need to consider how people understand and interpret feelings, sensations, and phenomena associated with the CRFS. This involves how they interpret the feeling and express it within themselves. In developing testing instruments for adults, we have jumped in and thrown words at them. *Our* words. In most cases, these words are inadequate and actually misleading. Moreover, they have selected those words because of words or phrases they heard from us to begin with. Descriptors (words or terms) may be as misleading as definitions (i.e., as in "The Word = the Word" problem). The answers to such fundamental questions as "How does it feel?," "How bad is it?," "Has it changed?," or "What does it mean to you?" may not lie in words. Age, gender, cultural background, peer group and lifestyle orientation, language sophistication, and actual levels of excitement and mental exhaustion or confusion can have a significant impact on communication.[5]
2. Etymology is the science that studies the historical origins and development of languages and how forms and meaning of words were transmitted from one language to another. To demonstrate the difficulty and diversity of verbal communication in terms of etymology alone, review the historical presentation of relevant words associated with the CRFS (see Table 1-1). In addition, techniques from the developing field of sociolinguistics may be able to facilitate our task.

   In Chapter 23, Tricia C. Corbett suggests that the word *fatigue* should be abandoned altogether. As she put it, "Sometimes you simply do not have the word to describe how you are feeling. You either dance around the problem in muddled explanations, or you use words like 'fatigue,' which are sort of close, but not close enough. Here the miscommunication starts. People think they know what the word fatigue means and don't really listen to what you are trying to say." She emphasizes that we should encourage the use of all types of communication, nonverbal as well as verbal (i.e., metaphors, art, poetry, gestures, descriptors) to communicate feelings and phenomena related to the CRFS. Another problem is that people with cancer often do not know how to communicate what is happening to them or what is different. They do not have the words that plug into the professional vocabulary. They are trying to communicate with us at a time when they are so exhausted. We should be facilitating them; they should not have to struggle to facilitate us. We need to conceptualize this in terms of a multidimensional model of translation, transliteration, and transformation of various kinds of information.

3. Finally, we need to work on communicating and integrating information between disciplinary specialties, especially those representing different philosophies of science.

The biggest problem in CRFS scholarship today involves communication deficits that can be traced to *us*. Fatigue has been a trendy word for decades, used by scientists of various disciplines depending on sociohistorial exigencies and on the sources of research funding. The use of the same word for multiple phenomena by multiple disciplines has contributed to the confusion and ignorance that currently inhibit an understanding of the CRFS.

Contemporary CRFS scholars do not seem to be aware of much of the historical precedents associated with the study of fatigue. There are several reasons for this: (1) The use of electronic database systems is partially responsible, since the contents of whole libraries of publications prior to the era of computerized reference databases have become relatively inaccessible. (2) Many older books and research articles were printed on high-sulfur-content paper, particularly during wartime and the 1930s depression era. This paper is now crumbling, and methods to preserve it or put the pages on microfilm are economically prohibitive for most libraries, particularly in the face of cutbacks. (3) Most older scholars who were familiar with this literature are retired or deceased. With their departure has gone a great deal of unrecorded experience and oral history. (4) The current approach to obtaining research funding and the emphasis on referring only to recent references have resulted in ignorance or repetition of quality research that was carried out as much as several decades ago. In some cases, today's research, although popular, is inferior in quality to that done in the past. (5) Today's researchers are demonstrating considerable neglect in tracing

> *They do not have the words that plug into the professional vocabulary. They are trying to communicate with us at a time when they are so exhausted. We should be facilitating them; they should not have to struggle to facilitate us.*

the origins of ideas, theoretical models, and research findings to their roots. The intellectual acknowledgment of the contributions of others in our work (including work done by researchers in other disciplines) through careful referencing of publications is more than an issue of honesty. This scholarly integrity helps us plot an orderly and productive course to the future by examining the road map of our past. As a result of all these factors, we are not taking advantage of considerable knowledge that has implications for the CRFS and could allow us to make faster progress toward finding effective interventions.

A Mathematical Model for Evaluating Fatigue in Cancer

Using a mathematical construct can help us categorize information in such a way as to contribute rapid, organized, and effectual progress in investigating the CRFS. We could start by placing a simple conceptual equation in the form of questions:

(A)   What is the experiential nature of a phenomenon?
(B) – What is the common experience of that phenomenon?
(C) = What is the unique/specific experience of that phenomenon?

When examining any clinical phenomenon or symptom, there is a need first to inquire about its overall characteristics and mechanisms. Do they exist in the healthy population in general? It is impossible to clarify the issues in the cancer experience in isolation (i.e., only in people with cancer). However, it is necessary to subtract the universal experience or phenomenon to isolate the issues specific to the subpopulation we wish to study. If the experience of a phenomenon is only known among specific clinical populations, we would benefit by examining the experience in those populations. Elsewhere in this book, issues related to cognitive fatigue are presented, and the effects of mild traumatic brain injury (MTBI) are compared with those of cognitive fatigue in cancer. There seem to be a number of similarities. Whereas little research has been carried out on intervention techniques for cognitive fatigue in cancer, some of the many techniques used in MTBI may be helpful. There are currently no data to indicate that the CRFS is different from the fatigue associated with any other debilitating chronic illness.·

Following are two approaches for applying these principles to the CRFS:

(A)   What is the overall experience of fatigue in people with cancer?
(B) – What is the experience of fatigue in healthy individuals?
(C) = What fatigue experiences are specific to people with cancer?

Alternatively, depending on what information is needed, the equation could be phrased as follows:

(A)   What is the overall experience of fatigue in people with cancer?
(B) – What is the experience of fatigue in people with chronic illnesses?
(C) = What fatigue experiences are specific to people with cancer?

Using this model, we can identify our first imperative: Separate out the causes or conditions of cancer-related fatigue from the causes of everyday, normal fatigue. Until we do that, we do not know how to address the issues specific to cancer. Dimensions can be added to this model to investigate the effects of time and interaction. To date, this has not been done. Hence, we need to undertake quality empirical research that separates and elucidates the experiences and mechanisms specific to cancer.

Research carried out by NASA demonstrating the dangers of bed rest in healthy individuals is a case in point. Since all humans are subject to the same physical and physiological influences, it is safe to assume that cancer patients who spend increasing time in bed or in recliners, for whatever reason, will experience similar effects. (These are discussed in greater detail in Chapter 2.) Greenleaf and Kozlowski (1982) presented the concept of a horizontal-vertical ratio as contributing to optimal health: Increased time spent in the horizontal position (increased rest or sleep) decreases time spent in the vertical position and affects the ratio unfavorably. This seems to contribute to deterioration of every organ system of the body. It would be neither efficient, beneficial, nor ethical to subject people with cancer to bed rest studies merely to test whether they respond the same as other humans. Just because they have cancer does not make them less than human! Because we already possess some information, we can continue with the next step, testing interventions. We know that NASA has carried out extensive studies looking at the ill effects of bed rest and how to prevent them. How much of what cancer patients experience is preventable by the same interventions, and how do we carry out those interventions safely, considering the complicating conditions of cancer? By comparing two control groups (a normal healthy group and a cancer control group) with the cancer intervention group, it will be possible to determine whether the cancer intervention group has an unexpected or differential response.

Proposing a Conceptual Matrix as a Basis for Research

Building on the mathematical model, we can organize what we already know versus what we do not know into a more complex conceptual matrix. In this way, we can break down how much we know into the appropriate category and start to focus on the most fundamental, critical areas. This is illustrated in Table 1-2.

Knowledge is entered into the matrix on the horizontal dimension with established, research-based knowledge on the right and complete lack of knowledge on the left. Specificity of information is entered on the vertical dimension with universal phenomena on the top and specific, qualitative information on the bottom. Each level contains more data from which applicable information can be drawn. As data accumulate, there is a synthesis of implications across disciplines (obviously requiring global thinking and interdisciplinary training). Each downward level not only provides more information but also provides data on which information is appropriate to the needs of any specific individual based on genetic,

| Table 1.2 | Conceptual Matrix for Categorizing the Knowledge Base Related to Cancer-Related Fatigue | | | |

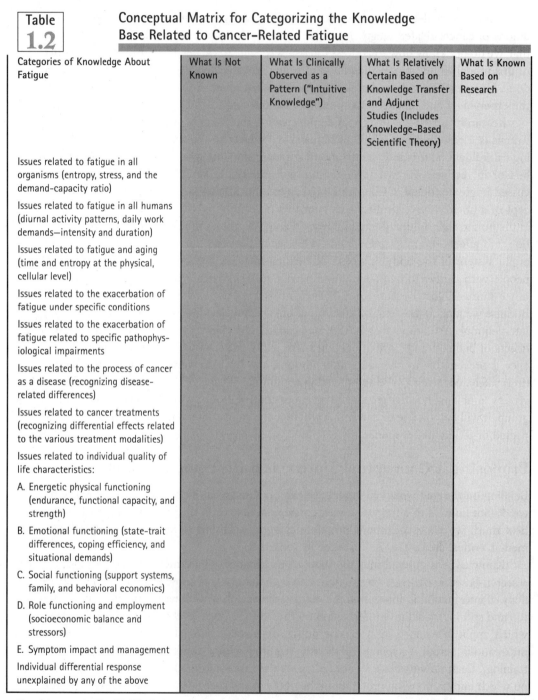

Categories of Knowledge About Fatigue	What Is Not Known	What Is Clinically Observed as a Pattern ("Intuitive Knowledge")	What Is Relatively Certain Based on Knowledge Transfer and Adjunct Studies (Includes Knowledge-Based Scientific Theory)	What Is Known Based on Research
Issues related to fatigue in all organisms (entropy, stress, and the demand-capacity ratio)				
Issues related to fatigue in all humans (diurnal activity patterns, daily work demands—intensity and duration)				
Issues related to fatigue and aging (time and entropy at the physical, cellular level)				
Issues related to the exacerbation of fatigue under specific conditions				
Issues related to the exacerbation of fatigue related to specific pathophysiological impairments				
Issues related to the process of cancer as a disease (recognizing disease-related differences)				
Issues related to cancer treatments (recognizing differential effects related to the various treatment modalities)				
Issues related to individual quality of life characteristics:				
A. Energetic physical functioning (endurance, functional capacity, and strength)				
B. Emotional functioning (state-trait differences, coping efficiency, and situational demands)				
C. Social functioning (support systems, family, and behavioral economics)				
D. Role functioning and employment (socioeconomic balance and stressors)				
E. Symptom impact and management				
Individual differential response unexplained by any of the above				

pathological, intellectual, emotional, social, and other needs. In summary, medical scientific knowledge should dynamically progress from the general to the specific, from the universal to the individual, to produce a more humanistic medicine. As each downward level provides information that can be strategically individualized according to the need of the individual, there should be a corresponding increased potential for enhancing quality of life.

We seem to have forgotten our heritage. The good science of today builds on the solid science of the past. How can this happen when students are penalized for using any references more than five or ten years old? Not only are young scholars in training ignorant of their heritage, but their mentors are equally ignorant. By encouraging graduate students to track the historical origins of their disciplines, they will make a grand discovery: Much of what is being called new today has a conceptual base that may go back 100 years or more.

A study of the philosophy of science among graduate students in most disciplines is rapidly becoming an anachronism. The fundamental rules of scientific inquiry are few; yet it is likely that few graduate students could repeat and explain even one of Newton's rules of science (see next section). Regardless of the disciplinary training we have received as scientists, a brief review of the following ideas that changed the world may guide us in rediscovering our common past and our quest of the mysteries of the CRFS.

The farther back we go, the more we discover our common scientific roots. That is also the basis for our understanding of one another. The innovation and creativity required to elicit the mysteries of the foundations of science in the late 1500s are the same as those required for the discovery of the foundations of cellular metabolism in the late 1700s, intracellular stability in the late 1800s, and genetic cellular mechanisms being elucidated at the end of this millennium. Those discoveries still speak to us today. Throughout these centuries, there were corresponding theoretical developments in the understanding of philosophy, probability, and statistics that eventually led to the development of the modern psychosocial disciplines.

Insights about fatigue are threaded throughout the development of the sciences. We need to go back to the greatest leader in the origins of science to be refreshed in the basics of what caused science to change the world.

Words From the Wise

Some attribute the birth of modern science to a single statement by William of Ockham (fourteenth century). "Ockham's Razor," as it is called, simply states, "What can be done with fewer is done in vain with more." In other words, keep it simple if simple will do. Sir Isaac Newton provided us with four rules of reasoning in philosophy. These are originally found in Book III of *Principia* written in 1687, but today can be found in various places (e.g., Modern History Sourcebook, Isaac Newton: *The Mathematical Principles of Natural Philosophy;* <http://www.fordham.edu/halsall/mod/newton-princ.html>). Newton started by acknowledging Ockham's logic:

1. *We are to admit no more causes of natural things, than such as are both true and sufficient to explain their appearances. . . . Nature does nothing in vain, and more is in vain, when less will serve; for Nature is pleased with simplicity and affects not the pomp of superfluous causes.* This concept of "true and sufficient" is a challenge to us: It has always been the basis for good science. Can we look for a simple explanation behind what appears to be complex phenomena?

2. *Therefore to the same natural effects we must, as far as possible, assign the same causes. . . . As to respiration in a man and in a beast.* In other words, don't waste time investigating the obvious. Nature is very efficient. It is not the similarity but the differences that are remarkable and warrant investigation (such as is presented in the section "A Mathematical Model for Evaluating Fatigue in Cancer").

3. *The qualities of bodies . . . which are found to belong to all bodies within the reach of our experiments, are to be esteemed the universal qualities of all bodies whatsoever.* The application of this third rule is not as easy as it appears. What are the "universal qualities of all bodies"? Where do our assumptions become presumptions? When are we wasting time reinventing the wheel? We can guard against violating this rule by careful reviews of the literature and prior work to see whether we find an exception that demands clarification. In the psychosocial sciences, the use of statistics tests how universal the outcomes are among a group being studied.

4. *In experimental philosophy we are to look upon propositions inferred by general induction from phenomena as accurately or very nearly true, notwithstanding any contrary hypotheses that may be imagined, till such time as other phenomena occur, by which they may either be made more accurate, or liable to exceptions.* In other words, "Good inductive reasoning may not be sabotaged by sloppy and poorly rationalized hypotheses."

Newton could not resist adding a clarification to the fourth rule: He warned against vain hypothesizing, something he found particularly irritating. He had no tolerance for windbags who liked to hypothesize without a responsible reference to facts or data. This

---

How are the healthy to understand the bone-wearying fatigue the ill live with? Again and again we are struck with the difficulty patients have in making others understand how much even the slightest exertions cost. A few days after the liberation of the Nazi concentration camp Bergen-Belsen, Fania Fenelon described their liberators . . . "We felt an absurd desire to finger them, to let our hands trail in their eddies as in the Fountain of Youth. . . . How alive they were, they walked quickly, they ran, they leapt. All of these movements were so easy for them, while a single one of them would have taken away our last breath of life. These men seemed not to know that one can live in slow motion, that energy was something you saved."

M. Gilbert, *The Holocaust: A History of the Jews of Europe During the Second World War*

prohibition against hypothesizing, of offering explanations not directly supported by experiments, defined the scientific method as it has been practiced since Newton's time and as it should be practiced today.

By following these simple rules, we can see that both biophysical and psychosocial sciences are best served. On this common ground, we can meet and bring our findings. On this meeting ground, we can make tremendous progress in jointly pursuing an understanding of the CRFS.

Where Do We Go From Here?

If we are going to make effective and coordinated progress toward an understanding of the CRFS, we need to carry out a six-point plan:

Fatigue is not a definition, nor is it a simplistic problem. It is an exploration. The magnitude of the problem presents exciting hopes for us all to work together to develop ways to alleviate the suffering of others. . . . the greatest gift we can both give and receive.

1. Form an interdisciplinary team of scholars to peruse the research literature dating back as far as the 1880s and earlier for clues relating to fatigue. A repository of key references and resources should be assembled for access by other scholars and especially to help in training graduate students in the art of following historical, scientific trails. These clues can then be inserted in the appropriate place on the matrix in Table 1-2 to provide a map for further work.

2. Place this initial matrix on an international Web site so researchers all over the world can submit their work for identified placement.[6] The matrix will need to be reformulated and expanded as the knowledge base increases. This should help all scholars and researchers to broaden their understanding of the CRFS and develop more creative approaches to investigation. It should help prevent unnecessary overlap between research done by various disciplines and institutions while encouraging efficiency and cooperation. This should also facilitate in identifying findings that need further investigation.

3. At the same time, carry out the development of a broad database of descriptors and other forms of communication used by people with cancer with respect to their fatigue. This should be across age groups and multinational in nature. Researchers who work on this database should be multilingual and have multicultural experience. Art, poetry, music, and sculptures should be included. It is important to emphasize that "talent" consists of the experience, not the polished professionalism of the product.

4. Encourage the formation of interdisciplinary teams in each clinic and medical center for the further investigation of the CRFS and how it interacts with other symptoms, syndromes, and outcomes in general. Established techniques for evaluating quality-control outcomes can be used to facilitate this task.

5. Establish an international quality-control database examining interventions that appear to have the greatest positive outcome with respect to individual functional independence and quality of life. This can help identify the places where third-party reimbursement policies can be focused to do the most good.

6. Make sure articulate, informed consumers are on every interdisciplinary research team.

Fatigue is not a definition, nor is it a simplistic problem. It is an exploration. The magnitude of the problem presents exciting hopes for us all to work together to develop ways to alleviate the suffering of others. To be able to alleviate suffering is the greatest gift we can both give and receive. Few researchers today have ever read the seminal works of science. Cumulative science, requiring an awareness of fundamental rules of scientific logic, must, of necessity, assemble and maintain a database that includes seminal works, and present it in an articulate progression through rigorous curricula and integrity in research mentoring. Science is about facts, about sound reasoning about solid facts. Reasoning without data quickly degrades into specious sophistry.

Endnotes

1. I have heard a number of women liken cancer fatigue with their experience of pregnancy-related fatigue. This may provide a unique subpopulation for study since they seem to identify a different perceptual baseline than the "healthy" who have no frame of reference. People experiencing an analogous, debilitating fatigue that accompanies other chronic illnesses, certain medications, or severe injuries also seem to use similar descriptive metaphors and comparisons. They also share comparative insights and reports of disruption in their lives.

2. Schweitzer conceptualized pain as anything that contributed to a "diminution of life." Certainly cancer fatigue is consistent with this. The origins of the word *fatigue* include torture, anguish, and pain.

3. Note to readers: Although many think Dr. Hans Selye coined the word *stress*, he actually applied it as a generalized expression (1956) based on Cannon's 1915 presentation of a unified sympathetic nervous system response to environmental threat through the "fight or flight" mechanism. The word *stress* as related to emotional distress dates at least to the days of Shakespeare! In the 1950s, Selye emphasized that threats were "stressors" and that threats could also come from within. Coping theory suggested that efficiency of adaptation to the stressor was really the critical issue. Selye's general adaptation syndrome theory also talked about an ultimate exhaustion from long-term stressors that exceeded the organism's capacity to respond and adapt. Also see J. Aistars excellent article on fatigue in cancer, which incorporates stress theory (1987).

4. I once witnessed a physician interrupt a patient who was trying to describe her pain: "You're too close to the problem to be objective. . . . *I'll* tell you when you're in pain"!

5. In my copy of Cannon's book, *Bodily Changes in Pain, Hunger, Fear, and Rage* (1929), an anonymous former owner wrote the following delightful annotation: "Even science palls before the

moods. Here is a book dealing with the bodily changes characteristic of the fundamental emotions of human and animal life–pain, hunger, threat, fear, and rage; yet the changes characteristic of sex are unmentioned. This cannot be due entirely to instrumental difficulties. The study of sex is not restricted to a study of the sex act. In humans, at least, instrumental difficulties may, to some extent, be overcome–as has been proven even by Columbia undergraduates. The difficulty appears to be in the chaste Harvard mind."

6. Some significant research related to the CRFS that has been published and is being carried out outside of the United States is not receiving the appropriate recognition or visibility. European publications, in particular, are often not accessible or acknowledged in the United States. This work should be recognized and appreciated.

References

Aistars, J. (1987). Fatigue in the cancer patient: A conceptual approach to a clinical problem. *Oncology Nursing Forum, 14*, 25–30.

The American Heritage dictionary of the English language, third edition (1992). Boston: Houghton Mifflin. Electronic version licensed from INSO Corporation.

Barton-Burke, M. (1998). *Fatigue and quality of life.* In C. R. King and P. Hinds (Eds.), *Quality of life: From nursing and patient perspectives* (pp. 255–283). Sudbury, MA: Jones and Bartlett.

Cannon, W. B. (1929). *Bodily changes in pain, hunger, fear, and rage.* 2nd ed. New York: D. Appleton (first edition published in 1915).

Cella, D., Peterman, A., Passik, S., Jacobson, P., and Breitbart, W. (1988). Progress toward guidelines for the management of fatigue. *Oncology, 12* (11A), 369–377.

The compact edition of the Oxford English Dictionary (1971). Oxford: Oxford University Press.

Crabb, G. (1879). *English synonymes* (p. 856). New edition. New York: Harper & Brothers.

Fatigue Coalition (1998). Fatigue most prevalent, longest-lasting cancer-related side effect. <http://www.plsgroup.com/dg/b090c.htm>.

Greenleaf, J. E., and Kozlowski, S. (1982). Physiological consequences of reduced physical activity during bed rest. *Exercise and Sports Science Review, 10*, 84–119.

Haylock, P. J., and Hart, L. K. (1979). Fatigue in patients receiving localized radiation. *Oncology Nursing Forum, 2*, 461–467.

Kaplan, A. (1964). *The conduct of inquiry.* San Francisco: Chandler.

Karnofsky, D. A., and Burchenal, J. H. (1949). The clinical evaluation of chemotherapeutic agents used in cancer. In C. M. MacLeod (Ed.), *Evaluation of chemotherapeutic agents* (p. 196). New York: Columbia University Press.

March F. A., Sr., and March, F. A., Jr. (1902). *A thesaurus dictionary of the English language* (p. 1192). Philadelphia: Historical Publishing.

Muscio, B. (1921). Is a fatigue test possible? *British Journal of Psychology, 12*, 31–46.

Nightingale, F. (1859). *Notes on nursing.* London: Harrison and Sons. (Reprinted in offset in 1946 by Edward Stern & Co., Philadelphia.)

Schweitzer, A. (1948). *Out of my life and thought: An autobiography.* C. T. Campion, translator. New York: Henry Holt.

Scott, G.R. (1952). *Swan's Anglo-American dictionary* (p. 1514). New York: Library Publishers.

Selye, H. (1956). *The stress of life*. New York: McGraw-Hill.

Tufte, E. R. (1997). *Visual explanations* (pp. 94–95). Cheshire, CT: Graphics Press.

Van Doren, C. (1991). *The history of knowledge*. New York: Ballantine.

World Health Organization (1992). *International diagnostic classification (ICD-10)*. Geneva: World Health Organization. Web site: <http://www.who.int/msa/mnh/ems/icd10/cliexamp.htm>

Wyld, H. C. (1939). *The universal dictionary of the English language* (p. 1440). Chicago: Standard American Corporation.

Resources

These are some classic references that every serious scholar of the CRFS should read. Most are out of print, but may be obtained through a medical library or a used bookstore.

Cannon, W. B. (1929). *Bodily changes in pain, hunger, fear, and rage*. 2nd ed. New York: D. Appleton (first edition was published in 1915).

Hart, L. K., and Freel, M. I. (1982). Fatigue. In C. M. Norris (Ed.), *Concept clarification in nursing* (pp. 251–261). Rockville, MD: Aspen.

Hockey, R. (Ed.), *Stress and fatigue in human performance*. New York: John Wiley.

Holding, D. (1983). Fatigue. In R. Hockey (Ed.), *Stress and fatigue in human performance* (pp. 145–167). New York: John Wiley.

Morris, M. L. (1982). Tiredness and fatigue. In C. M. Norris (Ed.), *Concept clarification in nursing* (pp. 263–275). Rockville, MD: Aspen.

Nicogossian, A. E., Huntoon, C. L., and Pool, S. L. (1989). *Space physiology and medicine*. 2nd ed. Philadelphia: Lea & Febiger.

Rhoten, D. (1982). Fatigue and the postsurgical patient. In C. M. Norris (Ed.), *Concept clarification in nursing* (pp. 277–300). Rockville, MD: Aspen.

Additional Resources

Following are various resources in etymology, linguistics, and sociolinguistics that may be of interest to some readers. Be aware that Web sites change rapidly and may no longer be valid.

American Dialect Society (ADS) <http://www.americandialect.org>. This is the only scholarly association dedicated to the study of the English language in North America–and of other languages, or dialects of other languages, influencing it or influenced by it.

American Dialect Society search site <http://filemaker.equinox.net:591/americandialect>. The DARE linguistic map is based on settlement history and population density.

American Dialect Society is the sponsor for the *Dictionary of American regional English* (Vol. I), Frederic G. Cassidy, chief editor, and *Dictionary of American regional English* (Vol. II D–H), Frederic G. Cassidy, chief editor, and Joan Houston Hall, associate editor. Copies should be available at any good bookstore, or order from Harvard University Press, 79 Garden Street, Cambridge, MA 02138. Sales phone: (617) 495-2480. Web site: <http://www.hup.harvard.edu>. ISBN 0-674-20511-1 (vol. I); 0-674-20512-X (vol. II); 0-674-20519-7 (vol. III).

Ammer, C. (1997). *The American heritage dictionary of idioms*. Boston: Houghton Mifflin.

Atwood, E. B. (1953). *A survey of verb forms in the eastern United States.* Ann Arbor: University of Michigan Press.

Carver, C. M. (1989). *American regional dialects.* Ann Arbor: University of Michigan Press.

Crystal, D. (1987). *The Cambridge encyclopedia of language.* Cambridge: Cambridge University Press.

Dykema, K. W. (1956). How fast is standard English changing? *American Speech 31*(2), 89–95.

Lighter J.E. (Ed.) (1994). *Random House historical dictionary of American slang.* (Vol. 1, A-G). New York: Random House.

Mathews, M. M. (1931). *The beginnings of American English.* Chicago: University of Chicago Press.

McDavid, R. I., Jr. (1963). *The American language by H. L. Mencken.* One-volume abridged edition. New York: Knopf.

North, M. (1998). *The dialect of modernism: Race, language, and twentieth-century literature.* Oxford: Oxford University Press.

Onions, C. T. (Ed.) (1983). *Oxford dictionary of English etymology.* Oxford: Oxford University Press.

Reed, C. E. (1977). *Dialects of American English.* Amherst, MA: University of Massachusetts Press.

Wilson, C. R., William, F., Haley, A., and Abadie, A. J. (Eds.) (1989). *Encyclopedia of southern culture.* Chapel Hill: University of North Carolina Press. Includes excellent references to African-American culture.

William Labov. Paper: *The Organization of Dialect Diversity in North America.* Web site: <http://babel.ling.upenn.edu/phono_atlas/ICSLP4/BW/ICSLP4BW.html>. This is from extensive work at the Linguistics Laboratory of the University of Pennsylvania. It addresses all English dialects and the extent of ongoing sound changes. This has been critical to the development of speech recognition software.

Select CD-ROM Dictionaries

Oxford English dictionary (1989). 2nd ed. CD-ROM. Oxford: Oxford University Press.

Webster's unabridged dictionary (1996). New York: Random House. Based on the second printed edition, newly revised and updated. ISBN: 0-679-44998-1.

Samuel Johnson: A dictionary of the English language. Anne McDermott, editor. Cambridge: Cambridge University Press Electronic Publishing.

Sociolinguistics

Sociolinguistics, an increasingly important and popular field of study, studies how language uses symbolically fundamental dimensions of social responsiveness interaction. Sociolinguistic techniques could contribute insight into how different age groups and persons with culturally diverse experiences communicate about the CRFS. All individuals working on quality of life or fatigue instruments should consult with a sociolinguistics specialist:

Trudgill, P. (1995). *Sociolinguistics: An introduction to language and society.* London: Penguin Books.

Wardhaugh, R. (1992). *An introduction to sociolinguistics.* Cambridge, MA: Blackwell.

Wen I git tird my fac felz flat

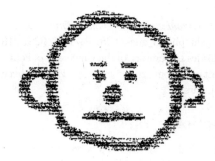

7-year-old boy with leukemia

The Foundations of Energetics: Fatigue, Fuel, and Functioning

Maryl L. Winningham

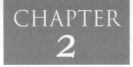

Sometimes you simply do not have the words to describe how you are feeling. You either dance around the problem in muddled explanations, or you use words like fatigue, which are sort of close, but not close enough. Here the miscommunication starts. People think they know what the word fatigue means and don't really listen to what you are trying to say.

Tricia Corbett, 10-year survivor, 1998

Background

Fatigue is best understood from the point of view of energetics. *Energetics* is the study of energy in its many forms and how it is used in organisms, specifically, the cells of the human body. As such, it is the underlying principle of how organisms live and function. In our bodies, we refer to the energetic dance of life as *metabolism,* with its anabolic (building up) and catabolic (tearing down) components. There is also a phenomenon—entropy—that works against all life, from conception to death. *Entropy,* the "dark side" of the metabolic process, is the ongoing process of energetic loss. Entropy ensures not only that we never win in life, but also that we cannot break even. It is like playing against the house in Monte Carlo. This influence has profound implications for every aspect of life as we know it, and it is perhaps the deepest and most pervasive law of nature. An understanding of fatigue and entropy also requires an understanding that fuel (foodstuffs broken down into usable molecules by the digestive system) and oxygen (which supports the breakdown of fuel into energy and by-products) are combined in the presence of specific enzymatic substrates in the cellular mitochondria.

Remember the old grade-school story about "the sun shines and causes the grass to grow, the cow eats the grass, and people eat the cow" or in the event of steak and salad, "the sun shines and causes the lettuce, tomatoes, and onions to grow and the people eat them." (Some of us are unrepentant omnivores!) The people then play, work, make love, laugh, cry, and sleep—all of life's functions, from the energy provided by the sun. It is all a matter of energy conversion, and we learned it so long ago, we probably forgot that it might have something to do with fatigue in cancer!

There is something incredibly poetic and philosophical about this phenomenon of energetics that came out of the realm of physics, biochemistry, and mathematics, for as surely as we are conceived and born, live, and love, so shall we die. Out of life comes death. We eat and work, but eventually we must sleep. There is something perverse about entropy: No human being has ever escaped its logic. It was this observation that was at the core of the question of the ancient Greeks, What is life?

This chapter discusses the phenomena that are the foundations of fatigue from an energetics perspective. This is a discussion of the basis of the energy of all life, the grand model that underlies all disciplines whether we recognize it or not.

It is quite remarkable when we hear comments like, "Little is known about fatigue in cancer." On the contrary, there is much that we know that could be brought to bear upon the science of fatigue in general, and cancer fatigue, specifically.

Graduate education in this century has become increasingly narrow. Most scholars and researchers have become less able to understand and synthesize global knowledge, let alone appreciate the specialized knowledge of other disciplines. Yet, global knowledge is exactly what is needed to discover the secrets of the cancer-related fatigue syndrome (CRFS) and develop effective interventions. Finally, some of the most basic and exciting discoveries in science must be revisited if there is to be a common ground for study and understanding. This chapter cuts across history and challenges belief systems, tracing the development of knowledge that contributes to an understanding of scientific laws and forces that are a part of fatigue-related phenomena that permeate nature.

Once again the question arises: If fatigue in cancer is such a serious problem, why has it taken so long for it to be recognized as such? As pointed out in Chapter 1, part of the problem is how we collect data in clinical decision making (i.e., the problem of clinician-induced artifact). Another part of the problem is communication about manifestations of fatigue. The multidimensional nature of fatigue presents another problem: Medical, surgical, and radiation oncology, nursing, physical energetics, biochemistry, immunology, exercise science, medical sociology, rehabilitation medicine, the rehabilitation therapies, kinesiology, pharmacy, psychiatry, medical nutrition, psychology, linguistics, ethics, theology, and sociology are but a few of the disciplines whose expertise is required for a comprehensive study of the CRFS. Of particular value are researchers who have had cross-disciplinary, multilingual, cross-cultural life experiences. Some of the most prominent leaders in the "hard sciences" in the twentieth century have also been philosophers and humanitarians who bridged disciplines: Among them are Albert Szent-Györgyi and Sir

---

I become so angry when I tell my doctor "I'm having this problem with my memory–it's like I can't keep track of things. I'm forgetting to pay bills–last week the electricity was shut off–I lost a big check I was supposed to deposit. I can't make decisions. I can't focus. I go to the store, but I can't remember what I'm there for." . . . And he pats me on the knee and says, "Well, you know, we're all getting older. I'm having those problems, too." How dare he! I feel a helpless rage. I know the difference between normal aging and how I feel. That fact is, this is very different. I've never been like this before. I know people think I'm being irresponsible. I'm working so hard, but it's like I'm spinning my wheels. It's like the Swiss cheese memory

Hans Krebs, Linus Pauling, Albert Einstein, and Hans Selye. Remarkably, each of these also contributed in some way to our understanding of energetic processes.

Unfortunately, throughout most of the twentieth century, the diverse academic research disciplines have viewed one another from a suspicious if not polarized perspective. The choice has often been presented as the hard science of forbidding, objective, cold, insensitive, quantitative measures of real science (as perceived by some psychosocial researchers) versus the touchy feely disciplines of psychosocial or qualitative research (as sometimes perceived by the biophysiological, qualitative researchers). This approach has been particularly counterproductive in investigating phenomena like fatigue. Historical developments linking medical education to the hard sciences have contributed toward a premed curricular bias in the past 80 years. This featured a narrow interpretation of the scientific method as it had been developed in the 1550s through the 1700s.

Lest the suggestion of adversarialism, as mentioned earlier, appear to be too harsh, notice the following description of true science as provided by Van Doren (1991):

1. Science is practiced by specially trained people—scientists—committed to being "objective, unsentimental, and unemotional."

2. Science deals almost exclusively with the external world, those things that can be concretely observed, measured, and described in mathematical terms.

3. The best-known method consists of an experiment, which consists of formulating an idea or problem as a hypothesis, then testing that hypothesis in a controlled environment to test its validity. It is the method used to do the work and the language of reporting results, particularly mathematics, that is distinctive.

Van Doren explained that because these characteristics are universal, scientists everywhere understand them. Van Doren went on to suggest that psychologists (implying the psychosocial sciences in general) do not practice "real science because they are investigating feelings."[1] This would suggest that only the "white coat" purists in the hard sciences have a corner on truth or the scientific method.

In order to gain perspective on the CRFS, it is necessary to retrace briefly the paths of discovery and to examine fatigue as part of historical and universal phenomena, scholarship that includes philosophical, behavioral, physical, and physiological concepts and processes. In Chapter 1, a model was presented for exploring the difference between normal fatigue, fatigue common to chronic illness, and those experi-

---

syndrome: He has little cheese holes like you find with normal aging–like baby Swiss–and he has the nerve to say it's like what I am experiencing. I'll tell you what I'm going through: It's like great big Swiss cheese holes. It's not at all like the baby Swiss. Things just seem to disappear in my mind. Important things are not at all connected and I know I'm missing something, but I don't know how to find it. I have this constant sense of lostness and confusion. Will my mind ever come back? I don't know. It seems to last forever. I hope, somehow, it will get better.

Breast cancer survivor, 49, undergoing chemotherapy and radiation therapy

ences and phenomena associated with the CRFS.[2] This chapter presents an approach to understanding the universal phenomena of normal fatigue and discusses basic areas where cancer fatigue–related phenomena may be similar or different. If we are to effectively investigate the CRFS, we must agree on the fundamental question, What is it we wish to know? This inquiry should involve all representative disciplines with something to contribute if we are to find an answer. The research methods used should reflect the nature of the question and the four basic rules of science, regardless of the discipline. As pointed out in Chapter 1, Newton's *Principia* provides a solid logical as well as historical framework for scientific reasoning and the theoretical basis for this process.

Historical Framework for Understanding Energetics and Fatigue

Investigating the nature of fatigue-related issues goes back at least two millenia to Hippocrates (350–400 BC) and is embedded in the questions, What is life? How do living and healthy bodies differ from dead or sick ones? What differentiates living from nonliving things? Continuing to investigate these questions, Aristotle, the father of biology, reasoned that every part of the body, everything served a purpose. His teaching that structure determined function was highly influential in the development of embryology and comparative anatomy. *Vitalism,* which considered life to be activated and maintained by some intrinsic, inestimable, and unmeasurable factor, was an outgrowth of Aristotle's philosophy. Vitalism was incorporated into what became medical dogma through the influential work of the physician Galen (ca 170 AD), who also introduced use of the pulse as a diagnostic indicator (this was the origin of the present clinical *vital signs,* the fundamental indicators of life and health today). Thus, breathing and a pulse were recognized to be characteristics of human life and significant indicators of illness or wellness.

As the Roman Empire crumbled, and libraries were demolished throughout Europe by the eastern tribes, Celtic and Arabic scholars became the protectors of ancient knowledge. Later, the Catholic Church of Rome took over political control from their more liberal Celtic brothers and designated the Arabs as "infidels." At its best, political control meant maintaining centers of learning and protecting manuscripts and documents written by scholars and philosophers of the past. The monopoly on learning followed two trends: (1) The guilds became the repository of the arts and crafts. (2) The universities became the repositories of literary documents. Both monopolies were tightly restricted. Teachers in the universities were largely doctors of theology and servants of the church. The study of medicine, the "exact arts of antiquity" (which included astronomy, mathematics, geometry, philosophy/science, and related areas) essentially involved the rehashing of knowledge laid down by the Babylonians, Egyptians, Assyrians, and Greeks (Neugebauer, 1957). The great cathedrals of Europe reflected the architectural concepts as passed along from Grecian geometry. Indeed, volumes were written on the spiritual symbolism of geometric shapes and numbers. Indeed, all the arts reflected these symbols. Despite a few intellectual "lights" of the Dark Ages, such as Thomas Aquinas, learning consisted of studying the past. Lest there were any who thought of deviating from it, there were occasional purges. The line between being a great scholar and an unfortunate heretic was sometimes very thin: Any hint of divergent and independent thought was closely scrutinized. The Inquisition is commonly thought of as Spanish in origin and religious in nature, as being the child of the Dark Ages. In fact, there were Protestant and Catholic inquisitions on the continent and England, the Spanish Inquisition in the Americas, and the New England witch trials that continued through the 1800s: They were often political and academic in nature, and independent thinkers were fair game.

The schism between schools of academic philosophy/theology and science began to crack in Newton's day. There is little question that the global contributions of Sir Isaac Newton were a major catalyst. It was not a question of god versus science, for Newton and many of those who developed modern science were devout Christians. It was a matter of challenging explanations about the existence of matter and science that the church, the source of educated men at that time, taught as absolute. Even in Newton's time, those who went too far in challenging religious and philosophical dogma (the two were, for all practical purposes, identical) were being persecuted by the Inquisition and even burned at the stake in some parts of Europe (Roth, 1996). Until Newton's era, science was philosophy. Indeed, the full name Newton gave his seminal *Principia* (*The Mathematical Principles of Natural Philosophy*), Book III (1687, translated from Latin to English in 1729) was *Rules of Reasoning in Philosophy*. It was subtitled *The System of the World, Phænomena, or Appearances*.

The real question is, What is it we wish to know? The inquiry should involve all representative disciplines with something to contribute toward discovering answers. The methods should reflect the nature of the question, regardless of the discipline.

The transition between philosophy/theology began through the pure science of mathematics and rigorous, unabashed observation, and accelerated with the development of research methods and designs. The interactive influence of philosophy/theology on scientific theories and thought still continues, with science having a counterinfluence on theological theories. Indeed, in this century, scientific theories and discoveries have had a powerful effect on the development of philosophical thought.[3, 4, 5]

The most powerful challenge to vitalism, as a scientific theory, came in the early 1600s when Descartes presented his philosophy of mechanics. This was a courageous and radical departure: Aristotelian vitalism was still being taught by the leading intellectual and spiritual leaders of the day. Like Newton, Descartes made many and varied contributions to science that are still having an influence today. Among his "children" were the ideas of conditioning affecting emotional responses and the influence of the mind on the body (this later contributed to the development of stimulus-response theory in the early part of the twentieth century and psychoneuroimmunology in the later half). In the meanwhile, explanations for the nature of the physical world were coming out of the laboratory as well as from mathematical theoreticians. Mystery was being challenged by fact.

From the mid-eighteenth century through the end of the nineteenth century, methods were developed to elucidate the mechanisms of life. Although vitalism generally fell into disrepute among scientists, vestiges remained. Those who held that there was a strictly mechanistic basis for life were called *mechanicists.* However, as late as the nineteenth century, invalids or sick individuals who showed fatigability, weakness, or cachexia were identified as lacking in "vital powers" or "vital force." (This was the era when illness was still attributed to "bad air" or "bad blood," and when "germs" were just a theory.) (Refer to Chapter 1, Figure 1-1 to trace the historical introduction of energy- and fatigue-related words into the English language during these centuries.)

Some philosophers and researchers were convinced something was still missing. The basics of cellular respiration and animal metabolism were being elucidated, but there were those who maintained that energy output from fuel/food and oxygen were not sufficient to initiate or sustain life:[6] On one hand, this question was pursued through the philosophy of Henri-Louis Bergson (1859–1941), a French philosopher and Nobel laureate, who proposed a theory of evolution based on the spiritual dimension of human life. He coined the concept of *élan vital* (life force), hypothesized to be a source of efficient causation and evolution in nature. This was what some also call a "soul," an essence of being and life that went beyond observations of life processes.

On a more sophisticated level, the idea of another source of energy was central to the development of Hans Selye's general adaptation syndrome ("stress") theory. He called it *adaptive energy* (Selye, 1976, 1978). Although this energy was not derived from nutrient utilization in metabolism, he acknowledged he had no idea what it was, just that it existed. Selye proposed that adaptive energy held the key to understanding fatigue and aging (Selye, 1976). In one of the earliest theoretical articles on fatigue in cancer, Aistars (1987) built upon Selye's stress and general adaptation syndrome concepts. Although it is beyond the scope of this chapter, a review of this work is essential to those who wish to be scholars of the CRFS.

Galileo Galilei (ca. 1600) was, in a modern sense, the father of critical thinking. He enjoyed using "thought experiments" to confound and enrage the Aristotelians, using their own assumptions. Thought experiments, drawing on common sense, rely on the concept of "necessary and sufficient." Indeed nearly all good scientific theories, regardless of their disciplinary origins, rely on some form of the "true and sufficient" argument, that is, (1) what is necessary for a condition or phenomenon to occur and (2) what is sufficient for that condition or phenomenon to come to fruition. These two concepts are not the same, as a consideration of thermodynamics, nutrition,g fatigue, and energy (discussed later) will demonstrate. Of course, the concept of true and sufficient was at the core of Newton's *Principia.* It acknowledged the need for an efficiency or economy of thought and action to develop viable theories and carry out research (see Olders' example in Chapter 11).

Statistics to the Rescue

Occasionally, researchers of the CRFS are heard to say, "There are no data to support. . . . More research is needed." Sometimes this is true, and sometimes it reflects ignorance or inability to transfer, apply, and synthesize knowledge rather than a lack of data. A study of basic elements of reasoning, defined as the ability to think logically and analytically, is also helpful. In both major types of reasoning, deductive and inductive, it is critical to identify and understand the assumptions before drawing any conclusions. The developments of modern science did not render the contributions of the ancient philosophers meaningless. Quite the contrary, those same arguments provided the foundation of various approaches to research.

Deductive reasoning, developed by the ancient Greek philosophers, was often expressed in syllogisms, depended on two premises, and involved drawing a logical conclusion from them. Deductive reasoning usually went from the general to the specific. Here is an example: All human beings have two arms, two legs, and a head. Ralph is a human being. Therefore, Ralph has two arms, two legs, and a head.

In contrast, *inductive reasoning*, developed by later philosophers such as Francis Bacon, David Hume, and John Stuart Mill, went from the particular to the general. Here is an example: Ralph has five fingers on each hand, five toes on each foot, and one head. Ralph is human. Therefore, all human beings have five fingers on each hand, five toes on each foot, and one head. For inductive reasoning to become scientifically useful, it became necessary to consider the issue of probability and formulate appropriate hypotheses accordingly.

The basic issue in probability involves the assumption, that what is true in a certain number of observed cases is also true in similar cases that were not observed. What if Ralph had a birth defect resulting in six fingers on each hand and six toes on each foot, and he was the single observation? Clearly, the accuracy of the projection from the specific to the general would be affected. More than one observation is obviously needed to confirm the truth of certain kinds of knowledge. The question becomes, How many observations are necessary to accept or reject the hypothesis that six fingers on each hand and six toes on each foot are the norm for human beings?

Inductive reasoning led to the development of *statistics*, the branch of mathematics that deals with collecting, organizing, and analyzing numerical data. It is also intrinsic to the problem of experimental design and decision making.[7] At the core of statistical reasoning is the theory of probability, which determines the likelihood of a particular outcome as a result of a given event or experiment. As this mathematical philosophy was developing, advances were also being made in physics, astronomy, chemistry, and biology. This brought about two divergent approaches in the search for "scientific truth": (1) scientific truth as a challenge to chance and probability, and (2) truth as revealed in certain laws of nature.

Universal Laws

In contrast to the idea of probability being the basis of science, the idea of universal laws, things that are generally assumed, may come as a shock for psychosocial researchers. For those trained in the psychosocial disciplines, where probability is an assumed approach, it is difficult to bridge this conceptual gap. For example, how many people have to be killed as a result of leaping off a very tall building before it is universally accepted and understood that leaping off a very tall building has consequences that are counterproductive to life and health? If the distance of the fall is sufficiently great and the surface landed upon sufficiently resistant, the reality of all manner of physical laws is conclusively demonstrated by a dead "N=1"! An eminent scientist once said, "You can do nearly anything . . . once" (A. E. Wilder-Smith, personal conversation; Basel, Switzerland, 1972). To volunteer to repeat the experiment to validate the outcome has nothing to do with probability and everything to do with remarkable stupidity! It is like the old joke about the inheritance pattern of death: It is 100%!

In contrast to statistically based sciences, it is common in the biophysical sciences to conduct research on a single subject or mechanism, such as with a single cell line. Sometimes very good experiments, when carried out in small numbers, are sufficient. Once again, an examination of the assumptions is critical. For instance, we know certain energetic pathways are universal throughout nature. On the other hand, there are issues in genetic probability within a given species that must be remembered. Through careful control and observation, it is not necessary to use the "Cecile B. DeMille approach," with a cast of thousands. Obviously, there are many approaches to science and we have to understand and respect the advantages and disadvantages of each approach. Our heritage has solid, common roots on which to build. This must be the goal in researching issues related to the CRFS. The complexity of clinical problems increasingly requires that basic scientists use more sophisticated statistical approaches to hypothesis testing. The complexity of behaviorally unexplainable variables demands that psychosocial scientists be more sophisticated in their understanding of the biological basis of life.

How does this relate to the CRFS? Why is the concept of energy and energetics critical to studying the CRFS? As shown in Table 1-1, the incorporation of words like *fatigue* and *energy* into the English language came from diverse sources. (The same respect must be accorded other linguistic sources, but discussion of this is beyond the scope of this book.) The selection of words to describe related feelings depends on many variables. Tricia Corbett even points out (in Chapter 23) that the very word *fatigue* may actually constitute a barrier to communication and understanding. There seems to be at least a 2,000-year link between perceptions of energy or vitality and lack of energy or fatigue. Indeed, how people perceive their energy seems to be the most important, the central factor, in how they assess their own health and well-being (Dixon, Dixon, and Hickey, 1993).

Fatigue is perceived as a loss, a deficit, a lack or inability as the result of an exertion or excess, a response to a stimulus. When left to their choice of words, patients tend to self-select words like "no energy" in preference to the word *fatigue,* thus reinforcing the concept of fatigue as a negative expression. A young person who has experienced no deficits has no frame of reference for understanding exhaustion and confusion of thought such as that found in the CRFS. Children engage in "puppy play," during which they run or play until they are exhausted, fall asleep, and get up feeling refreshed and run around again. After a nap, they are fully refreshed (with the exception of the phenomenon parents identify as not having enough sleep, or having too much sleep). Whence the origin of their energy? Using the background of history, we explore what is known to shed light on the profound experience of the cancer–related fatigue syndrome.

A Story of Energy

All life, all functioning cellular activity is built on cellular biochemistry, which is built on cellular genetics, which is ultimately built on the basic forces of atomic physics. Traditionally, physiologically based cancer research has assumed that effective cures and treatments for cancer would take place at these levels (see Chapter 13 for a brief history of cancer research). Everything we do at a behavioral, macroscopic level is supported by biochemical resources at the microcellular level; however, there is much we do not yet know about cellular biology.[8] Often, psychosocial researchers protest this approach as "reductionistic" and find it to be of minimal practical value in

> *It is absurd as well as counterproductive to erect intellectual barriers where none exist in nature.*

solving clinical problems like the CRFS. They have a good point. While the "secrets of life" are being elucidated, many people continue to suffer needlessly. For this reason, we must depend on the work of psychosocial researchers and knowledge established from the development of current interventions. Since it is absurd as well as counterproductive to erect intellectual barriers where none exist in nature, a review of some of the fundamental aspects of energetics may facilitate a common understanding.

Where Does Metabolism Get Its Energy?

In the later part of the eighteenth century, a breakthrough in an understanding of the source of energy for life was made with the discovery of oxygen by researchers Joseph Priestley and Antoine-Laurent Lavoisier. This was a time of exciting discoveries and national fervor in scientific work.[9] Lavoisier went on to establish the experimental evidence for the law of conservation of matter, as well as the role of combustion and oxidation in cellular respiration. In its most simplistic form, the chemical equation for this basis for animal life was:

$$\text{Oxygen} + \text{Fuel (Food)} = \text{Energy} + \text{Carbon Dioxide} + \text{Water}$$

As any school child knows, the ultimate source of fuel in our universe is the sun, which supports all life on earth through the production of food. From the above equation, the second requirement for life's energy is oxygen. In humans, oxygen is taken from the environment through the lungs and transported throughout the body to each cellular membrane by a specialized respiratory pigment called *hemoglobin*. At the cell membrane, myoglobin takes the oxygen to the mitochondria, sometimes called the powerhouses of the cell.

Energetics

In the body, energetics is expressed in terms of metabolism. Although the ability to convert energy for living from the breakdown of the molecular bonds of foodstuffs is not characteristic of living organisms alone (obviously, the sun is a nonliving case of energy conversion), it is the fundamental requirement for all aspects of life. *Metabolism* is defined as the sum of *anabolism* (processes that build up) and *catabolism* (processes that break down). Anabolic as well as catabolic chemical reactions are the means by which the cells of organisms transform energy, maintain their structure and identity, function to meet their own needs, and reproduce. This process is dependent on many hundreds of precise metabolic reactions, each of which is triggered, controlled, and terminated by specific proteins called *catalytic enzymes*. Further, each of these reactions is coordinated and balanced with many other reactions at a given time. It is analogous to a dance—the dance of life. *Anabolism* is the process by which new cells and tissues (structural elements) are built and maintained using carbohydrates, proteins, and fats. *Catabolism* is the process that breaks down foodstuffs for fuel to produce the energy required for all internal and external activity. Catabolism also involves the maintenance of body temperature and the degradation of more complex chemicals into simpler substances that are removed from the body as waste products through the lungs, kidneys, intestines, and skin. Aristotle's idea of the interdependence of structure and function comes through loud and clear.

The Myth of Homeostasis

There is an old assumption that continues to haunt physiology textbooks in the medical profession. A misplaced faith in this assumption has unwittingly contributed to the "get more rest" advice frequently given cancer patients when they complain of fatigue. It also explains why people have trouble understanding how therapeutic exercise can reduce fatigue and optimize energetic capacity. This myth is "homeostasis." It grew out of the work of Claude Bernard, a failed nineteenth-century playwright, who is considered the founder of experimental medicine. Building on the work of others, Bernard proposed the concept of "interior milieu," that is, how the body uses its complex mechanisms to maintain a state of internal balance. Following up on this work, Harvard medical researcher Walter Cannon (1967) gave this self-regulating process the name *homeostasis*. Somewhere in basic physiology courses, we were all taught about "the resting 70-kg male" (the 70-kg male, having been designated somewhere in the primordial past by long-departed sages as a "standard").[10] At rest, energy required by the body to maintain the processes essential to sustain life is called the *basal metabolic rate* (BMR). This rate is expressed and measured in terms of the minimum amount of heat produced by the body at rest. Crudely put, when anabolism exceeds catabolism, growth or weight gain occurs. When catabolism exceeds anabolism (e.g., in starvation or cachexia), weight loss occurs. The gain or loss in weight reflects a sum of metabolic phenomena in the body. Finally, the myth continues, when anabolism equals catabolism, the organism is said to be in a state of homeostasis or dynamic equilibrium.

Our professors were mistaken. There are two basic problems with homeostasis: (1) Over several decades, National Aeronautics and Space Administration (NASA) research demonstrated that the "*resting* 70-kg male" was neither ideal nor normal. Every single organ system of his body was deteriorating day by day. In other words, he was going to physiological hell in a handbasket. Beyond participating in the rest necessary for normal circadian rest and recovery, the resting 70-kg male (or anyone else) is subject to the laws of thermodynamics (more about these later). (2) No matter how healthy and long-lived a person may be, catabolism eventually wins out and we die, so no organism really experiences a true state of dynamic equilibrium (back to number 1).

These two points are significant because cancer is essentially a metabolic disease. Inappropriate interventions may unnecessarily facilitate catabolic processes. Several chapters in this book are devoted to concepts of rehabilitation and ways to negate the unnecessary catabolic processes. One more step is necessary to start pulling all this together into an understanding of the foundations of fatigability. That involves an introduction of the concepts of thermodynamics as they apply to the well-being of living cells.

The Laws of Thermodynamics and the Cancer-Related Fatigue Syndrome

Most fundamental in understanding cellular metabolism and fatigue is an understanding of the laws of thermodynamics[11] and cellular respiration, in other words, the source of metabolic energy. Genetics is also a metabolic process, since it is the means by which each organism passes on the specific instructions on how to intercept, transform, build structure, and pass on the characteristics unique to each species. Although the implications of the laws of thermodynamics are complex and permeate the entire world around us (they can be expressed in terms of mechanical, thermal, chemical, electrical, radiant, and atomic energy), their core concepts as they apply to the human experience are simple. They involved several key discoveries into how energy works. These discoveries in physics, physiology, and the biochemistry of energetics were dramatic. Parallels, such as systems theory, were quickly applied by theoreticians to phenomena in the psychosocial sciences. Thermodynamics is, first and last, about temperature, about energy as it relates to heat, about conversion of energy from one form to another.

The First Law of Thermodynamics

The first law of thermodynamics states that energy cannot be created or destroyed. This discovery implied a stability in our system, a god-like energetic eternal state.

The Second Law of Thermodynamics

The second law states that energy can only be transformed from one form to another. Although this law can be applied to many areas of physics, biochemistry, mathematics, and engineering, on earth the best example of this is in the energy-converting chlorophyll of plants. Chlorophyll is a magnificent organic structure that captures energy from sunlight to power the synthesis of living plant cells, the foundation of the food and energy transfer web, from inorganic substances like water, ammonia, and carbon dioxide. This energy is ingested first by herbivores and then by carnivores, providing the sole source of energy and anabolic chemicals. Except for a few recently discovered deep sea creatures that use sulfur to "oxidize" in this process of tearing down food into structural material and fuel, oxygen is essential to the catabolic process that releases energy for cellular use.

Based on this information, it is important to notice the following:

1. There is a predictive mathematical relationship between food taken in or stored, the oxygen taken in to oxidize it, and the energy produced as a result of cellular processes of building up and the work performed. By measuring the amount of oxygen used as well as the ratio of oxygen to carbon dioxide at a given level of exertion (physical work), it is possible to calculate (a) how much energy the person is using to do work and (b) whether the person is metabolizing primarily fats or carbohydrates to do that work. This ratio is called the "nonprotein R" because in normal states, the amount of protein the body utilizes to convert and produce energy for work is negligible. This is how the ratio looks:

$$R = \frac{\dot{V}_{CO_2} = \text{volume of } CO_2/\text{min}}{\dot{V}_{O_2} = \text{ volume of } O_2/\text{min}}$$

   The direct way to measure energy is by using a bomb calorimeter to measure heat production. Unfortunately, this is not practical. The indirect way to measure energy is through the measurement of oxygen consumption. This is done in laboratories and rehabilitation centers as an indicator of changed cardiorespiratory capacity and efficiency.

2. This relationship implies there is a sufficient provision of fuel and oxygen under the right conditions (enzymatic substrates in cellular mitochondria). In the absence of sufficient oxygen in the cell, there is incomplete fuel breakdown and its utilization becomes very inefficient.

Implications for Cancer

Decreased activity (deconditioning) promotes the breakdown and loss of the enzymes involved in cellular energy production. Fuel and oxygen utilization becomes less efficient. Further, lack of oxygen in anemia results in a metabolic shift to the lactic acid system instead of the aerobic (oxygen) system. Not only is this less efficient, but it also visibly affects everyday activities. Patients who have spent even several days in bed demonstrate profound deconditioning and changes in activity patterns. This can be seen in the rapid-onset breathlessness and the tendency to engage in brief bouts of activity, followed by a need for extended recovery. In addition, the effects of nutritional deprivation, treatments, and disease that promote nausea, vomiting, and gastrointestinal distress (which impairs nutritional intake) aggravate the process. Under optimal conditions, it is difficult to prevent the progressive loss that often characterizes cancer.

The Third Law of Thermodynamics

Now comes the bad news. The first two laws were exciting, but implications from the third law were overwhelming. Rudolf Clausius, the discoverer of the third law of thermodynamics, made the distressing finding that not only is energy interconvertible, but also it is constantly less available for work. That is, there is a guaranteed, built-in inefficiency in the system: Whenever energy is converted, in whatever state energy (heat) was, one always had to put in a lot more than one got out of the system. Heat always went to cold, order to disorder—never the reverse. In other words, no matter what we do, we cannot win; what's more, we cannot break even. He named this process *entropy:* It was the dark side of energy.

Like fatigue, no one has ever seen energy or entropy. They are something felt through their effects. Energy is known by its ability to accomplish something, to do work. *Work* is defined, according to physicists, as a force applied through a distance. Entropy is known by the change in energy available in one state in time versus another. Hence, entropy, like energy, is dynamic, always changing. Fatigue is known by its inability to accomplish something. This accounts for the difficulty measuring it.

As our cells apply energy to do work, to maintain their structures, and to maintain their genetic mechanisms, much of that energy is given off as various types of heat. If we place a warm hand on a cold surface, the hand cools until the two objects eventually reach a thermal equilibrium. The heat irretrievably goes from warm to cold, never the reverse. As a person works, friction is another irretrievable type of lost energy.

Figure 2-1 illustrates the four uses for energy in cells and demonstrates how most of it is lost to entropy (in the form of radiated heat) as part of the energy conversion process. In the beginning, at conception, it may be said, are the "messaging," the genetic mechanisms. This energetic process defines all aspects of life. As we age, there appears to be a self-destruct mechanism in cells that makes them less able to repair or reproduce themselves. The genetic mechanism is useless without fuel and nutritional resources to use as building

| Figure 2.1 | The Relationship Between Energy, Entropy, and Organic Functioning |

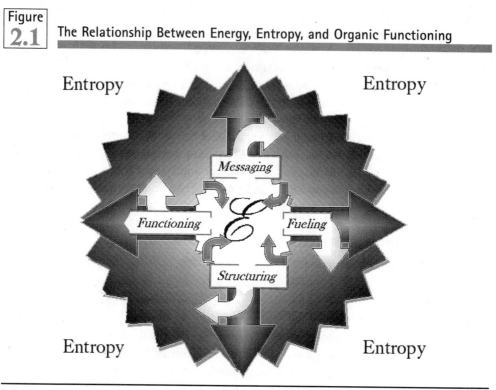

E=Energy

blocks. The building blocks are determined by species-specific as well as organism-specific codes that are organized into a cellular structure to carry out the cell's role. Finally, the genetic mechanism, the nutritional resources, and the structure enable the organism to function in a way to carry out its existence.

Although the value varies widely with each person, level of activity, and training, there is about a 25% efficiency associated with doing work (physical exertion). In other words, 75% of the energy produced by the person is lost.

$$\% \text{ Efficiency} = \frac{\text{Useful work output}}{\text{Energy expended}} \times 100$$

Efficiency depends on such variables as the gender of the individual, type of work or activity done, and how well trained the individual is (conditioning). For example, efficiency in horizontal walking can vary from 20% to 35%. As the person becomes less efficient as a result of aging, deconditioning, and cancer and treatment effects, even small amounts of exertion are perceived to be more stressful and more fatiguing. Indeed, as in the earlier example, the resting 70-kg male (or any other human) begins to experience metabolic changes resulting in increased inefficiency. Two thousand years ago, Hippocrates observed ⟵ that prolonged rest and inactivity had a profound effect on inducing weakness and ability to engage in activity (Chadwick and Mann, 1950). Scores of bed rest studies based on the NASA space program indicate that this loss begins to take place within the first 24 hours (Greenleaf and Kozlowski, 1982). On the other hand, space program researchers in the United States and the Soviet Union discovered that therapeutic exercise programs could counter much of that loss. The full ramifications of these observations have never been appreciated in oncology.

Using oxygen consumption as an objective energetic performance measure, the first prescriptive, aerobic exercise program designed to minimize loss in breast cancer patients undergoing chemotherapy successfully demonstrated an improvement in energetic performance while the women were still receiving treatment. The original Institutional Review Board papers indicated that the investigator hypothesized the exercise program could minimize loss or maintain functioning (Winningham, 1983). Follow-up research not only validated this intervention for functioning losses in breast cancer patients on chemotherapy, but also revealed improved functioning (MacVicar and Winningham, 1986; MacVicar, Winningham, and Nickel, 1989). Later research showed that there is a relationship between the highest energy-producing capacity in our bodies and the energy used in everyday activities (Berthouze et al, 1995). As mentioned earlier, with aging, every organ system of our bodies starts to deteriorate and we experience an entropic loss in functioning. Independent of illness or accidents, people who stay active do not deteriorate as rapidly as those who are sedentary. There is much about cancer and cancer treatment that accelerates the normal entropic losses; after all, cancer is essentially an accelerated entropic process.

Much of this may be preventable; some may not be. However, how do we know unless we test it? Heretofore, we have generally assumed that the losses we observe are directly related to cancer and treatment. Cancer and cancer treatments are also accompanied by nutritional and fluid deficits that aggravate the entropic processes. The increase in time in the horizontal position (bed rest) seen in many patients also predisposes to dehydration from the change in body water distribution. There is usually a change in lifestyle associated with cancer treatment, as patients try to accommodate the rigorous schedules of clinic visits, chemotherapy, and especially radiation therapy. Finally, confronting a potentially lethal disease and the changes in roles and expectations in life is its own stressor. No wonder Selye (1978) suggested that the emotional aspects of human existence were the most stressful, making the greatest demands on "adaptation energy."

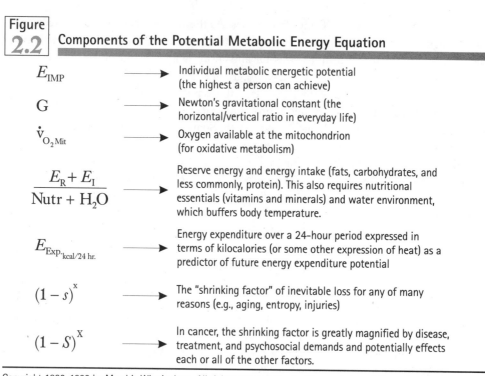

Figure 2.2   Components of the Potential Metabolic Energy Equation

E_{IMP} ⟶ Individual metabolic energetic potential (the highest a person can achieve)

G ⟶ Newton's gravitational constant (the horizontal/vertical ratio in everyday life)

$\dot{V}_{O_2 Mit}$ ⟶ Oxygen available at the mitochondrion (for oxidative metabolism)

$\dfrac{E_R + E_I}{Nutr + H_2O}$ ⟶ Reserve energy and energy intake (fats, carbohydrates, and less commonly, protein). This also requires nutritional essentials (vitamins and minerals) and water environment, which buffers body temperature.

$E_{Exp \cdot kcal/24\,hr.}$ ⟶ Energy expenditure over a 24-hour period expressed in terms of kilocalories (or some other expression of heat) as a predictor of future energy expenditure potential

$(1 - s)^x$ ⟶ The "shrinking factor" of inevitable loss for any of many reasons (e.g., aging, entropy, injuries)

$(1 - S)^X$ ⟶ In cancer, the shrinking factor is greatly magnified by disease, treatment, and psychosocial demands and potentially effects each or all of the other factors.

Unfortunately, it is not as easy to measure adaptation energy from a biophysiological perspective. This is the area that has largely been ignored in medicine. This is where people live their everyday lives, and this is where the psychosocial researchers can make their greatest contribution. Work on the burden of illness and treatment, quality of life, and caregiver burden is important if we are to comprehend more fully the emotional energy required in adapting to cancer and its treatments. We need to conceptualize these issues, too, in terms of thermodynamics. Entropy is a powerful concept. We expect patients to make lifestyle changes at a time they can scarcely place one foot in front of another. At a time they have less functional energy available to adapt (cope), we expect them to make enormously draining changes.

The factors that contribute to energy in our bodies are presented in Figure 2-2. Although there is some interaction, it makes the point that the contributing physiological factors are relatively few and simple. The focus is not on an ideal individual metabolic potential for athletes, but on what each person can accomplish. Since energy of activation could be hypothesized to be on both sides of the equation, it cancels out, and is not included in Figure 2-2.

Figure 2.3	Optimizing Individual Potential Metabolic Energy

The Conceptual Equation for Potential Metabolic Energy in a Healthy Person

$$E_{\text{IMP}} = G\left[\dot{v}_{O_2\,\text{Mit}}\right]\left[\frac{E_R + E_1}{\text{Nutr} + H_2O}\right]\left[E_{\text{Exp·kcal/24 hr.}}\right]\left[(1-s)^x\right]$$

The Conceptual Equation for Potential Metabolic Energy in a Person with Cancer

$$E_{\text{IMP}} = G\left[\dot{v}_{O_2\,\text{Mit}}\right]\left[\frac{E_R + E_1}{\text{Nutr} + H_2O}\right]\left[E_{\text{Exp·kcal/24 hr.}}\right]\left[(1-S)^X\right]$$

Gravity has a profound metabolic effect on humans. Newton's gravitational constant, as it is known, demonstrates the reciprocal gravitational effect of the relationship between the earth and each person living on it. G represents Newton's gravitational constant where

$$G = \text{CONSTANT} \times M \times m \div d^2$$

Oxygen available at the mitochondrial membrane commonly can be affected by cardiorespiratory disease and by anemia. The appropriate nutrition is critical. E_R stands for reserve fuel in the body. Conceptually, it is possible to be overnourished and undernourished. Both are equally threatening. In addition, the proper nutrients (vitamins and minerals) are essential–too many can be toxic, too few impede energetic metabolism. The right amount of water is also significant. Water acts as a solvent in the body, as a thermal buffer, and serves to maintain turgor in the muscles for optimal strength. Energy expenditure during a 24-hour period determines the enzyme substrates that produce energy in our bodies. Finally, the 1–s and 1–S shrinking factors account for the stressors that promote entropy and cause the person to slow down.

These factors are placed in the format of rough mathematical equations in Figure 2-3. It is the first four items in these equations–gravity, oxygen, nutrients, and energy expenditure–that determine the overall energy available for work in our bodies.

Notice that the value S varies. This is the shrinking factor based on entropy. Since cancer or any chronic illness tends to have more entropic features (including need to adapt to disease and treatment-related stressors, stigma, increased social and financial burdens, and increased physiological entropy), the other variables are all affected. If we can establish normal values, it would be possible to quantify abnormal declines and losses in functioning. In Figure 2-3, the assumption is made that the energetic process begins at conception and that the fetus is nearly a year old at birth. It also assumes the normal life span for a male, without medical intervention, to be about 70 years. The trajectory of change peaks at 25 years, initiating a gradual decline. A more precipitous decline occurs at age 50. In normal males, the value of x can be estimated to be 0.00383 in loss per month of life. Women tend to live somewhat longer; therefore, their *s* value is slightly lower. Note that these equations are about potential functional energy, not necessarily longevity.

Energy, Stress, Coping, Symptoms, Fatigue, and Functioning: All for One and One for All

All the above concepts can be wrapped up into the psychobiological entropy model (Figure 2-4). The sources of energy from Figures 2-2 and 2-3 fit into the upper left corner. Issues relating to adaptive energy and coping–emotional stressors–fit into the upper right corner. The many conditions and symptoms cancer patients have that can cause physiological as well as psychosocial distress are primary symptoms. The overriding principle is this: Whether fatigue is initially a cofactor or not, any symptom or condition (including well-intentioned medications) that causes the person to slow down will lead to increased fatigue and decreased functioning. This in turn can contribute to unnecessary impairment and disability. The possibility of preexisting conditions, treatments, environmental influences, and disease as contributing factors must also be considered. The good news is that areas represented by an arrow or an interaction in Figure 2-4 are where an intervention can be tested.

From the NASA studies, we know that a fractional increase in horizontal body position versus the normal vertical body position over a period of time contributes to proportional decrements in health and generalized breakdown in organic functioning. By engaging in mild to moderate activity interspersed with appropriate (prescriptive) rest, losses in biochemical determinants of functional capacity can be minimized. There is no question: Forty years of research has demonstrated that bed rest is hazardous to health.

Throughout this book are scattered quotes from Florence Nightingale. The descriptors of illness she poses sound very much like those related to deconditioning in the space program and in people who have spent time in bed. These patients exhibit a great deal of physiological and emotional lability. One explanation, the "white coat syndrome," causes patients to appear more functional than they are. People become excited when they interact with others. As long as the epinephrine is rushing, they truly do not feel fatigue or other distressing symptoms. In fact, they may honestly say they feel fine. It is like the story of the old lady carrying her piano out of the burning house. However, afterward, they feel an overwhelming exhaustion, an exhaustion that may last several days. With the epinephrine "rush" comes glycogen ("people starch") depletion. Normally, in well-nourished individuals, this is rapidly restored. However, many of our patients are not optimally nourished. In fact, people who say they are eating and drinking "just fine" may only be taking in between 600 and 700 kilocalories per day as a result of exhaustion, anorexia, or other related symptoms. Glycogen rebuilding is not easy under those circumstances.

Did you ever have an "almost accident"–a situation in which you had a very close call, such as a truck almost hit your car at an intersection? How did you feel afterward? Washed

Figure 2.4 The Winningham Psychobiological–Entropy Model of Functioning

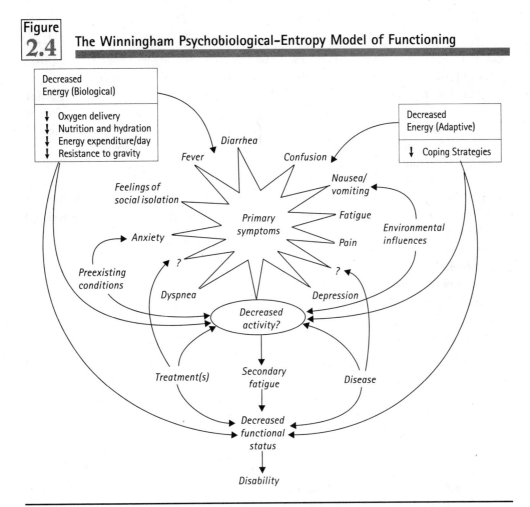

out? Weak? Shaky? Exhausted? Nauseated? That was not a time you felt like eating well; yet, the "fight or flight" of the epinephrine response caused muscle and liver glycogen break-down to produce instant energy. Later, you paid for it. How did you feel a few hours later, that night, and the next day? The aftereffects are not easily ignored. This is how many cancer patients feel much of the time. Their hearts are already beating faster than normal at rest, in compensation, because of deconditioning or anemia, or both. Even slight disturbances cause an epinephrine response. They are suffering from cognitive deficits, "chemo brain," "Swiss cheese memory," and "fuzzy thinking" that result in a constant "I lost my wallet" panic feeling.

Where Do We Go From Here?

This chapter examined a global approach to understanding the source of fatigue from the most fundamental laws of the world around us. This, plus the suggestions made in Chapter 1, can provide a unifying basis for all disciplines to understand and appreciate our common past. The imperative we face is to do what we can, based on knowledge of energetics, entropy, nutrition, oxygenation, activity, and rest. The goal must be to minimize loss of functioning, maintain what is possible, and promote gain if we can. It is likely that most of this will involve common sense rather than high-tech medicine. Ultimately, it could result in increased economical efficiency in medicine at a time when it is sorely needed. What is learned in work with cancer patients can be applied to other chronically ill populations. Much of the work has already been done—what remains is to catalog it, apply it, and see what interventions are the most appropriate for use in alleviating the suffering associated with the CRFS.

There is no question cancer survivors face a multitude of overwhelming and deenergizing problems. A common complaint is, "I just don't have any energy." That is a remarkably astute observation, with a sound scientific basis. As will be discussed by Henry Olders in Chapter 11, we need to differentiate between the acute effects of deconditioning, such as experienced by a bone marrow transplant patient, and chronic fatigue that may be linked to depression and sleep disturbances.

Other important steps we could take might include the following:

1. Identify biological mechanisms of fatigue specific to the different causes of cancer and the corresponding treatment (i.e., such as cytokines or neurotransmitters) and what may be done to minimize their side effects.

2. Conduct clinical trials on medications that may help manage manifestations of fatigue (such medications cannot, by definition, promote catabolism or feelings of lethargy).

3. Search for substitutes for medications that currently contribute to increased fatigue, muscular weakness, and feelings of lethargy.

4. Develop and promote rehabilitation techniques and model programs that can address survivors' adaptive issues:

   a. Develop improved screening and intervention techniques.

   b. Develop better techniques for monitoring changes.

   c. Develop a battery of testing protocols that routinely can be used to evaluate changes in functional status similar to the routine laboratory tests used for medical conditions.

5. Encourage graduate students to appreciate the history and philosophies of science so they can learn to ferret out the secrets of their past as a foundation for the future.

Endnotes

1. It is important to understand the historical development of twentieth-century medicine. Physicians are often referred to as "men of science." The strict, objective, scientific model that characterized medicine for most of the twentieth century is the result of a series of diverse forces. As early as 1870, highly rated universities like Johns Hopkins and Harvard began to place such a focus on faculty hard-science research that many feared there would be a precipitous loss of clinical practice skills and quality teaching. At the same time, American universities were trying to emulate the German academic model, emulating its departmentalization, concept of academic freedom, research productivity, and pursuit of the doctoral degree (doctor of philosophy) as a minimal faculty credential. Research, scientific publications in newly founded specialist journals, and grants were part of the objective, laboratory science that dominated the new era; in fact, Johns Hopkins led in the coup of the informal "annual page count" in the United States by founding the first official university press in 1891 (Rudolph, 1962; Starr, 1982). In contrast, a recent report, *Scholarship Reconsidered: Priorities of the Professoriate,* funded by the Carnegie Foundation for the Advancement of Teaching, has encouraged the creation of a new generation of scholars with an emphasis on the liberal arts at both the graduate and undergraduate levels (Boyer, 1990).

2. I (M.L.W.) experienced this difference when reviewing data from a study using a widely accepted instrument that examined psychosocial aspects of exercise in cancer. Statistics revealed that about 36% of the cancer patients reported difficulty sleeping. The next day, there was a newspaper article reporting that one-third of Americans had difficulty sleeping. Since there had been no "normal" control group, there was no way to determine if the experience of the cancer patients was different from usual.

3. The modern cost of creativity and professional courage that results in academic blackballing and denial of tenure pales in comparison with the determination and courage of the many-forgotten stalwarts who paved the way toward a whole new way of thinking.

4. The theory of relativity, Heisenberg's uncertainty principle, quantum theory, and chaos theory notwithstanding, laws of nature such as the law of gravity and the laws of thermodynamics describe absolute phenomena related to the interaction of our bodies with the world around us.

5. Despite our claim to modern scientific investigation and observation as the foundation of inquiry, philosophy (political systems, in particular) probably still influences science more than we would like to admit. We have only to be reminded of the thousands of scientists who labored under National Socialism (Nazism) and International Socialism (Communism), to produce and publish papers that were slavishly supportive of political correctness that had nothing to do with reality.

6. This is still acknowledged by some biochemists to be a problem. In essence, cellular life depends on the interaction of certain energy molecules that are dependent on one another. This problem of circuity cannot be ignored, even by the most sophisticated evolutionary theoreticians.

7. The earliest and most primitive forms of statistics involved census counts. Although practiced by the ancient Egyptians and Babylonians, one of the best historical examples lies in the Domesday Book, assembled by William of Normandy in 1086 AD after his conquest of England. Modern-day scientists will no doubt appreciate the Domesday Book as they struggle with gathering data and preparing statistical reports.

8. The study of cytokines is an excellent case in point. Cytokine researchers acknowledge that so little is currently known about cytokines that it is difficult to predict their behavior under various conditions. A change in a single variable, such as fever or the type of an infection, can result in an opposite cytokine response.

9. The nationalism that was sweeping Europe at that time resulted in fierce competition and competing claims for discoveries. This scarcely represented the ideal of objectivity that was supposed to characterize research. For a fascinating review of the events that led up to the presentation of Einstein's famous E=mc², read Michael Guillen's book *Five Equations That Changed the World: The Power and Poetry of Mathematics* (1995).

10. This value and values for men and women under various nutritional and metabolic challenges have been repeatedly challenged. For a more recent presentation of these issues, see *Energy and Protein Requirements: Report of a Joint FAO/WHO Ad Hoc Expert Committee* (1973).

11. Notice the word *laws*. We speak of the law of gravity. Science uses this term sparingly.

References

Aistars, J. (1987). Fatigue in the cancer patient: A conceptual approach to a clinical problem. *Oncology Nursing Forum, 14*, 25–30.

Berthouze, S. E., Minaire, P. M., Castells, J., Busso, T., Vico, L., and Lacour J-R. (1995). Relationship between mean habitual daily energy expenditure and maximal oxygen uptake. *Medicine and Science in Sports and Exercise, 27*(8), 1170–1179.

Boyer, E. L. (1990). *Scholarship reconsidered: Priorities of the professoriate.* The Carnegie Foundation for the Advancement of Teaching. New York: Jossey Bass.

Cannon, W. B. (1967). *The wisdom of the body.* (Rev. and enlarged ed.) New York: W. W. Norton.

Chadwick, J., and Mann, W. N. (1950). *The medical works of Hippocrates* (p. 140). Oxford: Blackwell.

Dixon, J. K., Dixon, J. P., and Hickey, M. (1993). Energy as a central factor in the self-assessment of health. *Advances in Nursing Science, 15*(4),1–12.

Greenleaf, J., and Kozlowski, S. (1982). Physiological consequences of reduced physical activity during bed rest. *Exercise and Sports Science Review, 10,* 84.

MacVicar, M. G., and Winningham, M. L. (1986). Promoting the functional capacity of cancer patients. *Cancer Bulletin, 38*(5), 235–239.

MacVicar, M. G., Winningham, M. L., and Nickel, J. L. (1989). Effects of aerobic interval training on cancer patients' functional capacity. *Nursing Research, 38*(6), 348–351.

Neugebauer, O. (1957). *The exact sciences in antiquity.* Providence, RI: Brown University Press.

Roth, C. (1996). *The Spanish inquisition.* New York: W. W. Norton (first printed in 1964).

Rudolph, F. (1962). *The American college and university: A history.* New York: Vintage Books.

Selye, H. (1978). *Stress in health and disease.* Boston: Butterworth.

Selye, H. (1976). *The stress of life* (p. 82). Revised edition. New York: McGraw-Hill.

Starr, P. (1982). *The social transformation of American medicine.* New York: Basic Books.

Van Doren, C. (1991). *A history of knowledge: Past, present, and future* (pp. 187–189). New York: Ballantine.

Winningham, M. L. (1983). "Effects of a bicycle ergometry program on functional capacity and feelings of control in women with breast cancer." Doctoral dissertation, Ohio State University, Columbus, OH.

Resources

Each of the following resources holds stimulating and intriguing ideas to challenge cancer fatigue scholars.

Brooks, G. A., Fahey, T. D., and White, T. G. (1995). *Exercise physiology: Human bioenergetics and its applications.* Mountain View, CA: Mayfield Publishing.

Cannon, W. B. (1929). *Bodily changes in pain, hunger, fear, and rage.* 2nd ed. New York: D. Appleton (first edition was published in 1915).

Cannon, W. B. (1984). *The way of an investigator: A scientist's experience in medical research.* New York: W. W. Norton (first published in 1945).

Groff, J. L., Gropper, S. S., Hunt, S. M., and Groff, J. (1995). *Advanced nutrition and human metabolism.* Belmont, CA: West/Wadsworth.

Guillen, M. (1995). *Five equations that changed the world: The power and poetry of mathematics.* New York: Hyperion.

Houston, M. E. (1995). *Biochemistry primer for exercise science.* Champaign, IL: Human Kinetics.

Joint FAO/WHO Ad Hoc Expert Committee (1973). Report. *Energy and Protein Requirements.* Rome: Food and Agriculture Organization of the United Nations.

McArdle, W. D., Katch, F. I., and Katch, V. L. (1996). *Exercise physiology: Energy, nutrition, and human performance.* 4th ed. Philadelphia: Lea & Febiger. (This may be the best all-around reference on your shelf.)

Nightingale, F. (1859). *Notes on nursing.* London: Harrison and Sons (reprinted in offset in 1946 by Edward Stern & Co., Philadelphia).

Salway, J. G., and Salway, J. D. (1994). *Metabolism at a glance.* Cambridge, MA: Blackwell Science.

Tipton, C. M. (1998). Contemporary exercise physiology: Fifty years after the closure of Harvard fatigue laboratory. *Exercise and Sports Science Review, 26,* 315–339.

Watson, R. R., and Eisinger, M. (Eds.) (1993). *Exercise and disease: Nutrition in exercise and sport.* Boca Raton, FL: CRC Press.

The following resources are especially valuable in examining issues relating to the CRFS, deconditioning, reconditioning, bed rest, and microgravity:

Nicogossian, A. E., and Parker, J. F., Jr. (1982). *Space physiology and medicine.* National Aeronautics and Space Administration, Scientific and Technological Information Branch. Washington, DC: U.S. Government Printing Office. NASA SP-447.

Nicogossian, A. E., Huntoon, C. L., and Pool, S. L. (1989). *Space physiology and medicine.* 2nd ed. National Aeronautics and Space Administration. Philadelphia: Lea & Febiger.

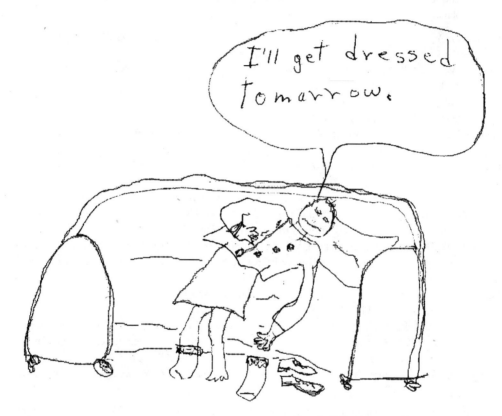

Brenda Heil, 33 years old, 9-year survivor

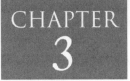

CHAPTER 3

Measurement and Assessment: What Are the Issues?

Claudette G. Varricchio

Before I decide what to do, I'm too tired to do it.
Brenda Heil, 33 years old, 9-year survivor

Background

Health care providers are showing a growing interest in cancer-related fatigue (CRF), its causes, incidence, and potential treatments. This is, to some extent, in response to increasing demands by cancer survivors that their symptoms be recognized and treated. Fatigue is not usually seen as a serious problem in healthy people because it is a temporary phenomenon and is not damaging. The slowness with which the research communities and health care providers have taken the phenomenon of CRF to heart may be related to several things:

- the subjective nature of the complaints
- the difficulty in assessing and measuring fatigue
- the assumption that it was just part of the disease and would get better with time
- the assumption that it presented no medical risk unless it reflected specific disease- and treatment-related pathologies
- the lack of a "magic pill" to effect a rapid cure

We are beginning to recognize that CRF is quite a serious problem: It is often chronic and relentless. The acknowledged difficulties in defining *fatigue* reflect the problems associated with determining etiology and, at present, with proposing interventions. A motivating factor involves the voices of the patients and families demanding recognition of, and attention to, this very troubling symptom.

Reports on wasting and debilitation associated with cancer can be traced back to ancient times. However, until treatments for cancer were developed and patients began to survive, it was a moot point: If you had cancer, you were sick, you became weaker, you went to bed, and you died. CRF was just part of the picture. Remarkably, expectations did not change among health care providers or patients, even after treatments began to be effective. Patients continued to suffer and health care providers continued to ignore it. It is remarkable that anything this prevalent and persistent could have been ignored for so long by the health care system.

It is generally agreed that fatigue is an abstract, subjective concept. In 1971, McFarland stated, "There is probably no single word in our vocabulary which has been less adequately described or understood, yet few people would deny personal acquaintance with it." In the intervening years, things have not improved. Definitions of fatigue are numerous, inconsistent, and varied according to the discipline of the author or the purpose of the research. Concept analysis would lead to explorations in a variety of fields, including medicine, physiology, ergonomics, physics, engineering, psychology, and biochemistry. *Impairment, loss of efficiency, weakness, boredom, muscle use, anxiety, depression, emotions, exertion, rest, exercise,* and *lifestyle* are terms associated with fatigue. Operational definitions vary. Considerations include measures of metabolism and muscular force, endurance and amount of sleep required or energy exerted, nutritional and hydration status, subjective reports of how much "pep" or vigor one has or how tired one feels, and mood and performance.

Recently, Schwartz, Jandorf, and Krupp (1996) described fatigue as a "frequent, albeit non-specific symptom encountered in a wide variety of clinical settings. It is a central diagnostic feature of chronic fatigue syndrome and a secondary symptom of major depression, rheumatoid arthritis, systemic lupus erythematosus, Lyme disease, many malignancies, renal failure and multiple sclerosis." Fatigue has not been measured routinely in patients with these disorders, despite its impact on them and the effect on quality of life (Glaus, Crow, and Hammond, 1996).

Fatigue manifests as an acute and chronic phenomenon. Acute fatigue can be the result of recent work performed that exceeded the energy resources available. Chronic fatigue is not relieved by rest or sleep, and its effect is cumulative. Chronic fatigue can be caused by a complex interplay of somatic and psychological factors (Jensen and Given, 1993). Some reports support the thesis that acute and chronic fatigue have different clinical courses (Nelson et al, 1987). Glaus, Crow, and Hammond (1996) suggested that fatigue should be viewed as a continuous dimension that is experienced as a subjective state. We are beginning to see reports from studies that describe fatigue as a symptom that persists for years after treatment ends, even when known causes have been resolved (Berglund et al, 1991; Dow et al, 1996).

Dimensions commonly encountered in the definitions and measurements of fatigue include the site and intensity of fatigue, the way and rate of change over time, the feelings that accompany fatigue, and

About the Contributor

Becoming a nurse was part of Claudette Varricchio's first memories. At the urging of an uncle who was a "family doctor," she attended a college that had a bachelor's degree in nursing. That was in 1971: Diploma programs were still thriving. It was almost by accident that she fell into a master's program: One day, she was standing in a student union cafeteria line behind the dean of a school of nursing who had just received military funding for physiologically based research in hyperbaric oxygenation. The dean offered an assistantship and Claudette jumped for it. Later, she had experience doing animal research with a group of French surgeons in Europe. After that, working in New York as head nurse of a radiation therapy department and being "mom" to two daughters was comparatively dull. She recognized relatively early that if she wanted to change things, she would have to get her doctorate and start with influencing students. By

the meaning patients attribute to fatigue. A review of the literature (Glaus, 1993) established fatigue as a "multidimensional experience that focuses not only on biochemical or pathophysiological causes, but also involves psychological and behavioral aspects." This description focuses on the dimensions that make the definition and measurement of fatigue problems for researchers and clinicians. In a study of fatigue among cancer patients after treatment, Irvine et al (1994) reported an incidence of 61% among cancer patients. Correlates were weight, symptom distress, mood disturbance, and changes in functional status. The authors reported that the best predictors of fatigue were symptom distress and mood disturbance. Fatigue and symptom distress were predictors of functional impairment related to illness.

What Do We Know About the Measurement of Fatigue?

Patients describe fatigue as a variety of problems: tiredness, lack of energy, generalized lassitude, inability to sustain exertion, loss of motor power, impaired mobility, sleepiness, drowsiness, confusion, apathy, poor concentration, helplessness, and a sense of inadequacy (Yasko, 1983). Because the definition of *fatigue* remains ambiguous, many attempts have been made to incorporate the measurement of fatigue into clinical assessments. Most commonly, fatigue is found as one item or scale in measures of functional status, or in the evaluation of mood, or as an item in a toxicity report. Recently, quality of life research has recognized the effect of fatigue and the interaction of fatigue with other symptoms or concepts that have an impact on quality of life. This has led to current efforts to determine what is to be measured, how, by whom, and when. There is a growing number of measurement tools reported in the literature (Tables 3-1 and 3-2). However, a significant amount of work is still required in the pursuit of developing reliable and valid measures that are appropriate to culturally, developmentally, and otherwise diverse groups of subjects.

Fatigue has both physiological and psychological components (Barofsky and Legro, 1991; Chen, 1986; Lee et al, 1994; Lewis and Haller, 1991; Potempa et al, 1986; St. Pierre

---

that time, she was commuting from Louisiana, where she taught, to Alabama, where she did her doctoral work. Two years after returning from a sabbatical at the National Cancer Institute (NCI), Claudette was drawn back to the NCI. Now, as she says, "I have an entire country to be my students and my mentors." She is not sure how she became interested in fatigue, but at some point she was asked to address the topic and became hooked.

This chapter is an expanded and updated version of an earlier work. It should be useful to those who want to explore fatigue in both research and clinical practice. More than another literature review, this chapter reflects the thought processes Claudette uses when evaluating a fatigue scale.

Table 3.1   Physiological Measures of Fatigue

Anaerobic metabolism (a cellular fatigue indicator of physiological processes) (Lewis and Haller, 1991; St. Pierre, Kasper, and Lindsey, 1992)

    Adenine diphosphate use

    Adenine triphosphate synthesis

    Anaerobic glycolysis (lactate production)

Change in body mass (especially muscle tissue) (Garn and Pesik, 1982)

    Loss of muscle protein (St. Pierre, Kasper, and Lindsey, 1992)

Energy expenditure (Winningham, 1990)

    Functional capacity (MacVicar, 1990; McCorkle and Young, 1978)

    Functional reserve (MacVicar, 1990; McCorkle and Young, 1978)

Exercise evaluation (Lewis and Haller, 1991)

    Bicycle ergometric test result (maximal oxygen uptake, peak oxygen uptake, or symptom-limited ergometric performance on cycle or treadmill ergometer) (Winningham, 1983)

    Cardiac output

    Perceived exertion during stepwise ergometric testing (Borg, 1970)

Muscle function as ability to perform work

    Accumulation of metabolic products to exhaustion (Sahlin, 1992)

    Repeated contractility to exhaustion (Allen et al., 1983; Winningham, 1983, 1990)

Nutritional status (Miller, 1978)

    Calorie intake and expenditure

    Hydration status

Oxidative metabolism (Lewis and Haller, 1991; Winningham, 1990)

    Maximal oxygen uptake vs. maximal work capacity

---

et al, 1992; Winningham et al, 1994). Most authors agree that fatigue is a subjective phenomenon. Therefore, it can be compared with the phenomenon of pain: It is what the person experiencing it says it is. Tables 3-1 and 3-2 list existing measures of fatigue, and Table 3-3 lists measures that include fatigue. These lists reflect the need to assess fatigue as a multidimensional concept. Fatigue assessment scales are most commonly visual analogue scales or numerical rating scales. Many have been validated on small samples, in patients with one kind of cancer or another disease state, and have no comparison data with healthy cohorts. This limits the usefulness in samples other than the original group. More psychometric evaluation is needed for most of the published scales.

Table 3.2	Self-report Measures

Cancer Fatigue Scale (Schwartz, 1998)

Diary/interview (Lee et al, 1994)

Fatigue Assessment Instrument (Schwartz, Jandorf, and Krupp, 1996)

Fatigue Assessment Inventory (Glaus, Crow, and Hammond, 1996)

Fatigue Body Scale (Glaus, 1993)

Fatigue Symptom Questionnaire (Wessly and Powell, 1989)

Functional Assessment of Cancer Therapy (FACT)—Anemia (Cella, 1997)

Functional Assessment of Cancer Therapy (FACT)—Fatigue (Yelien et al, 1997)

General Well-Being Schedule, Vitality Sub-Scale (Dupy, 1973)

Linear Analogue Scale (LAS) (Glaus, 1993)

Multidimensional Fatigue Inventory (MFI-20) (Smets et al, 1996)

Multidimensional Fatigue Inventory (Stein et al, 1998)

Multidimensional Measure of Fatigue Scale (Smets et al, 1995)

Pearson-Byars Fatigue Checklist (Pearson and Byars, 1956)

Piper Fatigue Scale, Revised (Piper et al, 1998)

Rhoten Fatigue Scale and Checklist (Rhoten, 1982)

SF-36 Vitality Scale (Ware et al, 1993)

Sickness Impact Profile (Bergner et al, 1976)

Symptom Distress Scale (McCorkle and Young, 1978)

Visual Analogue Fatigue Scale (Glaus, 1993; Rhoten, 1982)

Yoshitake Fatigue Symptom Checklist (Yoshitake, 1971)

How Does Fatigue Influence Quality of Life?

We have an intuitive knowledge that fatigue and quality of life are related. How highly will people who are constantly lethargic and tired, or who have difficulty in motivating themselves to do anything, rate their overall quality of life? Add to this other symptoms or effects of cancer or its treatment such as nausea, vomiting, or pain, and health-related quality of life will surely decline.

A relationship between fatigue and depression has been postulated by many authors. Visser and Smets (1998) showed only weak support for the relationship between these concepts. They reported that depressive mood appears to be an important predictor of quality of life.

Fatigue, when viewed from the patient's perspective, has a pervasive effect on health-related quality of life, manifesting symptoms and affecting physical function, mental health,

Table 3.3	Select Related and Indirect Measures

Activity and rest patterns

Anemia

Depression scales
   Beck Depression Inventory (Beck et al, 1961)
   CES-D (Radloff, 1977)
   Profile of Mood States (McNair, Lorr, and Droppleman, 1971)

Endurance
   Atrophy
   Strength
   Weakness

General health status

Performance status
   Karnofsky (Klein and Hart, 1978)
   (Zubrod, Eastern Cooperative Oncology Group [ECOG], and South West Oncology Group [SWOG]
      scales are based on the above)
   WHO scale (World Health Organization, 1990)

Single-item side effect checklists

Sleep patterns and duration

Toxicity scales

and other aspects of daily living such as sleeping, working, and socializing. Nelson and colleagues (1987) reported results of a study of 83 patients with the chief complaint of fatigue. Thirty-five patients (42%) reported problems with sleep; 27 (33%) with overall enjoyment of life; 22 (27%) with social life; 21 (25%) with sex life; 20 (24%) with their job and daily work; and 13 (16%), with family life. The subjects who complained of fatigue had substantially more bed days, disability days, and social role–related activity limitations than did their counterparts who did not complain of fatigue. The researchers concluded that "for the fatigue patients, this all adds up to a lower overall quality of life."

Influences on the Accuracy of Measurement

The conceptual and operational definition of fatigue used to identify the purpose of the assessment should determine how and when fatigue will be measured. Is fatigue defined clearly in the project? Does fatigue include, or is it limited to, sleep tiredness, strength, or level of activity? Is it seen as a physiological function, a psychological phenomenon, or a composite of both? To obtain a valid assessment, the choice of measure–physiological evaluation, paper-and-pencil assessment, or interview–must refer to the same definition of fatigue as the original question (Irvine et al, 1991). For example, a tool to assess mood may not be appropriate as a sole measure of fatigue when fatigue is defined as the ability to perform a physical task.

The purpose for measuring fatigue also plays a role in assessing it (Varricchio, 1990). For example, if the intent is to determine the effect on functional status, defined as the ability to perform daily chores, a measure of the functional ability is appropriate. If an assessment of health-related quality of life is the purpose, a multidimensional approach that includes fatigue as a measure is preferred. If the goal is to determine tolerance for a specific activity, measurement of a physiological parameter such as muscle fatigue is appropriate. Energy expenditure may be an acceptable marker of the overall disease trajectory and treatment effect.

Confounding variables present potential measurement problems. Factors that can influence fatigue scores and need to be controlled for or discussed in interpreting scores include age, disease severity, treatment intensity, and concurrent illness (Irvine et al, 1991). Patient burden and the timing of the measurement may also influence the validity of the data. These two factors are perhaps more important in measuring fatigue than in measuring other concepts.

To date, little attention has been given to the patterns of fatigue and the cause or rate of change in the experience of persons receiving chemotherapy or other cancer therapy (Richardson et al, 1998). Studies of fatigue have not looked at the trajectory of fatigue in relation to the cycles of treatment. These studies often do not report the number or intensity or pattern of the fatigue symptoms over time. They do not have a normal control group and mix chemotherapy protocols or disease stages.

A small exploratory study (Glaus, Crow, and Hammond, 1996) compared patterns of fatigue in healthy workers and cancer patients. The healthy workers felt fatigue as the day progressed, while the cancer patients reported continuous fatigue that may have been less in the evening. The authors proposed a circadian rhythm for fatigue in cancer patients.

Richardson et al (1998) reported a study of patterns of fatigue in 109 patients receiving chemotherapy. They used daily diaries and other measures to assess the patterns of fatigue. They observed the effect of the drug combination, the route of administration, and the time of administration on the reports of intensity and duration of fatigue. An unexpected finding was the apparent rise in fatigue before the subsequent cycles of chemotherapy. It has been commonly assumed that fatigue resolves after reaching its maximum around the nadir associated with the drug regimen.

One must be aware of the possibility that assessment influences the amount of fatigue reported by the subject. A complex, lengthy assessment instrument itself produces fatigue and respondent burden. Timing can introduce severe bias into the assessment: If the assessment is performed during or immediately following a procedure or other strenuous activity, the data will not represent the average fatigue state of that individual. Therefore, conscious, deliberate decisions must be made about the optimal time to measure fatigue, given the purpose of the assessment. If the purpose is to determine the amount of fatigue resulting from an activity, it may be appropriate to assess immediately after the activity is completed.

In an interview, or when one is developing an assessment tool, the structure of the questions that assess fatigue is important. Terms must be clearly communicated. If "fatigue" is used, it must be clear whether "tired," "exhausted," or "sleepy" is meant by the questioner or by the respondent. Clearly, educational background, age, culture, and primary language of the patient influence responses (Varricchio, 1997). What is the meaning of *fatigue?* What does it mean to admit to fatigue in the individual's culture? Is there a concept equivalent to the assessor's definition of *fatigue* in the patient's language or cultural frame of reference? Explorations of the concept of fatigue with bilingual and bicultural people help to determine an appropriate and valid assessment. Likewise, exploration of the concept of quality of life in the cultural and linguistic context is necessary for valid measures to be developed and used (McCabe, Varricchio, and Padberg, 1994).

The developmental stage, including age and physical condition of the patient, is an important influence on the assessment of fatigue and quality of life. Many existing measures of fatigue have been based on healthy, working adults. These norms may not apply to persons with cancer, older persons, the chronically ill, or children and adolescents (see Chapter 4). It is important to note the descriptions of the population or sample on which a given

Carry a Lighter Purse

The two biggest obstacles I have had to overcome are pain and lack of energy. Pain medications reduced the pain to a level I could tolerate. That left me the problem of adapting my lifestyle and processes to get the most out of the energy available and try to avoid pushing myself into exhaustion.

Now, let me explain something about myself. I am the sort of person who not only handled all my own problems, but also handled everyone else's, too. I was "Responsibler than Thou." If something needed to be done, I did it, and I did it right. It had never been any other way, and I found pride and pleasure in being that way.

But I was coming up against a big thick brick wall. Things were changing fast. Unbeknownst to me, through the years, my purse had gained weight. I realized how much it had gained when, on one particularly difficult morning, I discovered that I couldn't even pick it up and put it on my shoulder, let alone walk two steps with it. What was wrong? Everything in it was "essential"? Right? Right. I dug around until I found an old, small thin purse I had bought years ago in Mexico. It had about one-tenth the volume of my usual one. I put the bare necessities in the small purse and the remaining "essentials" in an insulated lunch bag in the car. That way I was never very far from the things I needed, but I don't have to carry them all the time.

Stairs became a problem. Doing a whole flight of stairs in one shot became impossible. I put a small barstool on the midway landing. Now, I can sit and rest a couple of minutes at the halfway point.

measure has been based: This is equally true of physiological and psychosocial measures. For example, measures that have been developed to assess fatigue in Japanese railroad workers or American jet pilots may not be appropriate for measuring fatigue in healthy Americans or those who have cancer. This is a problem to consider when weighing the decision to use an existing measure or to develop a new one.

Very few studies exploring fatigue in people with cancer have used comparison groups that comprise healthy subjects or people with other diseases or conditions. The comparison of subjects' current levels of fatigue with their precancerous or treatment levels of fatigue is also rarely reported. This makes conclusions about the cause of disease- or treatment-related fatigue difficult to reach.

The interaction and timing of medication on responses to the assessment must also be considered. Certain pain medications and tranquilizers may induce states that could be interpreted as fatigue by the subject. Chemotherapy-induced nausea and vomiting or other side effects as well as fatigue may influence responses. However, the purpose of the assessment may be to determine how much the treatment influences fatigue. Measurement closer to the time of treatment may be appropriate. If the purpose is not to assess the immediate effect of the treatment on fatigue and quality of life, a choice of assessment time consistent with the purpose must be planned.

I reviewed everything I did in my life to determine what was essential, like earning a living, because I enjoyed eating and having a roof over my head–especially the eating part. Those things that were not brutally essential, I had to stop doing. . . . No matter how much I really wanted to, the energy wasn't there. I had to learn to say a very hard word–"NO."

I began keeping track of my energy levels very closely, and I discovered that there were specific times during the day when my energy was higher and others when it was lower. Now I plan my days so that the things I absolutely have to do are scheduled for the times when my energy levels are high. Similarly, I make my plans to spend the low-energy times in the recliner.

I enlisted the help of my family to pick up a larger share of the chores. They each took a few of those things that I no longer had the energy, strength, or stamina to handle and worked out a way to do them for me. Now all I had to do was overcome the guilt when I watched them do those things instead of me. . . . I'm still working on that one. I'm lucky I have a family willing to cooperate. Some folks don't have that advantage.

Every day brings new challenges; there are things I either have found a way to do, or have found some way not to do. The one thing I am learning to do, however, is to be at peace doing nothing, when nothing is all I can do.

Surviving at last

Selecting a Measure of Fatigue

There are several issues to consider when selecting an instrument to study fatigue. This assessment of fatigue requires the following (Varricchio, 1985):

1. A clear definition of the concept must be provided.
2. The operational definition should be consistent with the conceptual definition.
3. The objective manifestations of fatigue must be identified.
4. The physiological and psychological components should be recognized.

The purpose of the assessment also influences the method of assessment. Does the purpose require a physiological measure, a psychological measure, a combination of both, an involved battery of tests, or a single-item subjective response (Winningham, 1990)?

Other issues must also be considered:

1. Does the assessment place a burden on the subject?
2. Is the fatigue being made worse by the choice of measure?
3. Does the measure correspond to the developmental stage of the subject?
4. Can the subject understand what is being asked?
5. Is acute or chronic fatigue being measured?
6. Does the approach chosen tap this dimension?
7. How sensitive to change is the assessment?
8. What is the subjective character of fatigue?

There is no "gold standard" for overall CRF assessment (Schwartz, Jandorf, and Krupp, 1996). Objective correlates have not yet been identified and agreed on. Related factors such as hopelessness, energy expenditure, and overall nutritional and hydration status warrant exploration.

Where Do We Go From Here?

The science of CRF assessment is in its teenage years. Much work has been done in developing a consensus on the definition of the concept and its interactions with other important, concurrently occurring states. There is much to be done to validate measures that will be consistent with the definitions and that are appropriate to specific groups of patients or to groups that have specific characteristics because of age, culture, or other variables. Early work relevant to interventions is emerging to address fatigue in the cancer patient. The problem is that it is difficult to promote the scientific basis of an intervention when the etiology of fatigue in the presence of cancer is not established.

Fatigue is a major problem for persons being treated for cancer or living with the effects of the treatment. It is a rich area for researchers who have the interest and the persistence to deal with the ambiguity and the difficulties of defining and controlling this subjective experience. There is much work to be done before we can say that the state of knowledge about fatigue is comparable to the current state of knowledge about pain or quality of life, for instance. Both of these concepts are also subjective and multidimensional. Both have evolved over time, with much discussion about definitions and the best way to assess and measure them. There is some consensus about these topics, but they are at a more advanced developmental stage than fatigue. They have a longer history of receiving scientific attention than does fatigue.

We can learn from the developmental experiences of pain and quality of life assessment and the translation of the assessments to interventions. Both are evolving areas of science. We know much about the assessment and interventions for pain, but pain is often not well managed in clinical practice. We are beginning to have options for the assessment of quality of life and the description of changes related to the experience of cancer and its treatment. We are not yet in the era of proposing and testing interventions to reduce the negative impact of cancer and therapy on quality of life. These are the goals that we who are interested in the phenomenon of fatigue have set for ourselves.

References

Allen, D., Westerbald, H., Lee, J., et al (1983). Role of excitation-contraction coupling in muscle fatigue. *Sports Medicine, 13,* 116–126.

Barofsky, K., and Legro, M. W. (1991). Definition and measurement of fatigue. *Review of Infectious Diseases, 13*(suppl 1), S94–S97.

Beck, A., Ward, C., Mendelson M., et al (1961). An inventory for measuring depression. *Archives of General Psychiatry, 4,* 53–63.

Berglund, G., Bolund, C., Fornander, T., et al (1991). Late effects of adjuvant chemotherapy and post operative radiotherapy on quality of life among breast cancer patients. *British Journal of Cancer, 27,* 1075–1081.

Bergner, M., Bobbitt, R. A., Kressel, S., et al (1976). The Sickness Impact Profile: Conceptual formulation and methodology for the development of a health status measure. *International Journal of Health Services, 6,* 393–415.

Borg, G. (1970). Perceived exertion as an indicator of somatic stress. *Scandinavian Journal of Rehabilitative Medicine, 2,* 92–98.

Cella, D. (1997). The Functional Assessment of Cancer Therapy–Anemia (FACT-AN) Scale: A new tool for the assessment of outcomes in cancer anemia and fatigue. *Seminars in Hematology, 34* (suppl 2), 13–19.

Chen, M. K. (1986). The epidemiology of self-perceived fatigue among adults. *Preventive Medicine, 15,* 74–81.

Dow, K. H., Ferrell, B. R., Leigh, S., et al (1996). An evaluation of the quality of life among long-term survivors of breast cancer. *Breast Cancer Research and Treatment, 39,* 261–273.

Dupy, H. (1973). The General Well-Being Schedule. In *National Center for Health Statistics, Plans and Operation of Health and Statistics.* Washington, D.C.: U.S. Government Printing Office. PHS series 1 (10b).

Garn, S. M., and Pesik, S. D. (1982). Comparison of the Benn index and other body mass indices in nutritional assessment. *American Journal of Clinical Nutrition, 36*, 573–575.

Glaus, A. (1993). Assessment of fatigue in cancer and non-cancer patients. *Supportive Care in Cancer, 1*, 305–315.

Glaus, A., Crow, R., and Hammond, S. (1996). A qualitative study to explore the concept of fatigue/tiredness in cancer patients and healthy individuals: Supportive care. *Supportive Care in Cancer, 4*, 82–96.

Irvine, D. M., Vincent, L., Bubela, N., et al (1991). A critical appraisal of the research literature investigating fatigue in the individual with cancer. *Cancer Nursing, 13*, 188–199.

Irvine, D M., Vincent, L., Graydon, J. E., et al (1994). The prevalence and correlates of fatigue in patients receiving treatment with chemotherapy and radiotherapy. *Cancer Nursing, 17*, 367–378.

Jensen, S., and Given, B. (1993). Fatigue affecting family caregivers of cancer patients. *Supportive Care in Cancer, 1*, 321–325.

Klein, E., and Hart, A. (1978). Assessment of quality of life: Scoring performance status in cancer patients. In N. Aaronson (Ed.), *The quality of life in cancer patients* (pp. 93–99). New York: Raven Press.

Lee, K. A., Lentz, M. J., Taylor, D. L., et al (1994). Fatigue as a response to environmental demands in women's lives. *Image–The Journal of Nursing Scholarship, 26*, 149–154.

Lewis, S. F., and Haller, R. G. (1991). Physiologic measurement of exercise and fatigue with special reference to chronic fatigue syndrome. *Review of Infectious Diseases, 13*(suppl 1), 98–108.

MacVicar, M. (Ed.) (1990). Functional assessment: Concepts and measurement. In *Altered functioning: Impairment and disability* (pp. 6–15). Indianapolis, IN: Sigma Theta Tau International.

McCabe, M., Varricchio, C., and Padberg, R. M. (1994). Efforts to recruit the economically disadvantaged to national clinical trials. *Seminars in Oncology Nursing, 10*, 1123–1129.

McCorkle, R., and Young, K. (1978). Development of a symptom distress scale. *Cancer Nursing, 1*, 373–378.

McFarland, R. A. (1971). Understanding fatigue in modern life. *Ergonomics, 14*, 1–10.

McNair, D., Lorr, M., and Droppleman, L. (1971). *Profile of mood states.* San Diego, CA: Educational and Industrial Testing Services.

Miller, H. W. (Ed.) (1978). *Plan and operation of the HANESII augmentation survey of adults 25-74 years, United States, 1974–1975.* Vital and Health Statistics. Series 1, No. 14. Washington, D.C.: U.S. Public Health Services. DHEW Publication No. (PHS) 78-1324.

Nelson, E., Kirk, J., McHugo, G., et al (1987). Chief complaint fatigue: A longitudinal study from the patient's perspective. *Family Practice Research Journal, 6*, 175–188.

Pearson, R. G., and Byars, G. E. (1956). *The development and validation of a check-list for measuring subjective fatigue.* Randolf AFB, TX: School of Aviation, USAF. Report No. 56-115.

Piper, B. F., Dibble, S. L., Dodd, M. J., et al (1998). The revised Piper Fatigue Scale: Psychometric evaluation in women with breast cancer. *Oncology Nursing Forum, 25*, 677–684.

Potempa, K., Lopez, M., Reid, C., et al (1986). Chronic fatigue. *Image–The Journal of Nursing Scholarship, 4*, 165–169.

Radloff, L. S. (1977). The CES-D Scale: A self-report depression scale for research in the general population. *Applied Psychological Measurement, 3*(1), 385–401.

Rhoten, D. (1982). Fatigue and the postsurgical patient. In C. M. Norris (Ed.), *Concept clarification in nursing* (pp. 277–300). Rockville, MD: Aspen.

Richardson, A., Ream, E., and Wilson-Barnett, J. (1998). Fatigue in patients receiving chemotherapy: Patterns of change. *Cancer Nursing, 21,* 17–30.

Sahlin, K. (1992). Metabolic factors in fatigue. *Sports Medicine, 13,* 99–107.

Schwartz, A. L. (1998). The Schwartz Cancer Fatigue Scale: Testing reliability and validity. *Oncology Nursing Forum, 25,* 711–717.

Schwartz, J. E., Jandorf, L., and Krupp, L. B. (1996). The measurement of fatigue: A new instrument. *Journal of Psychosomatic Research, 37,* 753–762

Smets, E. M. A., Garssen, B., Cull, A., and de Haes, J. C. J. M. (1996). Application of the Multidimensional Fatigue Inventory (MFI-20) in cancer patients receiving radiotherapy. *British Journal of Cancer, 73,* 241–245.

Smets, M. A., Garssen, B., Bonk, B., and deHaes, J. C. J. M. (1995). The Multidimensional Fatigue Inventory (MFI): Psychometric qualities of an instrument to assess fatigue. *Journal of Psychometric Research, 39,* 315–325.

Stein, K. D., Martin, S. C., Hann, D. M., and Jacobsen, P. B. (1998). A multidimensional measure of fatigue for use with cancer patients. *Cancer Practice, 6,* 143–152.

St. Pierre, B. A., Kasper, C. E., and Lindsey, A. M. (1992). Fatigue mechanisms in patients with cancer: Effects of tumor necrosis factor and exercise on skeletal muscle. *Oncology Nursing Forum, 19,* 419–425.

Varricchio, C. (1985). Selecting a tool for measuring fatigue. *Oncology Nursing Forum, 12,* 122–127.

Varricchio, C. (1990). Relevance of quality of life in clinical nursing research. *Seminars in Oncology Nursing, 6,* 255–259.

Varricchio, C. (1997). Measurement issues concerning linguistic translations. In M. Frank-Stromborg and S. Olsen (Eds.), *Instruments for clinical nursing research* (pp. 54–63). 2nd ed. Sudbury: Jones and Bartlett.

Visser, M. R. M., and Smets, E. M. A. (1998). Fatigue, depression and quality of life in cancer patients: How are they related? *Supportive Care in Cancer, 6,* 101–108.

Ware, J. E., Snow, K. K., Kosinski, M., and Dandek, B. (1993). *SF-36 health survey: Manual and interpretation guide.* Boston: New England Medical Center.

Wessly, S., and Powell, R. (1989). Fatigue syndromes: A comparison of chronic "post-viral" fatigue with neuromuscular and affective disorders. *Journal of Neurology, Neurosurgery, and Psychiatry, 52,* 940–948.

Winningham, M. L. (1983). "Effects of a bicycle ergometry program on functional capacity and feelings of control in women with breast cancer." Doctoral dissertation, Ohio State University, Columbus, OH.

Winningham, M. L. (Ed.) (1990). Physiological quantification of functional ability. In *Altered functioning: Impairment and disability* (pp. 85–90). Indianapolis, IN: Sigma Theta Tau International.

Winningham, M. L., Nail, L. M., Barton-Burke, M., Brophy, L., Cimprich, B., and Jones, L., Pickard-Holly, S., Rhodes, V., St. Pierre, B., Beck, S., Glass, E. C., Mock, V. L., Mooney, K. H., and Piper, B. (1994). Fatigue and the cancer experience: The state of the knowledge. *Oncology Nursing Forum, 21,* 23–36.

World Health Organization. (1990). *Handbook for reporting results of cancer treatment.* Geneva: World Health Organization.

Yasko, J. (1983). *Guidelines for cancer: Symptom management* (pp. 33–37). Reston, VA: Reston Publishing.

Yelien, S. B., Cella, D. F., Webster, K. et al (1997). Measuring fatigue and other anemia-related symptoms with the Functional Assessment of Cancer Therapy (FACT) measurement system. *Journal of Pain Symptom Management, 13,* 63–74.

Yoshitake, H. (1971). Relations between the symptoms and the feeling of fatigue. *Ergonomics, 14,* 175–186.

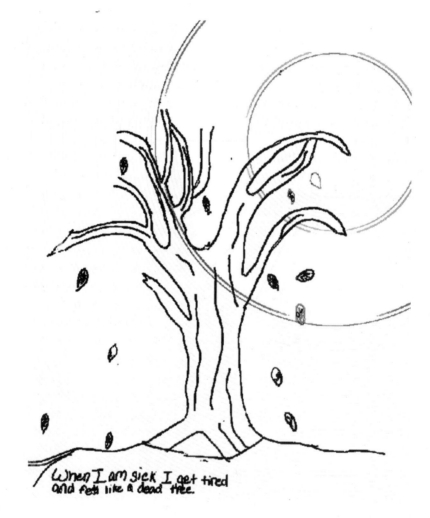

When I am sick, I get tired and feel like a dead tree.
Jessica Flores, 11-year-old leukemia survivor

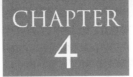

Fatigue in Children
and Adolescents With Cancer

Marilyn Hockenberry-Eaton

Pamela S. Hinds

Whenever I am home, like whenever I get to bed, I get rested. But whenever I'm in the hospital, I have to take vitamins [leukovorin] every 4 to 8 hours . . . you have to have blood drawn every 12 to 24 hours . . . and then you get the doctors coming in at 6:00 AM listening to your heart and stuff. So, at the hospital, I feel drained in the morning, not like I got any rest. But whenever I'm at home and I get a real night's sleep I feel a whole lot better.   Teen on fatigue in the hospital

Background

Cure rates for childhood cancer now exceed 55%. The success of treatment has occurred because of aggressive treatment regimens that are not without numerous side effects. Children with cancer experience problems associated with treatment including nausea and vomiting, which may cause weight loss, nutritional deficits, electrolyte imbalances, weakness, and lethargy. Infection and fever are common occurrences during treatment. While these side effects are discussed extensively in the literature, there is limited discussion of fatigue as a symptom experienced by children with cancer. No studies in the childhood cancer literature have evaluated fatigue. Bottomley, Teegarden, and Hockenberry-Eaton (1996) evaluated an instrument developed to measure childhood cancer stressors and found that over 50% of a group of 75 school-age children reported being tired, not sleeping well, and unable to do the things they wanted to do. More than half of these children were not as active as before the illness, and reported playing less.

Several articles published on chronic fatigue in children provide some insight into the concept of fatigue in children. Chronic fatigue syndrome (CFS) in children is defined as a severe, disabling fatigue that affects both mental and physical functioning and lasts for at least six months. Carter and colleagues (1995) examined symptoms of chronic fatigue in 20 children and found that these children experienced concentration changes, muscle weakness, depressed mood, decreased appetite, sleep disturbances, and a need for excessive sleep. A second article published in 1996 by Carter and associates evaluated certain psychological factors that discriminated chronic fatigue from depressive symptomatology in matched groups of 20 healthy, depressed, and chronic fatigue subjects. Characteristics of pediatric patients with chronic fatigue included multiple somatic complaints, excessive sleepiness, low energy, decreased appetite, loss of interest or pleasure in usual activities, loneliness, social isolation, and feelings of unhappiness. Depressed subjects reported more symptoms of affective disturbances; were more likely to have suicidal ideation and pronounced social isolation; and demonstrated acting out behaviors such as irritability, restlessness, trouble concentrating, anger, and aggression. Depressed subjects were significantly affected by feelings of tiredness, fatigue, and an excessive need for sleep.

Current Research: Fatigue in Children

Little is known about the occurrence, causes, conceptual and operational definitions of fatigue, and effective interventions in children and adolescents with cancer. The work that developed a fatigue research program for children was started in 1996, as the result of a research grant awarded by the Oncology Nursing Foundation (made possible through a grant by Ortho Biotec of Raritan, N.J.). Focus groups first were used to gain a contextual understanding of fatigue through discussions. Twenty-eight focus groups were held over a six-month period at two major children's cancer centers. Twenty-nine children participated in the focus groups; 14 were 7 to 12 years old and 15 were 13 to 16 years old. Twenty-two parents and 33 staff members also participated in the focus groups. Focus groups were held separately for each age group, lasted 30 to 45 minutes, and were tape-recorded. The audiotapes were transcribed verbatim, and Ethnograph software was used to number the data in order to sort and code the information. Researchers at both study sites coded the data independently within the context of the unit of analyses, which in this study were the study questions. Codes and descriptions were developed for the definitions, causes, and what helps fatigue (Hockenberry-Eaton et al, 1998).

Findings of the focus groups revealed that the definition of fatigue varies, depending on the developmental level of the participants. Teens used a noticeably larger vocabulary to

About the Contributors

Marilyn Hockenberry-Eaton has an exceptional ability for combining her advanced practice abilities with research. Pamela S. Hinds has combined her passion for research with administrative and educational talent and, as a Yankee transplanted to Tennessee, is fascinated by the works of Southern authors and about the Civil War. As mothers of children, both understand the worries of parents of children with cancer. Any observant parent can tell you that fatigue can affect every aspect of a child's life, including scholastic progress and social functioning. Marilyn and Pamela are pioneering the study of fatigue in children and adolescents with cancer. Although there have long been observations of malaise and difficulty with sleep

describe what fatigue is like and to discuss the differences between mental and physical symptoms. Teens described the causes of fatigue in much greater detail than children did and had many more factors associated with fatigue. The teen groups described more symptoms of worry and concern that resulted in fatigue compared to the children's groups. Teens were able to identify more interventions that helped decrease fatigue. Both children and teens described fatigue in terms of physical and mental symptoms, but children were unable to identify mental causes of fatigue. Discussion of the study results are presented in terms of the children's and teens' descriptions of fatigue, perceived causes of fatigue, and what helps when they are experiencing fatigue. Results of focus group discussions with parents and staff are also presented.

Children's and Adolescents' Perceptions of Fatigue

Children have described both physical and mental symptoms of fatigue (Hockenberry-Eaton et al, 1998). Physical fatigue was described as "it's hard to move and run" and mental fatigue as feeling "sad or mad." Children expressed their perception of fatigue in relation to changes that have occurred in their ability to perform activities they did prior to having cancer. One child stated, "Because I am tired, I don't have any energy. I can't run fast or anything." Significant changes in physical abilities occurred, such as playing sports or participating in activities with friends. A young boy with a brain tumor, when asked to describe fatigue, stated, "Well back before my surgery and I was kind of really active, but not very tired usually, and now I am very tired."

Several children described fatigue in terms of now doing more quiet activities such as watching television or reading books. One child stated, "When I am tired, I can watch a movie. I can't read too well anymore because I can't keep my eyes open." Children were able to describe physical symptoms related to their fatigue. One child described fatigue as, "I see a dull face when I look in the mirror." Another child responded, "I get tired all over." Some children were able to identify when fatigue occurred. Fatigue occurred most often in the mornings, on school days, and following treatment. The teen groups described physi-

and schooling in children with cancer, previously no one has studied the phenomenon of fatigue in these children. When the editors heard about this landmark work, they were impressed with its far-reaching clinical implications. They were even more intrigued with these contributors methods, because the techniques someday may be useful in studying fatigue across age groups and across cultural barriers. As this research is in its early stages, it provides an opportunity to watch it grow as the discoveries are published. It is our hope that you profit from the insights this chapter brings and appreciate the creativity of the contributors as well as the children who have taught them so much.

cal fatigue as "you don't feel like your normal self" and mental fatigue as "tired of everything that has happened."

Adolescents, like the children, frequently expressed fatigue in terms of physical activities they can no longer perform. One teen stated, "I used to play sports and play with my friends all the time, and now I am on crutches." Another teen reported, "You can't hang out with your friends and go to the skating rink." Mental fatigue was described in terms of feeling sorry for yourself, being mad at the world, or just not wanting to be bothered. One teen stated, "Sometimes you are tired and the mind doesn't do anything but shut off." Teens were able to describe the influence of mental and physical fatigue on each other. One teen stated, "You think about it, dwell on it, [and] it makes it worse. So, part of it's [fatigue] mental, part of it's physical." Another teen stated, "When you get cancer, your lifestyle has changed 100%, because you have to deal with getting cancer, understanding what you are about to go through. You have to mentally prepare yourself. I'm not going to let this take control."

Because I am tired, I don't have any energy. I can't run fast or anything.

When your counts are down, it's really bad.

Teens discussed being mad or upset during treatment. One adolescent discussed what it was like during treatment: "You're in there getting chemo . . . and you feel really bad . . . it makes you so mad." Another teen described what it is like to experience fatigue by discussing feeling sorry for oneself: "You see this nice beautiful sunny day and you're sitting there feeling, ugh, feeling your chemo." Adolescents were able to discuss specific times when fatigue occurs, describing it as usually following chemotherapy and when their counts were low. One adolescent said, "I just felt tired the days I get chemo." Another teen described fatigue as, "When your counts are down, it's really bad."

Children discussed the hospital environment as causing fatigue because of frequent disruptions in sleep. Some children also had trouble falling asleep in the hospital. One child stated, "When I am in the hospital, I am just so drained when I get home." Some children described low blood cell counts as causing fatigue and related it to altering their activities. A child stated, "I had to quit playing baseball. My counts were too low." Another child described having to stay home from school when the blood cell count was low. Children identified sleep changes as a cause of fatigue. Difficulty going to sleep was discussed as a cause of fatigue in the morning.

Pain was also identified as a cause of fatigue in one focus group. Treatment and its side effects were frequently described as causes of fatigue. One teen stated, "That's the worst, knowing what's going to happen . . . knowing that you have to go do it [chemotherapy], that it's going to wear you out."

Teens also discussed the hospital environment as a frequent cause of fatigue because of disruptions of sleep. Teen focus group participants discussed noises such as the nurses' station, younger patients, intravenous infusion pumps, telephones, shutting of doors, and frequent interruptions as causing fatigue because of lack of sleep. Sleep changes occurred when teens went to sleep late and were awakened in the middle of the night while in the hospital. One adolescent described being in the hospital as, "It's like jet lag." Another teen stated, "Whenever I am home, like whenever I get to bed, I get rested. But whenever I'm in the hospital, I have to take vitamins [leukovorin] every 4 to 8 hours . . . you have to have blood drawn every 12 to 24 hours . . . and then you get the doctors coming in at 6:00 AM listening to your heart and stuff. So, at the hospital, I feel drained in the morning, not like I got any rest. But whenever I'm at home and I get a real night's sleep I feel a whole lot better." One child also stated it was difficult to fall asleep because of problems getting comfortable in bed because of the intravenous line and needle placement.

In addition to the hospital environment disrupting sleep, lifestyle changes also altered the adolescents' previous sleep patterns. Teens who were on homebound education programs discussed staying up late at night and sleeping late into the morning. This made getting up early in the morning a problem, resulting in fatigue. Teens discussed being afraid to fall asleep at times, causing them to be tired the next day. One teen discussed being afraid to go to sleep in the emergency room, for fear of what might happen while she was asleep. Teens also discussed worrying about the future and being unable to fall asleep at night due to concerns that were on their minds.

Children described fewer interventions that helped decrease fatigue when compared to the adolescents. One child's description of how rest helps was, "I usually take two naps every day and that makes me feel better." A good night's sleep was described as something that helped the children when they were tired. One child who discussed not being tired at the time of the focus group stated, "I slept good last night." Children discussed quiet activities such as reading a book, or listening to music as helpful when they experienced fatigue. "Having someone come visit you" is an example of a child's description of how visitors can help distract them when in the hospital.

When you get cancer, your lifestyle has changed 100%, because you have to deal with getting cancer, understanding what you are about to go through. You have to mentally prepare yourself. I'm not going to let this take control.

The need for protected rest time in the hospital and for naps when at home were described as very helpful for most teens. One adolescent discussed how his mother provided a rest period when in the hospital. "My Mom normally will tell them not to come in and put a sign on the door . . . because I'm just so tired that I really can't talk to them." Participating in activities that keep adolescents busy and help take their mind off feeling tired were discussed as helping to decrease fatigue. One teen stated, "I don't know what it does for me but I've heard people say that if you're sick, laughter helps you . . . watching movies kind of relaxes you, and if it is funny and makes you laugh, then you feel better because you forget about being tired, hurting, and all that." Going outside when in the hospital also was described as helping to decrease fatigue by teens in one focus group. One teen expressed the need for sleeping pills at night to decrease fatigue, and one discussed that blood transfusions made him less tired. Several had participated in physical therapy while hospitalized and found this decreased their fatigue.

Parents' Perceptions of Fatigue

Parents' perceptions of fatigue were elicited through seven focus groups consisting of 20 mothers and two fathers who had children receiving treatment for cancer. The focus groups were tape-recorded and the tapes transcribed, similarly to the children and adolescent groups. Data from the groups were sorted and coded by two research teams. Codes and descriptions were developed for the parents' perceptions of the definitions, causes, and what helps fatigue.

Parents' descriptions of fatigue included physical and mental indicators. Parents observed that children had no desire to participate in usual activities or even special activities. One parent stated, "The week following [chemotherapy] she would be a couch potato. She didn't want to move." Parents observed mood changes, with children becoming more easily frustrated, angered, or worrying more. A mother stated, "Mine is more prone to break into tears as well when he's really tired and he gets very irritable and you can hurt his feelings very easily."

Parents described feeling weak as a manifestation of fatigue, with children needing frequent rest periods when walking. One parent discussed a recent trip to Disney World: "He must have walked about five feet and had to sit down on the grass and rest." Children were also less communicative when really tired, often refused to make eye contact, and often denied anything was wrong. One parent said in describing this, "It's like a curtain comes across."

Parents described numerous causes of fatigue in the children. These causes included treatment-related symptoms such as low blood cell counts, infection, and pain. Parents observed children being tired when blood cell counts were low. One mother stated, "They get anemic too, so when his red blood cells are really low, he's of course, especially tired."

An interesting observation by parents was labeled "interaction fatigue." Parents observed that children became fatigued by having to communicate with so many people in the hospital. One parent described it as, "At the end of the day, he is tired, and is tired of being talked to." Parents, like children and adolescents, described hospital disturbances as a cause of fatigue. These disturbances included noises in the hospital, interruptions during the night, and constant interactions with staff during the day. One mother described lack of a night's rest: "He didn't sleep real well because they were in and out very, very frequently."

Parents used several descriptions to reflect children's sleep and rest patterns. Children were most tired in the morning upon awakening, or in the afternoon, especially following school. Most children took naps during the day and parents perceived the rest periods as helpful. Older children stayed up later at night and slept in the next day. This "summer schedule" was enhanced for children receiving home school because teachers often came to their home in the afternoon. Most parents felt children developed a new sleeping routine during treatment, and often slept in a different location at night, most often the parents' bed.

Parents discussed their children reacting to parents' attitudes. Children tended to cue into their parents' state of mind and observe their parents' attitudes. If the parent was upset or tired, the child was aware of the parent's mood and also became upset or tired. One parent stated, "If you are easily upset and stressed out all the time, that child is going to be upset and stressed out right along with you." Another parent stated, "If you stay calm, they stay calm." Parents realized that children are aware of their attitudes and thought they should try to remain positive. One parent explained, "Watching the stress level of the parents go up and up and up, their energy level go down and down and down, and so if that child loves their parents at all, they're also feeling that. So, yeah, that's all got to contribute. It's got to be factored in."

Parents discussed that their child's inability to sleep throughout the night caused them to be tired as well. One parent stated, "Every 30 minutes, 'I got to go to the bathroom Mom.' Last night I was so tired that when she saw me breathe, she said, 'Mom, this is the last time, I'm not going to ask you again.'" Another parent said, "She'll just start screaming that something's wrong. She never gets any sleep, then I get mad, because I'm tired and I'm tired of getting up and running to her room."

> *Watching the stress level of the parents go up and up and up, their energy level go down and down and down, and so if that child loves their parents at all, they're also feeling that. So, yeah, that's all got to contribute. It's got to be factored in.*

Parents discussed numerous interventions that helped the children's fatigue. Allowing children to set their own pace was described as important. One mother said, "We just don't push him to do anything." Parents stressed the importance of allowing children to express their feelings. One mother expressed her concern for this by stating, "If you communicate with your child and let them communicate with you and it's okay that they express their feelings to you, whether or not they're mad, hurt, or whatever, maybe they need to talk, maybe they're worried, or they're struggling. . . . I think it helps a lot." Parents often altered discipline when children were fatigued. One mother said, "I'm not going to worry about it [behavior] because I know she normally wouldn't act like that." Adjustments to the child's changing sleep patterns and the psychological strain of dealing with the situation accounted for a difficult period for most parents. One parent stated, "It's the emotional and psychological end of it. That's where the real problem lies. I think it is a mental attitude that makes you physically tired, physically worn out."

Parents' discussion of fatigue in children with cancer reflected the significant impact this symptom has on the child and family. The lived experience of the parents' struggles captures the significance of this symptom in a child or adolescent with cancer.

Staff's Perceptions of Fatigue and Suggested Potential Interventions

Staff's sensitivity to the symptom of fatigue in children with cancer may promote more accurate staff assessments of the fatigue and more effective interventions. Our research has helped us to determine that staff's perspectives on children's fatigue differ from that of the child who is experiencing the fatigue. We hope to use these discovered differences plus the detailed descriptions from both staff and children to help correct perceptions that hinder staff efforts to decrease the intensity or even the duration of fatigue in these patients. To address this issue, we conducted focus groups with staff members from different disciplines who worked directly with children receiving treatment for cancer. Staff who participated included nurses, advanced practice nurses, nurse managers, nutritionists, chaplains, physicians, and social workers. Our findings clearly indicate that staff members believe that fatigue in children is multidimensional, has multiple causes, and is responsive to intervention. Staff viewed themselves as having definite roles in both causing and diminishing the intensity and duration of the child's fatigue (Hinds et al, 1999).

Staff identified three assumptions about fatigue in children being treated for cancer that prevented them from effectively diminishing the child's fatigue. First, staff do not expect children to be significantly affected by fatigue. This assumption diminishes the clinical and developmental significance of the fatigue. In turn, the low significance given fatigue in children reduces its priority for clinical intervention. The second limiting assumption is that fatigue is a natural outcome of having treatment for cancer. Staff are less inclined to attempt interventions to diminish fatigue when it is an expected occurrence. Third, staff assume that parents are a reliable source for estimating the presence and intensity of symptoms, including fatigue, experienced by their child. The difficulty with relying on the parents' perceptions of their child's subjective experience is that the parents may not recognize the symptom, or may not attribute change in their child's behavior to the symptom. The unfortunate outcome of these assumptions is that a treatable symptom (fatigue) which can seriously interfere with the ill child being able to accomplish developmental milestones is not addressed.

We have assumed in our research that fatigue in children occurs within the context of human and family development. This means that how fatigue is perceived by the individuals who surround the child during treatment will influence whether fatigue in the child is identified and assessed accurately. These perceptions will also determine whether or not attempts are made to diminish the child's fatigue. Staff are a part of the ill child's context. Therefore, the staff's perspective on fatigue needs to be considered when fatigue in these children is being assessed. In our research, staff readily acknowledged that fatigue is not included in their standard assessments of children during treatment. Staff indicated that fatigue is a low priority for them, as they believed it could be treated easily by asking the child to take a nap and that it did not last long and did not have long-lasting effects. Staff described being far more concerned about pain, nausea, and vomiting. Fatigue in a child is not as visible as these other subjective experiences. Perhaps because of this less visible presence, fatigue does not typically evoke uneasiness or urgency in staff. It is these kinds of reactions that prompt assessments and interventions by staff. The result of fatigue being a quiet symptom is that it is likely to be underestimated in occurrence, intensity, and impact on the developing child.

Because of the unknown qualities of fatigue in children, we began our research with staff by asking them to recall clinical examples. Using the concept analysis techniques of Wilson (Avant, 1993; Avant & Abbott, 1993), we used staff reports to develop a definition of fatigue in 7- to 12-year-old children with cancer: "Fatigue is a state of diminished to complete loss of energy and/or will." The outcome for the child experiencing fatigue was an inability to participate in usual social, academic, physical, or even self-care activities at the child's typical intensity level or duration. The fatigue could be acute, episodic, or chronic but is almost always accompanied by emotional or mental withdrawal, a mood change that usually shows itself as increased irritability, decreased cooperation, occasional spiritual distress, and a common desire to rest or lie down. Staff also reported observing patterns that included differences in the child's fatigue by time of day, by course of treatment, or by diagnosis.

Staff also identified in the environmental category the causative factor of cognitive demands. They defined this as the child being surrounded by noise, diverse personalities, and multiple–at times simultaneous–interactions with others, all of which contribute to mental fatigue.

In our research, we also asked staff to identify causes of fatigue and were impressed by the number of causes (15) they identified. Equally impressive were the 22 helpful or alleviating factors (those believed to diminish the child's fatigue) identified by staff. We grouped the causes and alleviating factors by similarity into the following categories: environmental, personal, cultural, and treatment-related (see Table 4-1 for definitions of the categories and for examples of the factors).

In the first category of causative and alleviating factors, environmental, staff identified four negative influences that contributed to fatigue. One factor was waiting. Staff described children as sitting while waiting to be seen for their appointments in the outpatient care center, or lying down in their inpatient beds while waiting to be examined. Staff perceived that sitting or resting rather than moving their bodies caused the children to become more weary. A second factor, according to staff, was that children did not have a schedule or routine. Lacking a schedule, in the staff's mind, led to the child being in limbo, without a plan, and more tired. Staff also identified in the environmental category the causative factor of cognitive demands. They defined this as the child being surrounded by noise, diverse personalities, and multiple–at times simultaneous–interactions with others, all of which contribute to mental fatigue. Staff from both the outpatient and inpatient care settings also identified the repeated interruptions that occur in a hospital environment as contributing to a child's sense of fatigue. Such interruptions occur throughout day and night and disrupt the child's usual sleep and eating patterns.

Table 4.1	Factors Perceived by Staff as Causing or Alleviating Fatigue in 7- to 12-Year-Olds Receiving Treatment for Cancer

Causing Fatigue	Alleviating Fatigue

Category: Environmental

Factors include the child reacting to a return or a continuing stay in the treatment setting, experiencing long waits involving prone positions or activities without physical movements, altered schedules or routines that do not reflect a defined beginning and ending of each day, and multiple situations of high cognitive demand such as information exchange and decision making.

Staff-initiated efforts include protecting rest or sleep periods of the child by organizing care into concentrated blocks rather than as continuous and intermittent care efforts, implementing a schedule that reflects a defined waking time and bedtime, abbreviating a clinic visit to allow the child to leave as quickly as possible, and minimizing noise levels and other forms of stimulation around the child.

Category: Personal and behavioral

Factors include the experience of altered or interrupted sleep patterns (i.e., changing sleep locations, hours of sleep, depth of sleep), the patient's age, and lack of sufficient cognitive stimulation, leading to boredom, the child's negative belief about being able to function in usual ways, or negative thoughts.

Staff-initiated efforts include emphasizing what the child is capable of doing rather than what the child cannot do, providing additional support for the child and encouraging expression of any concerns or fears, attempting to persuade the child to try to participate, allowing choices, being firm (at times) to involve the child in self-care activities, discovering ways to work with each child (such as slowly wakening the child), and encouraging the child to participate in exercise and other distracting activities as tolerated.

Category: Cultural, family, or other

Factors include the child's being adversely affected by the emotions, moods, concerns, and expectations of others, such as relatives or friends, and being urged by others to engage too vigorously in activities or to unnecessarily avoid participation in activities.

Alleviating factors observed by staff but initiated by families or friends include rearranging family schedules to do activities at times when the child is likely to have more energy or to include more quiet activities and rest periods. Staff-initiated efforts with family members include encouraging them to examine their expectations of the child (whether too demanding or too minimal) and to not unnecessarily limit the child's activities or efforts so as to avoid dependency, and teaching parents relaxation strategies and emphasizing the importance of maintaining their own health.

Category: Treatment related

Factors include the child's experiencing invasive examinations or procedures, repeated courses of treatment without sufficient days between to recover strength, inadequate nutrition or metabolic changes, adverse effects of therapy (such as inadequately functioning bone marrow), and diagnosis-related factors, such as stage of treatment.

Staff-initiated efforts include careful monitoring of the child's nutritional and hematological status; administering ordered blood products; and evaluating nutritional, hematological, and pharmacological interventions to make certain that they effectively meet the child's needs.

The alleviating factors in the category of environment included protected rest time. Staff described how they attempted to control the number of times they entered the child's clinic or inpatient room, particularly trying to honor the times identified by family members as the usual rest times for the child. Staff added that when it was necessary to interrupt, they attempted to make the interruptions both brief and quiet. Staff also indicated they purposely planned to minimize the time required for an outpatient stay such that the child could be seen quickly and exit quickly. Staff described attempting to interact with a fatigued child in a subdued manner, hoping that their quiet demeanor helped to decrease the amount of stimuli impacting the child.

The second category of causative and alleviating factors is labeled "personal and behavioral." The first factor in this category named by staff is changes in the child's sleep habits. Boredom is a second causative factor, and the third factor is the child believing that he or she could not tolerate participating in a certain social or academic activity. The fourth factor is depression.

These included emotional support and empathy from others, providing encouragement, presenting a positive attitude, allowing choices, staff firmness, allowing the child to awaken slowly, providing opportunities for the child to exercise, and providing something new in the child's environment.

The staff identified twice as many alleviating factors in the category of personal and behavioral factors than causative factors. These included emotional support and empathy from others, providing encouragement, presenting a positive attitude, allowing choices, staff firmness, allowing the child to awaken slowly, providing opportunities for the child to exercise, and providing something new in the child's environment such as unfamiliar activities that are helpful distractions. In addition, staff recommended offering positive instructions and completing assessments that distinguished the type of fatigue the child was experiencing (physical, mental, or a combination of the two).

The third category of causative factors as perceived by the staff was "cultural, family, or other." The staff identified only two factors within this category: when the child is pushed too hard to participate in activities or interactions, and inaccurate cues given to the child from others such as "you should not be tired," or "you shouldn't be involved in certain activities because you are too tired to handle them."

However, in the same category, the staff identified more than twice the number of alleviating than causative factors. These included helping the parent to relax and not be as intense, maximizing the child's energy, changing expectations of the child by making them more flexible, controlling for overprotectiveness, allowing the child to at least attempt involvement, and modifying activities to match the child's energy levels.

In the final category of both treatment-related causative and alleviating factors, the following causative factors were identified: (1) inadequate recovery time between courses of treatment, (2) adverse effects of treatment, and (3) the disease. Diagnostic procedures in particular were identified as contributing to a child's fatigue, as was inadequate nutrition.

Staff believed that they decreased the child's fatigue by carefully figuring out the best dosages of certain medications, providing nutritional supplements, and carefully administering ordered blood products.

In summary, staff acknowledged not anticipating fatigue as significantly and adversely affecting pediatric oncology patients. They admitted they did not routinely assess for the presence or intensity of fatigue in these patients. However, they indicated they were receptive to new information about fatigue in 7- to 12-year-old children receiving treatment for cancer. Staff view themselves as contributing to the children's fatigue and as responsible for helping to alleviate the fatigue. Almost half of all alleviating factors identified by staff could be staff initiated.

Interventions by Health Care Providers

Fatigue in children and adolescents with cancer is a symptom that often remains forgotten in the midst of other more obvious side effects of treatment. The work discussed in this chapter is the first to provide insight into the occurrence of fatigue in children and adolescents with cancer. Children as young as 7 years are aware of physical and emotional indicators of fatigue. This finding supports the importance of careful assessments that include questions reflecting the descriptions of fatigue by the participants in this study. Changes in activity and in participation in sports and play are common occurrences in the younger children experiencing fatigue. Mental descriptions such as feeling sad or mad may be reflective of fatigue and should be evaluated in children and adolescents. Mental symptoms such as altered mood, decreased communication with others, and not wanting to be bothered may be mistaken for depression instead of fatigue. Astute observation of the child or adolescent may assist the care provider in differentiating between symptoms of fatigue and those of depression.

Several causes of fatigue described by children and adolescents in this study are found in the adult literature. These causes included treatment such as chemotherapy, radiation therapy, and surgery. Side effects of treatment such as low blood cell counts and fever were also associated with fatigue. These contributing factors, while obvious causes of fatigue, are often not considered when providing education to the pediatric patient and family regarding what to expect following treatment. It is important for health care professionals to discuss fatigue as a symptom following treatment and to develop an awareness of interventions that will decrease fatigue while in the hospital and at home. Accurate assessment of other contributing factors that are associated with fatigue will allow for education of the patient and family related to expectations regarding other lifestyle changes. Sleep disturbances brought on by altered schedules, staying up late at night, and not sleeping in one's own bed may need to be discussed with the child or adolescent and parents.

Realization that the hospital environment is a major contributor to the occurrence of fatigue in children and teens is important. Knowledge of the impact a noisy hospital unit has on the sleep patterns of patients provides insight into changes that may need to occur

| Table 4.2 | Summary Comparison of Child, Teen, and Parent Descriptors About Fatigue or Definitions of Fatigue | | |

Descriptor/Source of Fatigue	Children	Teens	Parents
Variety of words	Fewer	Greater	
Vocabulary in describing physical and mental experiences	More limited	Larger vocabulary, finer differentiation	
Causes and factors relating to fatigue	Fewer	More factors Greater detail	
Worry and concern as basis for fatigue		Greater	
Physical and mental symptoms	Described symptoms	Greater differentiation reported	
Physical and mental causation	Unable to identify	More reported	
Number of coping/adaptive interventions used		Greater number reported	
Effect of laboratory values (abnormal)	Reported	Reported	Reported
Change in activities	Reported	Reported	Reported
Environmental disturbances	Reported	Reported	Reported
Mood changes			Reported
Disruption in sleep and rest patterns	Reported	Reported	Reported
Change in sensitivity to parents' emotional state			Reported
Protective emotional/communicative withdrawal (interactive fatigue)			Reported
Reactionary fatigue in parents			Reported
Change in behavioral/ disciplinary patterns			Reported

in hospital settings. Awareness that fatigue during hospitalization occurs because of disruptions in sleep due to noises, frequent interruptions, and even the location of the room can stimulate thoughts and ideas on how to make the hospital setting more conducive to rest and sleep. Grouping necessary nursing activities together so as to disturb the child or adolescent less frequently is an important consideration. Providing protected rest periods during the day and at night was helpful for the children and adolescents in this study. Increased awareness that the nurses' station should have quiet hours at night may also impact patients' ability to sleep at night.

Boredom brought on by having nothing to do created fatigue for participants in this study. Children and teens described participating in fun activities as helping their fatigue. Hospital activities may be used as an intervention to prevent fatigue in the future. Teens discussed worry or fear as sometimes causing fatigue, providing insight into the importance of nurses spending time with them and listening to their concerns.

Where Do We Go From Here?

Conceptualizing fatigue as a physical, mental, emotional, and spiritual experience in children and adolescents that is perceived differently by them, their parents, and their health care professionals (and in turn, is affected by those different perceptions) allows us to develop new approaches to identifying and reducing this fatigue (Table 4-2). An intervention will be most effective when directed at all three groups (patients, parents, and health care professionals). Different combinations of caregivers (patient, parent, and health care provider) and dimensions of fatigue (physical, mental, emotional, and spiritual) will further direct development of interventions. Future directions that will help to make this quiet yet powerful symptom more recognized and thus susceptible to intervention include the following:

1. Incorporate fatigue in routine assessments of children and adolescents who are being treated for cancer or being followed after completing treatment. The assessment will be most complete if it seeks details about both physical and mental fatigue.
2. Teach patients, parents, and health care professionals about the symptoms and impact of fatigue and the treatable nature of fatigue.
3. Intervene simultaneously with patients and parents using humor, distraction, nutrition, self-monitoring of hematological and immunological systems, and reviewing family schedules for ways to better match the patient's energy levels.
4. Intervene with health care professionals regarding ways to pace care with patients' energy levels, including grouping care activities to lessen the number of times needing to approach or involve patients in such activities, and ways to diminish environmental stimuli including one's own voice level.
5. Study the effectiveness of interventions by age of patient to determine type and intensity of intervention needed.

References

Avant, K. (1993). The Wilson method of concept analysis. In B. Rogers and K. Knafl (Eds.), *Concept development in nursing: Foundations, techniques, and applications* (pp. 51–60). Philadelphia: W.B. Saunders.

Avant, K., and Abott, C. (1993). Wilsonian concept analysis: Applying the technique. In B. Rogers and K. Knafl (Eds.), *Concept development in nursing: Foundation, techniques, and applications* (p. 61–72). Philadelphia: W.B. Saunders.

Bottomley, S., Teegarden, C., and Hockenberry-Eaton, M. (1996). Fatigue in children with cancer: Clinical considerations for nursing. *Journal of Pediatric Oncology Nursing, 13*(3), 178.

Carter, B. D., Edwards, J. F., Kronenberger, W. G., Michalczyk, L., and Marshall, G. S. (1995). Case control study of chronic fatigue in pediatric patients. *Pediatrics, 95,* 179–186.

Carter, B. D., Kronenberger, W. G., Edwards, J. F., Michalczyk, L., and Marshall, G. S. (1996). Differential diagnosis of chronic fatigue in children: Behavioral and emotional dimensions. *Developments in Behavioral Pediatrics, 17,* 16–21.

Hinds, P. S., Hockenberry-Eaton, M., Quargnenti, A., Martha, M., Burleson, C., Gilger, E., Randall, E., and O'Neill, J. B. (1999). Fatigue in 7 to 12 year old pediatric oncology patients from the staff perspective. *Oncology Nursing Forum, 26*(1), 37–45.

Hockenberry-Eaton, M., Hinds, P. S., O'Neill, J. B., Howard, V., Gattuso, J., and Taylor, J. (1998). Fatigue in children and adolescents with cancer. *Journal of Pediatric Oncology Nursing, 15*(3), 172–182.

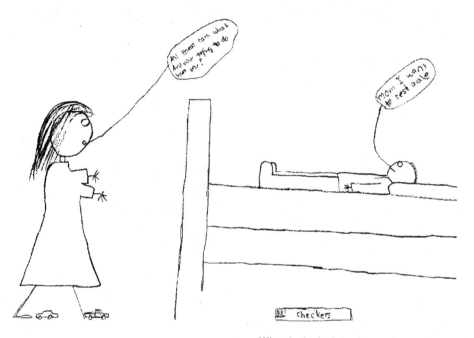

When he is tired, he does not want to play.
Drawing by Keith Grace, 11 years old, diagnosed with T-cell lymphoma.

A Behavioral
Medicine Perspective

Marjorie H. Royle

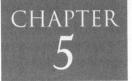

I think it is a very common error among the well to think that "with a little more self-control" the sick might, if they choose, "dismiss painful thoughts" which "aggravate their disease," etc. Believe me, almost any sick person, who behaves decently well, exercises more self-control every moment of his day than you will ever know till you are sick yourself. Almost every step that crosses his room is painful to him; almost every thought that crosses his brain is painful to him; and if he can speak without being savage, and look without being unpleasant, he is exercising self-control.

Florence Nightingale, *Notes on Nursing*

Background

The emerging field of behavioral or "mind-body" medicine provides some important insights and tools for enlisting the whole person, mind and emotions as well as body, in the healing process (Seago and Conn, 1996). This chapter examines fatigue from the point of view of a behavioral scientist. Chapter 7 examines many of the same phenomena from the perspective of a biochemist or a physiologist.

Behavioral medicine considers the patient as "actor," rather than "acted upon." It addresses the interactive effect of lifestyle, beliefs about health and illness, mental states, and stress and coping strategies on medical outcomes. It also considers the effects of the health care system itself, including patient-provider communication, outreach efforts, and the way health care is organized. It enlists the patient as participant through interventions such as relaxation and stress reduction, cognitive-behavioral therapy, and support programs. Such interventions impact both quality of life and medical outcomes such as longevity (Fawzy et al, 1995; Taylor and Aspinwall, 1990), and would be expected to affect fatigue as well.

According to cancer survivors, fatigue is one of the most common and debilitating aspects of cancer and its treatment (Irvine et al, 1991; Love et al, 1989; Vogelzang et al, 1997). For example, Vogelzang and colleagues found 61% of patients saying that fatigue had a greater effect on their daily lives than pain, while 31% said that pain had a greater effect. Oncologists, however, had opposite opinions, with 61% saying that pain had a greater effect. In spite of its importance to cancer survivors, fatigue has not been a major focus of study in behavioral oncology and has been the object of study in relatively few research studies. Some studies have examined fatigue as one among many symptoms, while others have examined fatigue with respect to quality of life or limitations in daily activities, both of which may be related to fatigue. In addition, much can be said by extrapolation from other areas of research that are similar to the experience of cancer.

One problem with studying fatigue is in defining it because it is, in essence, a subjective experience. Even the word *fatigue* is not usually used by cancer survivors. They are more likely to describe the phenomenon in terms of what they cannot do, what they used to do, being exhausted, or having no energy. To complicate the issue, fatigue and depression are closely linked and share many of the same characteristics. Depression is a common reaction to chronic or life-threatening illness, with fatigue often seen as a symptom or characteristic of depression. Conversely, fatigue may cause depression or exacerbate it when it forces survivors to limit many of life's important activities, a limitation that they fear may be permanent. Also, survivors may be both fatigued and depressed, each making the other worse (Moyer and Salovey, 1996; Winningham et al, 1994).

Many patients, particularly the less educated, may not be able to articulate the distinction that textbooks do between the phenomena of fatigue and depression. The same subjective state, described as "I'm always tired, I never have any energy," could be labeled as either fatigue or depression: The treatment team should consider the possibility that either or both may be present.

Meta-analyses, statistical methods that combine data from many studies, have demonstrated that depression is associated with increased risk of physical illness. This is particularly true of diseases of the immune system such as cancer and infection with the human immunodeficiency virus (HIV); indeed, depression has specifically been associated with decreased functional measures of immunity such as T-cell counts and natural killer cell activity (Herbert and Cohen, 1993). Treatment of depression has also been linked with better compliance with medical treatment (Halkitis, 1998). Therefore, survivors who report finding treatment increasingly burdensome should be evaluated as possibly suffering from depression. In addition, survivors who report fatigue should be evaluated and treated for depression where it is appropriate. Treating depression may help patients feel less fatigued, as well.

The Significance of Fatigue

Two major areas of behavioral medicine research literature are helpful in understanding the importance of fatigue in illness.

About the Contributor

Dr. Marjorie Royle describes herself as having had a "checkered career." After working as a civilian personnel research psychologist with the U.S. Navy for 17 years, she managed the research office of a large Protestant denomination. Afterward, she worked in a medical center setting on issues of compliance in mental health patients. She is currently involved in research for the state of New Jersey. She admits that

1. *Fatigue and quality of life.* As health care research is expanding from measuring mortality and morbidity due to a specific illness to a more general concern for the whole person, concerns for quality of life are becoming increasingly important. Researchers have developed many scales to measure the impact of the illness and the degree to which the survivor has returned to pre-illness levels. These include such areas of functioning as physical abilities (particularly with respect to the strength and endurance to pursue everyday activities); psychological, emotional, or sense of well-being; social and role alterations or strain; and spiritual well-being. Two approaches have been taken (Guyatt, Feeny, and Patrick, 1993). The first is demonstrated in the Medical Outcomes Study Short-Form Health Survey (SF-36) (Ware, Kosinski, and Keller, 1994), a brief instrument useful for patients with diverse diseases. A second approach measures the impact of specific diseases, usually with longer surveys containing more detailed questions about specific disease- or treatment-related problems. Cancer-related examples include the Quality of Life–Bone Marrow Transplant (QOL-BMT) scale (Grant et al, 1992); the various Functional Assessment of Cancer Therapy (FACT) instruments developed by Cella and colleagues; and specific to anemia-related fatigue, the Functional Assessment of Cancer Therapy–Anemia (FACT-An) scale (Cella, 1997).

> *For many survivors, the fatigue associated with cancer treatment causes significant disruptions in functional performance and has a negative impact on quality of life.*

For many survivors, the fatigue associated with cancer treatment causes significant disruptions in functional performance (Irvine et al, 1994) and has a negative impact on quality of life (Eller, 1995).

Even when specific research has not yet been done in cancer survivors, we can learn from studies on individuals suffering from other, similar diseases with long-term debilitating consequences. For instance, Karazc, Bochnak, and Ouellette (1994) found that role strain, the inability to perform social roles, moderated the relationship between disease activity and psychological well-being among women with lupus. That is, their sense of well-being was only affected by the disease progression if they perceived role strain to have occurred (i.e., they had difficulty doing the things they thought they should be doing). This suggests an interesting proposition with respect to cancer survivors: Fatigue may be significant, or most

---

her passion is for applied research, that is, "research that is practical in developing information for professionals to use in real-life settings." Her involvement in cancer became both personal and professional when her mother developed breast cancer. Because she herself has had endometrial cancer, she shows the insight unique to professionals who are also survivors.

significant in terms of well-being or quality of life, if it contributes to increased role strain. This critical issue should be studied in cancer survivors.

Kaplan and colleagues developed the General Health Policy Model, which provides a helpful way to measure disability. They categorized disability as temporary or permanent, and on a continuum expressed as a decrement from living at optimum functioning due to health-related limitations (Kaplan, 1991). This model is useful because it recognizes the significance of measuring the impact of subjective side effects like fatigue as well as traditional medical indicators in affecting medical decisions and outcomes. As people consider treatment options, they appear to utilize an internal self-made model that takes into account decrement in quality of life, duration of the decrement, and its meaning in term of their own values. Quality of life instruments may help people make these treatment decisions in a more informed and intentional manner.

It is important to note that while the concept "quality of life" is currently in vogue, much of the quality of life research is not novel. Related concepts have been studied for many years under various terms and in conjunction with such problems as disability, functioning, health outcomes, medical outcomes, well-being, and other concepts in medical sociology. The philosophical and theoretical roots of quality of life go back to early in this century and warrant in-depth study, particularly by graduate students and developing scholars.

It is important to note that while the concept "quality of life" is currently in vogue, much of the quality of life research is not novel. Related concepts have been studied for many years under various terms and in conjunction with such problems as disability, functioning, health outcomes, medical outcomes, well-being, and other concepts in medical sociology. Researchers would do well to review work done over the past two or three decades under related terms to keep from wasting time and resources in understanding aspects of how fatigue relates to life. In addition, they would profit from studying the historical development of different constructs that relate to quality of life. Quality of life is not a new concept: The philosophical and theoretical roots of quality of life go back to early in this century and warrant in-depth study, particularly by graduate students and developing scholars.

2. *Fatigue and adherence to treatment.* Fatigue is also important because it can affect adherence to treatment. The literature on compliance, or adherence to medical treatment and advice, found that factors important in adherence have much more to do with the medical system itself, the patient's experience of it, his or her perception of the disease, and the extent and nature of the social support the patient receives from family and friends than with personality or demographic characteristics (Carroll, 1992, p. 80). Kaplan (1991, p. 79) also said that patients "comply with treatment when they perceive a net benefit in terms of a general health outcome, and they fail to comply when the consequences of compliance appear to outweigh the expected benefits." In other words, they comply when they think it is worth it. When treatment increases fatigue, it may tip the balance in

favor of noncompliance. Not surprisingly, fatigue has been related to discontinuance of chemotherapy (Winningham et al, 1994).

Fatigue may affect adherence in another way as well. Adherence is higher when patients understand the need for treatment and believe it is beneficial. When treatment-related fatigue makes the cancer survivors feel weaker each day, the belief that the treatment is efficacious is difficult to maintain. Increased attentional fatigue, that is, the loss of ability to focus one's mind and concentrate (Cimprich, 1993), may also interfere with survivors' developing and maintaining understanding of and belief in the importance of treatment. Long-term fatigue interferes with the classic "institutionalized expectation system relative to the sick role" (Parsons, 1964, pp. 436–443, 445–447). At present, fatigue has neither objective markers to legitimize it, nor any magic means by which it is acknowledged, let alone medically treated or cured. Hence, fatigue may be difficult to understand or justify, and may be interpreted by the survivor, as well as others, as malingering or laziness for secondary gain. The emotional conflicts that result from trying to compromise between fatigue-imposed needs for lifestyle changes and the desire to appear normal can contribute to exhaustion and despair.

Prevention and Treatment

The behavioral health literature also provides important clues that may help mitigate fatigue. In addition, some interventions that may help fatigue may have other benefits as well, such as improved survival, immune function, and psychiatric symptomatology, including depression (Ironson, Antoni, and Lutgendorf, 1995; Meyer and Mark, 1995). These interventions also have some advantages over treatment using medications for cancer and HIV-infected patients, particularly reducing the burden of additional drugs. This is especially important because additional drugs often interact with the ones patients are already taking, which risks worsening problems of fatigue, lethargy, and interference with daily routines (Sikkema and Kelly, 1996).

Seven types of interventions have been identified—education, cognitive-behavioral therapy, coping skills training, individual psychotherapy, relaxation and imagery, social support, and exercise. Programs employing group processes may serve in multiple ways by combining education, cognitive-behavioral therapy, help with coping skills, and social support. Flint (1995) examined characteristics of women who attended support groups versus those who did not. She discovered that the coping styles of attenders was different from that of nonattenders. Attenders appeared to grieve losses associated with breast cancer, were more inclined to search for meaning in their experience, and actively worked to regain control over their lives. Of particular interest was her note that "cancer occurs within the context of living," something rarely addressed in the literature and in clinical settings. Clinicians and researchers often have no idea what patients have to deal with on an everyday level. Hence, several of the interventions, artificially provided by health care professionals, may spontaneously occur in a support group setting as individuals share how they adapt to their disease and treatment; explore expectations and outcomes, change in social roles, and their sense of self; and acquire information from one another.

Education

Educational or informational programs on what to expect or what others have experienced comprise one frequently used behavioral health intervention that can decrease disruption in activities and anxiety and increase quality of life for cancer survivors (Jacobs, et al, 1983; Johnson et al, 1988, Rainey, 1985). Although fatigue was not directly measured in the studies, it can be hypothesized that survivors may have experienced less disruption in activity due to decreased fatigue. These educational interventions typically provide information on what to expect from the treatments, how they work, what side effects may occur, and what measures may be taken to counter the side effects. Various modes of delivery have been used, including one-on-one or group presentation, audiotapes, and videotapes.

Johnson and colleagues (1988, p. 51) suggested that informational intervention is effective because it "supports an unambiguous cognitive representation of the experience, increases the predictability of the experience and focuses attention on the concrete objective aspects . . . [freeing people] to focus their efforts on solving problems" and increasing their confidence in their ability to cope. Specific information about how much fatigue to expect and when to expect it in the course of treatment allows the patient to plan accordingly. In other words, people like to know what is going on and what is reasonable.

Health care providers often hesitate to provide information on possible side effects, such as fatigue, for fear of increasing the likelihood that patients will develop them (power of suggestion). For fatigue, which is experienced by most people, this fear seems unnecessary. Research suggests, instead, that people are fearful of unexpected side effects and angry and disappointed with physicians who do not inform or warn them in advance (Vogelzang et al, 1997; Wortman and Dunkel-Schetter, 1979).

Because survivors undergoing cancer treatment also have heightened sensitivity to bodily changes, including fatigue, information that defines fatigue as normal and transitory and not as a character flaw or a sign of impending death may reduce anxiety. Information acknowledging that some people, especially older ones, may never return to their precancer levels of energy may also help them not interpret continued fatigue as a sign of recurring cancer.

Research suggests that survivors currently are not being informed adequately about fatigue, at least not in a way that they can hear or understand. Love and colleagues (1989) found that while only 8% of people undergoing therapy expected tiredness, 86% experienced it. They cited several barriers to complete communication, including resistance "due either to wishful thinking or the massive amount of other information that was also provided during [a] clinic visit" (p. 610). Additional barriers included still being in shock over the diagnosis or the severity of their illness, unwillingness to trust the source, and fatigue itself, especially attentional fatigue.

Communications research suggests the importance of the source of the information on fatigue being credible. For example, people may find it more beneficial to talk with another experienced survivor rather than a young and terminally cheerful health care provider. Excessive cheeriness in health care staff is often perceived as irritating and exhausting, rather than positive and encouraging. Use of several modalities, oral and written, repetition, and provision of materials that people can take home to review when they are less fatigued or emotionally stressed may also improve communication of information.

Education of families and caregivers about fatigue and other likely side effects of treatment is important as well (Jensen and Given, 1991). This allows them to assist the survivor with daily activities, to help set limits on exertion, and also to not panic when fatigue and other symptoms occur. Education of families may remove the burden from the survivor of putting up a good front, which may be another cause of fatigue. It may also help them cope better with their own fatigue.

Education of employers may help them understand what to expect from returning workers or those going through treatment. This might, in turn, remove some barriers to continued employment and help employers plan work schedules.

Patients comply with treatment when they perceive a net benefit; they fail to comply when the consequences of compliance appear to outweigh the expected benefits. In other words, they comply when they think it is worth it.

Cognitive–Behavioral Therapy

Cognitive-behavioral interventions have become important tools in addressing many health problems. These therapeutic sessions, often held in groups, use techniques of reframing, developing specific strategies for problem situations such as behavioral modifications that address specific problems, for example, nausea or eating disorders. Several studies and meta-analyses have documented their effectiveness in contributing to both psychological and physical positive health outcomes, often with greater effectiveness than interventions such as informational or support groups or traditional psychotherapy (Fawzy et al, 1995; Meyer and Mark, 1995). Sikkema and Kelly (1996) applied these techniques to address pain management, nutrition, and sleep disorders in people infected with HIV and provided many suggestions for further study and clinical practice in these areas. In a meta-analysis, Morin, Culbert, and Schwartz (1994) found that behavioral interventions improved sleep disorders by 50% to 60%. Although those with sleep disorders were not cancer survivors, such interventions show promise in addressing the part of fatigue due to sleep problems. Similarly, behavioral interventions for eating problems may address the nutritional component of fatigue.

In addition to these indirect effects, some studies suggested that cognitive-behavioral techniques can increase vigor and decrease fatigue (Bottomley et al, 1996). Specific fatigue-related interventions such as helping cancer survivors be aware of when they are likely to be most fatigued, and plan their daily activities accordingly, may be helpful (O'Brien and Pheifer, 1993). Interventions are needed to help give people the permission and tools to ask for help. For example, because fatigue is likely to increase as the treatment week progresses, one assignment might be to plan for meals later in the week by asking a friend who has offered to help to bring dinner. Because a cancer diagnosis can interfere with getting support (Moyer and Salovey, 1996; Taylor and Aspinwall, 1990; Wortman and Dunkel-Schetter, 1979), patients may need to be encouraged to ask for the help they need. Having a confirmation of the reality of fatigue may assist them in asking for help. Indeed, some patients are relieved by a diagnosis of cancer because their ongoing fatigue had been minimized as "in your head" or "laziness."

Finally, interventions to help survivors cope with problems caused by fatigue of directed attention may be useful. These might include prioritizing, narrowing focus, and putting issues in a "parking lot" to be picked up at a later time when fatigue has lessened. Cimprich (1993) found a different approach to be effective in restoring patients who had suffered from attentional fatigue. She found that breast cancer survivors who contracted to spend 20 to 30 minutes three times weekly in a restorative activity involving the natural environment such as watching nature or gardening, or pursuing arts and crafts or other hobbies, had a significant improvement in attentional capacity.

Coping Skills Training

Coping styles can affect the immune system and such medical outcomes as longevity with cancer, HIV infection, and other diseases (Fawzy et al, 1993; Greer et al, 1990; Stone and Porter, 1995). Positive coping, including positive reframing and the use of humor, was related to less emotional distress in breast cancer survivors (Carver, Scheier, and Pozo, 1992) and to decreases in depressive symptoms in people with acquired immunodeficiency syndrome (AIDS) (Fleishman and Fogel, 1994). Acceptance of the reality of the diagnosis was also strongly correlated with less emotional disturbance in breast cancer survivors (Carver, Scheier, and Pozo, 1992), possibly because acceptance releases emotional energy for moving forward in a positive way. This is discussed in more detail in Chapter 21.

If positive coping releases emotional energy, it may be associated with less fatigue. In one study of melanoma survivors, a program that provided specific training in coping skills as well as other behavioral health techniques resulted in the participants not only employing more active coping methods but also reporting less fatigue and more vigor. Less depression and improved general mood disturbance were also reported (Fawzy et al, 1990).

Individual Psychotherapy

Individual psychotherapy appears to be helpful in reducing negative emotional states that may be related to cancer (Fawzy et al, 1995; Meyer and Mark, 1995). Trijsburg, van Knippenberg, and Rijpma (1992) reported on three studies in which individual counseling tailored to the needs of the participants decreased fatigue during radiation therapy. In addition, Pennebaker (1992) found in a series of studies that writing or talking about stressful events or traumas improved active coping and self-esteem as well as health and immune function. He theorized that disclosure released the energy that had been used in inhibiting thoughts and feelings about the traumas. If this theory is correct, individual therapy may decrease fatigue by helping people release the energy used in coping both with the trauma of cancer or other medical diagnosis and with other traumas from their past.

It should be emphasized that this therapy should be undertaken by trained professionals only. Some individuals have had abusive backgrounds or prior violent experiences that require special treatment, especially since the experience of cancer and the associated treatment may open up old wounds and memories. Cancer sometimes is perceived as a retraumatization, whether consciously or unconsciously. That is, the effects of past trauma or powerfully hurtful events in their lives exacerbate the current response to cancer. Individual therapy may help patients deal with the past trauma and diminish the multiplicative effect. Regardless, the basis for the effectiveness of psychotherapy may be to increase the effectiveness of coping mechanisms.

> *Acceptance of the reality of the diagnosis was also strongly correlated with less emotional disturbance in breast cancer survivors, possibly because acceptance releases emotional energy for moving forward in a positive way.*

Relaxation and Imagery

Relaxation training can decrease anxiety and nausea from chemotherapy and pain in cancer survivors and may decrease depression and fatigue as well (Arathuzik, 1995; Carey and Burish, 1988; Taylor and Aspinwall, 1990; Wallace, 1997). Stress-management training was effective in reducing fatigue, at least when coupled with a mild physical therapy exercise program (Quested et al, 1982). Positive effects of both progressive relaxation training (PRT) and guided imagery on fatigue have been found in people with HIV infection. One study that randomly assigned subjects to either guided imagery, PRT, or a control group and administered the treatments using one training session and audiotapes found a significant decrease in fatigue in the group using guided imagery. In addition, there was a significant increase in CD4 cell count (a measure of immune function) in the group using PRT, while both groups demonstrated decreased depression and increased quality of life (Eller, 1995). Because most studies used small samples and did not control for other concomitant factors, the effectiveness of such therapies might be considered promising rather than proved.

Some patients object to relaxation training, guided imagery, or meditation on religious grounds. It is helpful to restructure the practice of this experience for them in terms of their spiritual framework. For instance, meditation on psalms or religious themes or images may be acceptable for them and may even be experienced as a form of prayer.

Regardless of the framework in which this occurs, it is critical to remember that even these activities may be exhausting for individuals who may be terminally ill. Meditation, imagery, prayer, worship, and even the use of music require significant energy for concentration. Hospice nurses report that these activities further the exhaustive state of their patients. Hence, careful assessment of the status and capabilities of the individual is necessary, and interventions should not be forced.

Social Support

Extensive literature has linked social support with decreased morbidity and mortality, as well as with improved immune function (Reifman, 1995; Uchino, Cacioppo, and Kiecolt-Glaser, 1996); support groups are one way to increase social support. Spiegel (1994) found decreased fatigue and other positive outcomes among metastatic breast cancer survivors who had one year of weekly support groups. Different types of support–informational, emotional, and tangible–are perceived as differentially helpful, depending on the type or stage of illness or their source (Martin et al, 1994). Tangible support might be expected to be most helpful in alleviating fatigue; however, when that support increases the burden, such as when an offer to clean house requires some "tidying up" before the offer can be accepted, it can make things worse!

Exercise

Nearly 50 years of research on bed rest clearly demonstrated the disastrous mental and physical health consequences of bed rest and inactivity. Despite this, cancer survivors are often told to get more rest. In a survey of cancer survivors who were athletes or identified themselves as physically active, exercise was a means by which they coped with the stress of cancer (Winningham and MacVicar, 1983). A follow-up study of breast cancer survivors undergoing chemotherapy indicated that participation in an individualized, supervised, prescriptive rehabilitative energy exercise program (PREEP) was beneficial in reducing feelings of fatigue (MacVicar and Winningham, 1986). This program used the Winningham Aerobic Intermittent Training (WAIT) protocol designed to gently stimulate all three metabolic energy systems without inducing physiological fatigue.

> *Tangible support might be expected to be most helpful in alleviating fatigue; however, when that support increases the burden, such as when an offer to clean house requires some work "tidying up" before the offer can be accepted, it can make things worse!*

Data are needed to investigate further how much rest is necessary versus how much activity is essential for optimal all-around functioning in people with cancer. Later work by MacVicar, Winningham, and Nickel (1989) demonstrated dramatic improvement in objective, physiological measures of functional capacity in response to the WAIT protocol. In addition to facilitating coping, exercise may be a means by which role strain is reduced because patients report more energy. Unpublished data from this study also demonstrate profound improvement in multiple measures relating to quality of life.

Powerful interventions also carry attendant risks. While exercise may be one of the most potent means of mitigating fatigue and achieving certain positive emotional as well as physiological gains, it also carries attendant risks. Recommendations and guidelines for safety in exercise for cancer survivors have been published and should be followed in any clinical intervention or research study using exercise (Winningham, 1991, 1994; Winningham, MacVicar, and Burke, 1986).

Where Do We Go From Here?

Getting people to engage in and stay in treatment has been a theme running through my research. Some of the questions I have examined include: How do you improve appointment keeping and prevent dropouts in mental health services? How can you engage the "hard to reach," whether they are the poor with few medical resources, the seriously and persistently mentally ill, or drug abusers with HIV infection?

In June 1994, I was diagnosed with endometrial cancer. In the process of my therapy I learned a lot about adherence to treatment regimens from the other side. I hated every day of my radiation treatment. No matter what I was told, the process felt like rape, an invasion of my body by a malevolent force. I seriously considered dropping out, and only completed the course of treatments under protest, acting as the bad patient as well as I knew how.

That experience taught me many things, two of which brought me to writing this chapter. First, the effect of medical treatment may be enhanced by enlisting the patient's mind in the process of healing. The turmoil in my mind over the illness and its treatment was more overwhelming than the trauma to my body. Behavioral medicine made sense, not just as an academic discipline, but also in my lived experience.

A follow-up study of breast cancer survivors undergoing chemotherapy indicated that participation in an individualized, supervised, prescriptive rehabilitative energy exercise program (PREEP) was beneficial in reducing feelings of fatigue.

Second, the fatigue accompanying my radiation was the worst part of the process, far worse than the surgery or my perceptions of the disease itself. The pats on the head that I received from medical care providers, however well intended, were irritating and did nothing to reduce the fatigue.

What can behaviorists do to help with fatigue? My behavioral medicine perspective as well as my personal experience suggests a need for change in four areas.

1. *Measuring fatigue.* Problems related to how to measure fatigue as well as the timing of measurement in fatigue have been discussed by Winningham and her colleagues (1994). Perceptions of fatigue may vary radically, depending on state of excitement, time of day, and status with respect to treatment. One additional consideration that may be equally important is the communication climate in which the questions are asked (DiMatteo, 1979). Love and colleagues (1989) demonstrated that patients often underreport side effects and fail to discuss their thoughts about discontinuing treatment. The Fatigue Coalition (Vogelzang et al, 1997, p. 11) concluded that "patients and oncologists have difficulty communicating about fatigue and perhaps are not exploring viable treatments." One possible reason for underreporting, which was true in my own experience, is the lack of energy to

make clinicians understand symptoms or effects, particularly when they show little interest in or concern about them. In addition, the rush and excitement of the clinical environment may cause patients to forget about significant issues they wanted to discuss until afterward when they get home.

Research techniques such as checklists and rating scales may improve clinical as well as research information gathering because they (1) validate fatigue (i.e., "It is normal to acknowledge it, you don't have to be stoical"); (2) give a frame of reference for comparison (more, less, a lot more, etc); (3) question patients in words that are familiar; and (4) allow questions about fatigue to be repeated at each visit. This is significant: Even though the treatment may not have changed, the way the person experiences the fatigue may well have changed. For example, the fatigue-related effects of treatment may manifest gradually or in a cyclic pattern. Questions about fatigue can also be embedded in the context of other questionnaires or models. For instance, the General Health Policy Model developed by Kaplan (1991) is also a useful way of quantifying the meaning of fatigue, in addition to its duration and severity, to the individual.

2. *Research needs.* Clinically oriented research is needed to test many of the laboratory-developed behavioral medicine interventions presented in the literature. Only a few studies have examined fatigue directly, and most of these need to be replicated with respect to the many different kinds of diseases and treatments. Other studies were extensions from research examining quality of life or limitation of daily activities or other outcomes, and need to be tested explicitly with measures of fatigue. Tailored interventions for people having different types of cancer in varying treatment protocols, as well as those from different cultural backgrounds, need to be developed and tested. Fatigue interventions need to be tested with respect to duration of treatment and delivery mode (individual, group, print, audio, or video materials), and combinations of techniques should also be examined.

My buddy told me, "Come on–it's just a matter of will power. Pull yourself out of it."

I replied, "That's not what this is like. Tell me, how hard would it be for you to climb one flight of stairs?"

He snorted, "Hey, no problem. I do it all the time."

I continued, "How about seven flights of stairs? How easy would it be for you to run up seven flights as fast as you can without stopping for rest?"

He said, "No way–I'm pretty out of shape. My legs would give out."

I told him, "Right now, climbing a single flight of stairs is, for me, more impossible than it is for you to run up seven flights."

Cancer survivor

3. *Delivery of care.* Cancer treatment should be planned with the assumption that fatigue may be a major factor. Information and intervention programs should be provided in short segments, early in treatment when the individual is not as tired. However, the first treatment session probably is not the best time for this because the person may be overwhelmed by the diagnosis and the newness of the treatment environment. During treatment visits, clinical staff should meet with patients before they receive treatments such as radiation, rather than afterward when they are more tired. Patients should be permitted to engage in adjunctive programs in interrupted segments, allowing for pauses and rests, to allow for the ups and downs in energy level and the need to recuperate (Kwasnik, Moynihan, and Royle, 1997).

Telephone therapy should be considered as an inexpensive, convenient, and less fatiguing adjunctive support (Fawzy et al, 1995). To fatigued people, behavioral health interventions to address fatigue may appear to be one more tiring and burdensome task. Those interventions may need to be clarified as ways to decrease fatigue or as integral and important to their treatment as radiation or chemotherapy is, and patients should be supported in attending them. Building on the suggestion to use telephone therapy, the interventions may also need to be delivered in a less fatiguing manner, such as counseling by telephone rather than an in-person support group, or giving take-home information like the *Dimensions of Caring* program (developed by Ortho Biotech of Raritan, N.J.) to review according to the person's readiness and energy level.

Some very exciting research has related amount of stress and preparedness for learning. It is clear that stress and learning readiness are a result of and have a profoundly different effect on brain chemistry. Since overstress contributes to fatigue, these relations should be considered in the development of educational programs. (This is discussed in more detail in Chapter 7.) Those of you engaged in patient education will find plenty of ideas for research on the delivery of educational information with specific implications for patient care situations.

4. *Health care systems issues.* Systems of health care delivery need to be redesigned so they do not contribute to further exhaustion by already fatigued people. This means removing physical and procedural barriers to care by providing more one-stop shopping, more outreach, and fewer assumptions that people are able to do tasks for themselves, such as calling to arrange for appointments or obtaining x-rays and carrying them by hand to appointments. While patients may be able to rally themselves and appear to be "up to the task," they often require up to several days afterward to recover from clinic visits and exhausting procedures.

Redesigning health care delivery also means changing the attitudes of health care professionals to enlist cancer survivors and their families in care, so they do not have to fight for information about possible side effects, treatment effectiveness, and alternatives. It means sensitizing young, healthy staff to how fatigued people feel so they do not appear callous. It means clearing up the exhausting insurance and billing problems that are widespread in health care today. There is no way an energetic, healthy person can begin to imagine the physical and emotional costs that may be required for even the simplest tasks; hence, cancer survivors should be included at every level of logistical and environmental planning.

In an exciting recent development, a virtual reality program called "In Their Steps" permits physicians and other health care providers to experience what cancer-related fatigue feels like as they go through their tasks of daily living. For the first time, instead of hearing how patients describe their experiences, health care providers can feel for themselves what the experience is like.

Many of these recommendations require more resources for research and for treatment; however, many require only consideration, compassion, and common sense. In an era of health care cost containment, such changes may be difficult to implement, but they may prove to be cost-effective once strategies are tested and established. The biggest barrier may turn out to be the attitude of health care providers. If changes result in less fatigue among survivors and better adherence to treatment, they may also demonstrate that customer satisfaction, improved quality of life, and cost containment do not have to be mutually exclusive.

References

Arathuzik, D. (1995). Effects of cognitive-behavioral strategies on pain in cancer patients. *Cancer Nursing, 17,* 207–214.

Bottomley, A., Hunton, S., Roberts, G., Jones, L., and Bradley, C. (1996). A pilot study of cognitive behavioral therapy and social support group interventions with newly diagnosed cancer patients. *Journal of Psychosocial Oncology, 14,* 65–83.

Carey, M. P., and Burish, T. G. (1988). Etiology and treatment of the psychological side effects associated with cancer chemotherapy: A critical review and discussion. *Psychological Bulletin, 104,* 307–325.

Carroll, D. (1992). *Health psychology: Stress, behaviour and disease.* Washington, D.C.: Falmer Press.

Carver, C. S, Scheier, M. F., and Pozo, C. (1992). Conceptualizing the process of coping with health problems. In Howard S. Friedman (Ed.), *Hostility, coping and health.* Washington, D.C.: American Psychological Association.

Cella, D. (1997). The Functional Assessment of Cancer Therapy–Anemia (FACT-An) scale: A new tool for the assessment of outcomes in cancer anemia and fatigue. *Seminars in Hematology, 34* (3, suppl 2), 4–12.

Cimprich, B. (1993). Development of an intervention to restore attention in cancer patients. *Cancer Nursing, 16,* 83–92.

DiMatteo, M. R. (1979). A social-psychological analysis of physician-patient rapport: Toward a science of the art of medicine. *Journal of Social Issues, 35,* 12–33.

Eller, L. S. (1995). Effects of two cognitive-behavioral interventions on immunity and symptoms in persons with HIV. *Annals of Behavioral Medicine, 17,* 339–348.

Fawzy, F. I., Cousins, N., Fawzy, N. W., Kemeny, M. E., Elashoff, R., and Morton, D. (1990). A structured psychiatric intervention for cancer patients. *Archives of General Psychiatry, 47,* 720–725.

Fawzy, F. I., Fawzy, N. W., Arndt, L. A., and Pasnau, R. O. (1995). Critical review of psychosocial interventions in cancer care. *Archives of General Psychiatry, 52,* 100–111.

Fawzy, F. I., Fawzy, N. W., Hyun, C. S., Elashoff, R., Guthrie, D., Fahey, J. L., and Morton, D. L. (1993). Malignant melanoma: Effects of an early structured psychiatric intervention, coping and affective state on recurrence and survival 6 years later. *Archives of General Psychiatry, 50,* 681–689.

Fleishman, J. A., and Fogel, B. (1994). Coping and depressive symptoms among people with AIDS. *Health Psychology, 13,* 156–169.

Flint, T. A. (1995). "Breast cancer support groups: Differences between attenders and nonattenders." Doctoral dissertation, University of Utah, City, Salt Lake City, Utah.

Grant, M., Ferrell, B. R., Schmidt, G. M., Fonbuena, P., Niland, J. C., and Forman, S. J. (1992). Measurement of quality of life in bone marrow transplantation survivors. *Quality of Life Research, 1,* 375–384.

Greer, S., Morris, T., Pettingale, K. W., and Haybittle, J. L. (1990). Psychological response to breast cancer and 15-year outcome. *Lancet,* 335, 49–50.

Guyatt, G. H., Feeny, D. H., and Patrick, D. L. (1993). Measuring health-related quality of life. *Annals of Internal Medicine, 118,* 622–629.

Halkitis, P. N. (1998). Advances in the treatment of HIV disease: Complexities of adherence and complications for prevention. *Health Psychologist, 20,* 6–7, 14–15.

Herbert, T. B., and Cohen, S. (1993). Depression and immunity: A meta-analytic review. *Psychological Bulletin, 113,* 472–486.

Ironson, G., Antoni, M., and Lutgendorf, S. (1995). Can psychological interventions affect immunity and survival? Present findings and suggested targets with a focus on cancer and human immunodeficiency virus. *Mind-Body Medicine, 1,* 85–110.

Irvine, D. M., Vincent, L., Bubela, N., Thompson, L., and Graydon, J. (1991). A critical appraisal of the research literature investigating fatigue in the individual with cancer. *Cancer Nursing, 14,* 188–199.

Irvine, D. M., Vincent, L., Graydon, J. E., Bubela, N., and Thompson, L. (1994). The prevalence and correlates of fatigue in patients receiving treatment with chemotherapy and radiotherapy. *Cancer Nursing, 17,* 367–378.

Jacobs, C., et al, (1983). Behavior of cancer patients: A randomized study of the effects of education and peer support groups. *American Journal of Clinical Oncology, 6,* 347–353.

Jensen, S., and Given, B. A. (1991). Fatigue affecting family caregivers of cancer patients. *Cancer Nursing, 14,* 181–187.

Johnson, J. E., Nail, L. M., Lauver, D., King, K. B., and Keys, H. (1988). Reducing the negative impact of radiation therapy on functional status. *Cancer, 61,* 46–51.

Kaplan, R. M. (1991). Health-related quality of life in patient decision-making. *Journal of Social Issues, 47,* 69–90.

Karazc, A. K., Bochnak, E., and Ouellette, S. C. (1994). Role strain and psychological well-being in women with systemic lupus erythematosus. *Health Psychology, 13,* 184.

Kwasnik, B. C., Moynihan, R. T., and Royle, M. H. (1997). HIV mental health services integrated with medical care (pp. 209–223). In M. G. Winiarski (Ed.). *HIV mental health for the 21st century.* New York: New York University Press.

Love, R. R., Leventhal, H., Easterling, D. V., and Nerenz, D. R. (1989). Side effects and emotional distress during cancer chemotherapy. *Cancer, 63,* 604–612.

MacVicar, M. G., and Winningham, M. L. (1986). Promoting the functional capacity of cancer patients. *Cancer Bulletin, 38,* 235–239.

MacVicar, M. G., Winningham, M. L., and Nickel, J. L. (1989). Effects of aerobic interval training on cancer patients' functional capacity. *Nursing Research, 38,* 348–351.

Martin, R., Davis, G. M., Baron, R. S., Suls, J., and Blanchard, E. B. (1994). Specificity in social support: Perceptions of helpful and unhelpful provider behaviors among irritable bowel syndrome, headache, and cancer patients. *Health Psychology, 13,* 432–439.

Meyer, T., and Mark, M. (1995). Effects of psychosocial interventions with adult cancer patients: A meta-analysis of randomized experiments. *Health Psychology, 14,* 101–108.

Morin, C. M., Culbert, J. P., and Schwartz, S. M. (1994). Non-pharmacological intervention for insomnia: A meta-analysis of treatment efficacy. *American Journal of Psychiatry, 151,* 1172–1180.

Moyer, A., and Salovey, P. (1996). Psychosocial sequelae of breast cancer. *Annals of Behavioral Medicine, 18,* 110–125.

O'Brien, M. E., and Pheifer, W. G. (1993). Physical and psychosocial nursing care for patients with HIV infection. *Advances in Clinical Nursing Research, 28,* 303–316.

Parsons, T. (1964). *The social system* (pp. 436–443, 445–447). New York: Free Press.

Pennebaker, J. W. (1992). Inhibition as the linchpin of health. In Howard S. Friedman (Ed.), *Hostility, coping and health.* Washington, D.C: American Psychological Association.

Quested, K., Malec, J., Harney, R., Kienker, K., and Romsaas, E. (1982). Rehabilitation program for cancer related fatigue: An empirical study. *Archives of Physical Medicine and Rehabilitation, 63,* 532.

Rainey, L. C. (1985). Effects of preparatory patient education for radiation oncology patients. *Cancer, 56*(5), 1056–1061.

Reifman, A. (1995). Social relationships, recovery from illness, and survival: A literature review. *Annals of Behavioral Medicine, 17,* 124–131.

Seago, M., and Conn, C. (1996). Mind-body partnering for clinical practice. *Journal of Psychosocial Oncology, 14,* 47–63.

Sikkema, K. J., and Kelly, J. A. (1996). Behavioral medicine interventions can improve the quality-of-life and health of persons with HIV. *Annals of Behavioral Medicine, 18,* 40–48.

Spiegel, D. (1994). Health caring: Psychosocial support for patients with cancer. *Cancer, 74,* 1453–1457.

Stone, A. A., and Porter, L. S. (1995). Psychological coping: Its importance for treating medical problems. *Mind-Body Medicine, 1,* 46–54.

Taylor, S. E., and Aspinwall, L. G. (1990). Psychosocial aspects of chronic illness (pp. 3–6). In Paul T. Costa, Jr., and Gary R. VandenBos (Eds.), *Psychological aspects of serious illness: Chronic conditions, fatal diseases, and clinical care.* Washington, D.C.: American Psychological Association.

Trijsburg, R. W., van Knippenberg, F. C. E., and Rijpma, S. E. (1992). Effects of psychological treatment on cancer patients: A critical review. *Psychosomatic Medicine, 54,* 489–517.

Uchino, B. N., Cacioppo, J. T., and Kiecolt-Glaser, J. K. (1996). The relationship between social support and physiological processes: A review with emphasis on underlying mechanisms and implications for health. *Psychological Bulletin, 119,* 488–531.

Vogelzang, N. J., Breitbart, W., Cella, D., Curt, G. A., Groopman, J. E., Horning, S. J., Itri, L. M., Johnson, D. H., Scherr, S. L., and Portenoy, R. K. (1997). Patient, caregiver, and oncologist perceptions of cancer-related fatigue: Results of a tripart assessment survey. *Seminars in Hematology, 34* (3, suppl 2), 4–12.

Wallace, K. G. (1997). Analysis of recent literature concerning relaxation and imagery interventions for cancer pain. *Cancer Nursing, 20,* 79–87.

Ware, J. E., Kosinski, M., and Keller, S. D. (1994). *SF-36 physical and mental health summary scales: A user's manual.* Boston: Health Institute, New England Medical Center.

Winningham, M. L. (1991). A walking program for people with cancer: Getting started. *Cancer Nursing, 14*(5), 270–276.

Winningham, M. L. (1994). Exercise and cancer (pp. 301–305). In L. Goldberg and D. Elliot (Eds.), *Exercise for prevention and treatment of illness.* Philadelphia: F. A. Davis.

Winningham, M. L., and MacVicar, M. G. (1983). Exercise as a tension reduction mechanism in cancer patients. [Abstract]. *Ohio Journal of Science, 83*(2), 75.

Winningham, M. L., MacVicar, M. G., and Burke, C. A. (1986). Exercise for cancer patients: Guidelines and precautions. *Physician Sportsmedicine, 14*(10), 124–134.

Winningham, M. L., Nail, L. M., Barton Burke, M., Brophy, L., Cimprich, B., Jones, L. S., Pickard-Holley, S., Rhodes, V., St. Pierre, B., Beck, S., Glass, E. C., Mock, V. L., Mooney, K. H., and Piper, B. (1994). Fatigue and the cancer experience: The state of the knowledge. *Oncology Nursing Forum, 21,* 23–36.

Wortman, C. B., and Dunkel-Schetter, C. (1979). Interpersonal relationships and cancer: A theoretical analysis. *Journal of Social Issues, 35,* 120–155.

Resources

The *Dimensions of Caring* includes a "Taking Control of Fatigue" module with a videotape, informational booklet, and workbook. The videotape contains vignettes of interviews of cancer survivors and their families, who represent a particularly credible source of information to other survivors. The various vignettes demonstrate that fatigue is a normal concomitant of cancer treatment; some make suggestions regarding ways to deal with it. These vignettes can help people articulate their experience with fatigue. They are also useful in training health care providers to become more sensitive to patient-fatigue issues. This program was developed in 1996 by ProEd Communications, for Ortho Biotech of Raritan, N.J. It is available through your local Ortho Biotech product specialist to your clinic or physician's office. Ask for it by name if you have not seen it.

Fatigue is like carrying a tremendous weight on my shoulders; therefore, the energy I use to dress or prepare a meal is equal to the energy I used to apply to carry luggage (& full) or moving a 40lb rock. I wear my activities of the day mentally and physically.

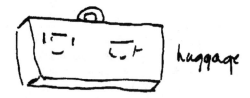

luggage

Linda Jimison, 50, myelodysplastic syndrome patient

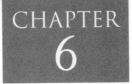

Physiological and Psychological Foundations of Fatigue Research: An Historical Perspective

Sandra J. Smeeding

It's not that you can't hear us. You don't want to hear us. To hear would mean you must do something. And most of you don't want to face what that means!

Cancer survivor

Background

Fatigue is a common medical complaint; however, it is difficult to clearly delineate it from confounding variables such as depression and anxiety. It is equally difficult to measure. Private as well as public financing has encouraged research in industry, the military, aerospace, sports science, and medicine to find ways to measure fatigue as the key to understanding it in the context of human performance. Fatigue research historically passed through several major phases of interest that involved different disciplines and methods of study. Today, fatigue research continues, under one of four general areas:

1. Building on past work, aerospace and military science is interested in the significance of fatigue syndromes as they affect health and performance. Periodic accidents in the commercial airline as well as trucking and automotive industries continue to challenge the role of fatigue in travel safety.

2. Sports physiology, sports psychology, athletics, and sports medicine have become highly competitive and polished in their use of research-based techniques that refine athletic training and enhance performance; in addition, sports medicine continues to examine the effects of psychological state and trait on fatigue and performance outcome.

3. Business and industry are taking a fresh look at fatigue as it influences workmanship and quality control. Even "power naps" are getting attention as possible productivity enhancers.

4. Health care is becoming aware of the effect of long-term, illness-related fatigue and its relationship to functional independence, performance, cost of living with chronic conditions, and quality of life.

Initial interest in the measurement of fatigue was in discerning the effect on work performance or decrement in conditions of stress. This interest was particularly significant during World War II when it became necessary to understand the point beyond which workers in assignments such as flying bombers long distances or watching radar started making significant, even fatal, errors. Prior to this time, research had focused more on physical fatigue; however, in these tasks, it became critical to identify the limits of attentional fatigue in making fatal errors. Figure 6-1 compares historical influences and trends in research.

Qualities of fatigue include mental and physical components as well as weakened motivation and activation. This is particularly significant to the cancer-related fatigue syndrome (CRFS) because cancer patients often remonstrate with themselves about being "lazy" or "unmotivated." Moreover, employers and casual observers—even family members—may make the same assumptions. This can contribute to such problems as unnecessary guilt on the one hand, and loss of employment on the other.

Traditionally, the study of fatigue took on one of two approaches: fatigue as an objective phenomenon and fatigue as a subjective phenomenon. Some studies looked at the interactive effect of both kinds of fatigue. *Objective* studies of fatigue usually addressed biochemical or physiological measures of physical or muscular performance. For instance, an objective measure of fatigue would be blood lactate or respiratory oxygen uptake levels in subjects undergoing a specific physical stressor such as endurance running, sprinting, or weight lifting. *Subjective* studies of fatigue involved psychological measurement of self-perceived fatigue or the effect on an individual's performance in response to various challenges and under specified conditions. An example of subjective fatigue may be difficulty concentrating when an individual performs repetitive tasks over a long period of time. An example of combining objective with subjective measures would be to assess how well athletes are able to make critical decisions after several hours of competitive cycling, as in the Tour de France. Another example of this might involve determining how well an individual can cognitively perform after working under hot, humid conditions for several hours.

Researchers in industry, the military, aerospace, sports science, and medicine studied fatigue within the context and boundaries of their disciplines. Each discipline added insight into the ongoing process of other areas of fatigue research. Understanding the more than 90-year history of inquiry into fatigue, in general, may shed light on the unique aspects of the CRFS. Hence, anyone who wishes to study or understand the CRFS should first become intimate with prior fatigue research in the various disciplines. The contextual development of both physiological and psychological approaches to research in industry, the military, aerospace, sports science, and medicine is represented here. A few of the major, confounding variables that have hampered the ongoing study of fatigue are also presented.

About the Contributor

Sandra J. Smeeding, a family nurse practitioner residing in Salt Lake City, Utah, received her bachelor's degree in nursing from the University of Wisconsin at Oshkosh. She is a seasoned practitioner with an analytical mind for addressing clinical problems. For instance, she conducted a demonstration project showing it is possible to cut costs and increase efficiency in an intensive care nursing unit without compromising quality care. Her special interest is the problem of fatigue in clinical populations, which dates back more than ten years, culminated in her pioneering development of a postsurgical fatigue measurement

Fatigue as a Clinical Problem

Fatigue and lack of energy have been identified as common complaints heard in clinical practice (Friedlander, 1962; Jerrett, 1981; Kaye, 1980). The National Ambulatory Medical Care Survey (1975) found fatigue to be the seventh most frequent initial complaint in U.S. medical offices (Solsberg, 1984). In 1975, there were 10.5 million visits for this problem, and 25% of the time it was a new concern (Solsberg, 1984). Medical evaluation, however, is frequently frustrating to physicians because of fatigue's wide variety of causes, its attributed psychosocial origins, inadequate means of testing for it, and its resistance to traditional medical therapies. Indeed, Harms and Soniat (1952) listed the following conditions associated with the fatigue complaint: debilitating illness, lack of motivation, nervous tension and anxiety, depression, hypertension, and chronic inhibition of ego function.

Confounding Variables in Clinical Fatigue Research

Clinical research into the origin of fatigue is confounded by its close association with other conditions, such as depression. Fatigue is often listed as one of the preeminent presenting symptoms of depression (American Psychiatric Association, 1980). However, whether fatigue causes depression or depression causes fatigue is not clear. Fatigue, although it can be identified, can scarcely be isolated from conditions associated with it, and which often form a basis for it (Bartley, 1965).

Certain physical symptoms are characteristic of depression. The most prominent are lack of energy and fatigue, particularly in women: Everything is an effort; the patient tires easily and may feel tired all the time (Hamilton, 1982). Some patients say they feel completely exhausted all the time. Depressed individuals usually display at least three of the following symptoms (American Psychiatric Association, 1980; Hamilton, 1982; Tourney, 1970):

1. alterations in body weight due to either increased or decreased appetite
2. difficulty sleeping or hypersomnia
3. loss of energy, easily fatigued, or tired
4. agitation or retardation of psychomotor activity
5. loss of interest in normal activities
6. decreased mentation, concentration, or slow thinking

scale in 1986. She was clearly ahead of her time! She continues to be interested in how emotional and spiritual energy influences a person's physical well-being, social integration, and survival. She was asked to contribute this chapter because her global, historical perspective could contribute a sense of history and proportion to this book. Her favorite out-of-work activities include being a mother, hiking in the canyons of southern Utah, and skiing, which is why she finds Utah such a congenial place to live.

Figure
6.1

Historical Timeline of Scientific Inquiry Into Fatigue

Process of inquiry	ERA							
	200 BC // 1800 AD 1900	1920	1940	1960	1980	2000		
	RELATED WORLD EVENTS							
	Increased scientific competition among nations	WW I	WW II	Bedrest studies	Vietnam conflict / Manned space flight	Computers in research	Increased aging and chronic illness in Western populations	
Philosophy and gross observation								
Physiological research defining life								
Physiological research defining homeostatis and stressors								
Applied research on human performance								
Navigation and aviation								
Aerospace/NASA								
Sportsmedicine and athletic performance								
Energy and fatigue in health care								
Physical and occupational rehabilitation								
Cardiac/ pulmonary rehabilitation								
Cancer energetic and fatigue research								

Nixon declares "War on Cancer"

Two retrospective medical studies were conducted to obtain data to support the hypothesis that roughly one-half of individuals seen in a general practice setting who listed fatigue as their chief complaint (CC) had a problem of psychological origin. In the first series of 176 patients whose CC was fatigue, depression was undoubtedly the most important cause (76 patients [43%] were diagnosed as clinically depressed) (Solsberg, 1984). The other study of 57 patients concluded that in 21 (37%), fatigue had a psychological basis (Morrison, 1980). Remarkably, it is significant to note that over half of the patients in both groups were *not* determined to be clinically depressed.

Anxiety is another confounding variable in the study of fatigue. In examining anxiety, researchers proposed a close relationship between anxiety and fatigue. They believed that anxiety delays feelings of fatigue and that it may be possible to be too busy or distracted to feel tired until it becomes overwhelming. In this case, the perception of fatigue may be postponed. The anxiety component in fatigue is theorized to interfere with rest and recuperation, leading to a chronic experience of fatigue. Cameron (1973) suggested that a broad conceptualization of fatigue should include reference to anxiety.

Focus on Fatigue Research in Medicine

Although there was some inquiry into muscle physiology and fatigue versus psychological fatigability as early as the turn of the century, the origins of most twentieth-century fatigue research occurred on the battlefields of World War I. Physician researchers from the United States such as Walter B. Cannon became involved in treating the effects of arousal and shock in the trenches. In Europe, they had the opportunity to meet men with brilliant minds like Sir William Osler and John Haldane. In England, physiological research focused on problems like tetanus, surgical techniques for battlefield injuries, or fatigue and efficiency in munitions workers. Upon their return, the American medical physiologists continued to develop these areas of research (Cannon, 1984).

The major focus of fatigue research in the medical field was on metabolic (biochemical) responses to determine the cause of, or minimize damage on, the organism. One of the earliest efforts to study the causes of fatigue manifested itself in the development of the Harvard Fatigue Laboratory at Harvard University in 1926. The Fatigue Laboratory was developed because of interest in the physiological differences between individuals, applied physiological differences, and studies of "what is vaguely called fatigue and fatigue's influence in industrial psychology and physiology" (Dill, 1967, p. 160). The Harvard Fatigue Laboratory was dissolved in 1946 due to financial pressures in the era after the war; however, work accomplished during that 40-year period influenced the disciplines of exercise physiology, industrial medicine, psychology, aviation medicine, research in environmental stress, ergonomics, the aerospace sciences, and clinical medicine.

It is no surprise that the same themes running through fatigue theory also run through stress theory (Selye, 1974, 1976). In his discussion of exhaustion, adaptive energy, and stress, Selye made a bold prophecy: "Further research along these lines would seem to hold great promise, since here we appear to touch upon the fundamentals of fatigue and aging" (1978, p. 82). In this same context, he suggested that each of us may be born with a certain amount of adaptive energy at birth: "In any case, there is just so much of it, and (we) must budget accordingly."

Select Theories of Metabolically Induced Muscular Fatigue

There are essentially two theories of muscular fatigue: chemical (peripheral) and central nervous system (CNS). The chemical theory states that the loss of performance results from the consumption of energy-producing substances and an accumulation of waste products as muscle fatigues, with the electrical phenomena in muscles and nerves playing only a secondary part (Grandjean, 1979). Although recent discoveries of local as well as central neurohormonal influences on fatigue suggest a more complex interaction, much can still be learned by examining the literature relating to these two theories.

Peripheral Mechanisms of Muscular Fatigue

The ability of muscle fibers to contract depends on the muscle's ability to supply adenosine triphosphate (ATP) to the contractile proteins. ATP performs three major functions in muscle contraction and relaxation (Grandjean, 1970):

1. The energy released from ATP splitting is directly coupled to the movement of cross-bridges.
2. ATP binding to myosin is necessary to break the link between the cross-bridges and action, allowing the cross-bridges to operate cyclically.
3. Energy released from ATP splitting is utilized by the sarcoplasmic reticulum to reaccumulate calcium ions, resulting in relaxation.

Note that both contraction and relaxation are both necessary for the cycle. For a muscle to continue to contract, an adequate supply of oxygen and nutrients from which ATP is produced is required. A deficit of either oxygen or nutrition (foodstuffs) results in a reduced capacity to do work.

There are three sources for ATP in the body:

1. creatinine phosphate
2. oxidative phosphorylation in the mitochondria
3. substrate phosphorylation during glycolysis

Different muscle groups are better at producing more of one kind than another, depending on their performance specialty.

Creatinine phosphate provides the most rapid means of forming ATP in the muscle cell. The combined energy of both the stored ATP and the creatinine phosphate in muscle is capable of causing maximal muscle contraction for no longer than a few seconds (Guyton, 1981). The next energy sources used to reconstitute both creatinine phosphate and ATP are glucose, fats, and proteins. Glucose is the most immediate source of energy for contracting muscle. However, the total quantity of glucose in extracellular fluid is only 20 grams; thereafter, glucose is released from the liver to prevent hypoglycemia (Newsholme, 1981). The liver also produces glucose from noncarbohydrate sources through a process called *gluconeogenesis* (Fehlig and Wahren, 1975; Newsholme, 1981). Only about 2% of the energy is obtained from protein (Bartley, 1965).

At moderate levels of muscle activity (moderate rates of ATP breakdown), most of the ATP needed can be formed by the process of oxidative phosphorylation using fatty acids as the predominant source of nutrient and to a lesser extent carbohydrates (Vander, 1980). Triacylglycerol, which is stored in adipose tissue, is a long-chain fatty acid and is the largest fuel reserve in the body. Triacylglycerol, after it is released into the bloodstream, is taken up and oxidized by muscle tissue (Newsholme, 1981).

When muscle activity reaches and exceeds about 50% of maximum (50% of the maximal rate of ATP breakdown), glycolysis begins to contribute an increasingly significant fraction of the total ATP production (Newsholme, 1981; Vander, 1980). The glycolytic pathway, although producing only small quantities of ATP from each molecule of metabolized glucose, can operate at a high rate and can also proceed in the absence of oxygen. Thus, during muscle activity, if the oxidation rates of blood-borne fuel (fatty acid and glucose) are insufficient to meet demands, glucose stored as muscle glycogen must be used to supplement the blood-borne fuels. Obviously, these resources are very limited and lead to fatigue. The onset of fatigue is closely correlated with the depletion of muscle glycogen stores and the ability of the fibers to replace ATP rapidly by glycolysis (Bartley, 1965; Guyton, 1981; Hermansen, Hultman, and Salten, 1967; Newsholme, 1981; Vander, 1980).

As we near the end of this century, clinical science–nursing, medicine, the therapies, nutrition–has just begun to realize the significance of this common, seemingly mundane symptom or syndrome of fatigue as an alert to imbalances in mind, body, and spirit.

At intense levels of muscle activity, fatigue may occur before the glycogen supplies have been depleted because the very high rate of ATP breakdown is faster than the rate at which new ATP can be supplied by glycolysis (Vander, 1980). This theory proposes that the sensation of fatigue is a result of a depletion of substrate at the cellular level. This area of research has focused increasingly on the roles, the activity and inhibition, of specific enzymes in producing energy in the cell. In August 1998, the work of hundreds of researchers for more than 20 years culminated in the exciting announcement, by two independent laboratories, of the discovery of the structure of cytochrome oxidase, the specific enzyme that drives the cells. It is this enzyme that actually converts oxygen and nutrients in the cell to water, carbon dioxide, and energy.

In every case, oxygen is required for recovery of the cell's energetic capacity, regardless of the metabolic system involved in the exertion. Under conditions of acute anemia, as well as in cellular starvation, the potential for activity (physiological work) as well as metabolic recovery is impaired. Although there are comparatively few data that can explain how cancer and its associated treatment(s) interact with cellular energetic metabolism in a way that would contribute to cellular fatigability, this is a promising area for future research.

The Central Nervous System Theory of Muscular Fatigue

The CNS theory of muscular fatigue regards the biochemical depletion of substrate merely as a releasing stimulus for sensory impulses that travel along the nerves to the brain and cerebral cortex. The cortex is where muscular fatigue makes itself evident as a sensation of weariness; in addition, the afferent impulses inhibit the center of the brain responsible for motor control of movements and thus bring about a reduction in the number and frequency of impulses along the motor neuron. This, in turn, produces the external sign of muscular fatigue—namely, the reduction in muscular power and, where rhythmic movements are concerned, shortening and retardation of muscle movement (Grandjean, 1979).

General Central Nervous System Influence on Fatigue

Early work on CNS mechanisms focused on arousal and inhibition as functions of the integrative action of the diencephalon (Hess, 1948; Moruzzi, 1960), specifically the thalamic reticular system (Jasper, 1949; Mogoun, 1946; Moruzzi and Mogoun, 1949). This work approached fatigue as being related to sleep (Jouvet, 1967).

In the past decade, as more sophisticated techniques of studying brain function have evolved, CNS neurotransmitter activity and metabolic functions in various parts of the brain have been the targets of exciting research. This area of study may have the most promising implications with respect to the attentional fatigue reported in patients with the CRFS and the development and possible use of effective pharmacological agents.

Toward a More Holistic Understanding

Neither of the two theories explains everything. Both the CNS phenomena (recruiting of motor neurons and neurotransmitter activity) and the biochemical processes in the muscles (depletion of energy reserves) contribute some understanding to the concept of fatigue. Fatigue cannot be considered a simple physiological condition resulting from sustained muscular activity. In considering the body as a whole, fatigue cannot be defined solely in terms of biochemical changes in the muscles or nerves or by the exhaustion of energy reserves (McFarland, 1971).

Physical and Attentional Fatigue Research in Industry and Aerospace

Fatigue research, like most trends in science, has generally followed the demands of money and war. In the periods during and after World War I, extensive research was carried out in England by the industrial Fatigue Research Board (Cameron, 1973). The board's area of interest was productivity in industry. The guiding theme of this work was the notion that output of the worker was limited in some way by fatigue, and that alleviation of fatigue, by whatever means, would enable production to be maintained at a high level (Cameron, 1973). Many of these earlier researchers were primarily concerned with fatigue effects following muscular work and fatigue's effect on nerve fibers (McFarland, 1971).

The second major wave of interest in fatigue effects occurred during the 1940s and 1950s (Cameron, 1973). The focus of these works was on aviation, especially military aviation. The classic works on fatigue by Bartlett (1943), Drew (1940), and Davis (1946, 1948) date from this period and employed more complex criteria than simple output figures (Cameron, 1973). The pattern of breakdown in skilled performance that occurs in fatigue, and indeed under the influence of other types of stress conditions, was clearly established as a result of the work (Cameron, 1973).

Immediately after World War II, attempts to extend the wartime fatigue research to commercial civil flying operations began. The works of Bartlett and Davis were essentially operational: They emphasized output and did not concern themselves with subjective feelings of fatigue. However, during the era after World War II, fatigue studies became broader and more humane in their approach.

Often, fatigue is the symptom of a major medical disorder that brings individuals to see a health care provider. They do not know what is wrong, but know something is wrong; they feel they are at the point where they cannot go on.

In a 1947 publication, Bartley and Chute emphasized the complex nature of fatigue. They distinguished three distinct facets of the problem (Cameron, 1973). They contended that *fatigue* should be used only to describe the subjective feelings of lassitude and disinclination toward activity that characterized the individual response to fatigue. They went on to suggest that the term *impairment* should be used "to identify the true reduction of physical capacity which resulted from an accumulated oxygen deficit in muscle tissue" (Bartley and Chute, 1947, p. 46). They designated deterioration in quality of performance as *work decrement*. Bartley and Chute (1947) also introduced a new and important emphasis on the chronic effects of fatigue. They pointed out that in clinical practice, chronic fatigue that was not dispelled by the normal processes of rest and recuperation was a common problem. Impairment or work decrement that responded to rest was unlikely to present a serious, practical problem.

The third area of interest in fatigue research also had its beginnings in the 1940s. The area of interest was in fatigue's effect on driving and accident involvement. Research in this area tended to follow the patterns set by earlier investigators in aviation. As in other investigations, fatigue was associated with deterioration in physical or mental performance to the exclusion of subjective feelings. Research in this area has continued to the present.

Measurement of Fatigue in Industry and Aerospace: Objective Measures

Researchers in industry and aerospace have spent a great amount of time and energy attempting to measure and study the effects of fatigue on human productivity. This has been a mechanistic model with a focus on the human as a production device. Attempts to measure fatigue effects generally employed three different methods of measuring performance:

1. The most common method, the interpolated test, consists of some special, quantifiable task that the subject is required to perform for a brief period during the performance of his or her usual task (Bartlett, 1943; Cameron, 1973).
2. The second method, employed by Davis (1948) and by Jackson (1958), measures some segment of performance at a task and plots its variation as a function of time (Cameron, 1973).
3. A third method, developed by Brown (1967), utilizes the idea of limited channel capacity. At intervals during a long period of driving a car, subjects are required to perform a subsidiary or secondary task of information processing. The theory is that the amount of spare capacity would be reduced by fatigue and would result in poorer performance on the secondary task (Cameron, 1973).

Stress theory and research began having an influence on fatigue research. Several industrial researchers later attempted to move away from the method of measuring fatigue in terms of performance measures such as elapsed time and activity (Appley and Trumbull, 1967; Cameron, 1973). They took another direction and were of the opinion that the appropriate methods for the measurement of fatigue effects were similar to those used for studies of the stress response. Their approach was that the human stress response involved the

---

By the end of the day I was exhausted. There was nothing left. I couldn't even remember large parts of my day because most of it was spent on autopilot, putting one foot in front of the other and hoping I would survive. I was in a fog. On Friday evening, I fell into bed. All weekend I lay around, too exhausted to do anything, as I tried to gather the strength to get through another week. It took so much energy just to do the everyday things others do without thinking. You have no idea what that's like. I try to remember the days when it used to be different, but that seems like another person, another life, another world. I can't quite seem to grasp it. . . . You know, I used to be athletic!

Former hospice patient

whole system of biological emergency mechanisms and implied an abnormal demand on the energy resources of the system, resulting in fatigue (Appley and Trumbull, 1967). Furthermore, they hypothesized, although the degree of the fatigue experience may depend to some extent on the level of the stress response, duration would be the variable having the greatest effect (Austin, 1968; Cameron, 1968). This was similar to the concept of chronicity proposed by Bartley and Chute in 1947 as well as the prevailing stress theory.

Austin (1968) and Cameron (1968, 1969) proposed that the length of time needed to return to a normal arousal level could be used as an index of the severity of fatigue resulting from the stress state. The use of recovery time as an index permitted the separation of chronic and acute effects of fatigue (Cameron, 1968, 1969). Although measurement of fatigue recovery time and the suggested strong relationship to stress added a new dimension to the study of fatigue, the emphasis was still primarily on objective aspects of fatigue rather than on the subjective state of the individual.

Fatigue as Subjective Experience

Ways to measure the subjective qualities of fatigue generally relied on two methodologies: (1) psychophysical techniques and (2) rating scales (Kinsman and Philip, 1976). The psychophysical techniques involved "ratio scales," which were thought to be more precise in describing relationships between objective stimulus levels and perceptions (Kinsman and Philip, 1976). Rating scales have a wider application because of the ease with which the ordinal or interval scale may be used (Kinsman and Philip, 1976). More recently, a third methodology, involving a multivariate statistical procedure, was developed to identify categories or dimensions of symptomatology related to work performance and fatigue (Holsti, Loomba, and North, 1968; Kinsman and Philip, 1976).

The scaling techniques other than the ratio scale can be grouped into (1) nondimensional, single-point measures, (2) unidimensional rating scales, and (3) multidimensional rating scales (Kinsman and Philip, 1976).

The nondimensional measurement of subjective fatigue employs the simplest methods of measurement and generally requires a single verbal report during work performance (Kinsman and Philip, 1976). Most often an attempt is made to identify factors displacing the fatigue point toward or away from the initiation of work (Kinsman and Philip, 1976). The various nondimensional studies reveal little consistency between the qualities measured (tiredness and undifferentiated fatigue), tasks used, or subject populations selected (Kinsman and Philip, 1976). Single-point, nondimensional measures of fatigue are open to criticism. Fatigue is conceptualized in these studies as an all-or-none event: Either the individual is experiencing a certain degree of fatigue or they are not (Kinsman and Philip, 1976).

Unidimensional rating scales attempt to quantify dimensionally a single subjective quality (i.e., feeling tone, undifferentiated fatigue, tiredness, or perceived effort). The studies utilize 4-point to 15-point rating scales. Nussbaum (1963) used a 9-point rating scale to evaluate subjective undifferentiated fatigue in 80 male college students (Kinsman and Philip, 1976). The testing program encompassed six test sessions with a control group and an experimental group. The rating scale ranged from no fatigue (1) to extreme fatigue (9). Pulse rate was measured before the work task, at the end of the work task, and after 10 minutes of recovery (Kinsman and Philip, 1976). Nussbaum (1963) concluded from his study that "physiological changes are not directly related to fatigue" (Kinsman and Philip, 1976).

As early as 1928, Poffenberger reported the use of a simple rating scale to evaluate the feeling of tiredness during prolonged mental work. Poffenberger used a 7-point ordinal scale ranging from extremely good (1) to extremely tired (7) with a midpoint defined as medium (4). Poffenberger's results indicated a fairly clear relationship between tiredness and performance in prolonged mental work (Kinsman and Philip, 1976).

Pearson and Byars (1956) reported the development of a ten-item unidimensional scale measuring the subjective quality of tiredness. Their interval scale represents the most thorough effort to devise a measurement of subjective fatigue as a unidimensional feeling of tiredness (Kinsman and Philip, 1976). They followed the procedures for scale construction recommended by Edwards and Kilpatrick (1948). In their scale, a set of adjectives is arranged in a continuum, with equidistant adjacent items, so the subject can report a level of tiredness by pinpointing a position along this continuum (Kinsman and Philip, 1976). As a unidimensional measure of tiredness, Pearson and Byar's (1956) interval scale is unsurpassed, as it was constructed systematically, according to sound psychometric principles (Kinsman and Philip, 1976).

McNelly (1976) used Thurstone's (1929) scaling techniques to develop a 9-point rating scale of tiredness. An attempt was made to construct an interval scale with adjacent scale points of equidistance (Kinsman and Philip, 1976). The validity of the scale was tested on 80 male and female undergraduates using a block-turning task with heavy (11 ounces) or light (4 ounces) blocks either with massed practice (without rest) or spaced practice (rest after each trial). Rating of tiredness showed a significant change from before to after work. However, similar to the Pearson-Byars scale, the composition of McNelly's scale includes colloquial items (e.g., "fagged," "in gear," etc) that are unique in regard to culture, time, and geographic location (Kinsman and Philip, 1976).

Multidimensional analysis of subjective qualities added a new dimension to the measurement of subjective fatigue. Multidimensional analyses, such as factor analysis or key cluster analysis, provided ways to identify sets of symptoms that group together to form symptom categories (Kinsman and Philip, 1976; Weiser and Stampes, 1973).

The Japanese Industrial Fatigue Research Committee (Kashiwagi, 1971) developed a 30-symptom subjective fatigue list (Kinsman and Philip, 1976). The initial inventory included three symptom categories–physical, mental, and neurosensory fatigue–arranged in a checklist so that an individual could indicate the presence or absence of each symptom. The initial inventory was formulated on a conceptual, rather than an empirical, grouping of items within the symptom categories.

An empirical derivation of this early scale was presented in 1970 by Saito, Kogi, and Kashiwagi. Kashiwagi (1971) incorporated the results of the Japanese Fatigue Scale so fatigue could be judged by observation, that is, by how the subject looked. Twenty-eight items were prepared for the fatigue rating scale (appearance, combined with 20 items from the Japanese Fatigue Scale). Kashiwagi (1971) placed one-half of the 20 items on the factor dimension "weakened activation" and the other half in "weakened drive or motivation."

Fatigue in Medicine

Fatigue has long been recognized as a complex postsurgical problem regardless of the surgical site (Megued and Egdahl, 1977; Rhoten, 1982). Examples of surgeries associated with postoperative fatigue include abdominal surgery (Christensen, Bendix, and Kehlet, 1982) and gynecological surgery (Rose and King, 1978). In Chapter 22, McDade gives an excellent presentation on the clinical implications of this problem.

As a clinician, I learned to consider fatigue an important symptom related to environment as well as part of many medical conditions. I had a hunch it required far more attention than it was getting because of its obvious link to quality of life.

Where Do We Go From Here?

Most current research pursuits are based on some conceptual variation of the historical developments described here. From the work on human techniques to measure productivity, studies of human performance in athletics and sports have developed. Some of these techniques have been applied to rehabilitation. Research in aviation and aerospace continues, with some of the latest space research being in immunological responses to microgravity and activity/inactivity. In looking for answers to the CRFS, we can look to the past for ideas. We can establish what did not work and what kinds of research led to dead ends and for what reasons.

For years, I observed fatigue in many patients. It was a symptom usually overlooked or not treated seriously in the patient's history and physical examination. As a clinician, I learned to consider fatigue an important symptom related to environment as well as part of many medical conditions. I had a hunch it required far more attention than it was getting because of its obvious link to quality of life. With fatigue, senses were dulled, concentration was altered, people seemed to be out of balance, and there appeared to be a deficit in overall feelings of well-being.

As I searched the literature and talked with patients, I tried to get a better understanding of this phenomenon. Fatigue appeared to have both positive and negative significance. First, it appeared to be a means by which the body communicated information on the state of being. It seemed to function as a biofeedback mechanism, trying to get through to the conscious mind: "Something is wrong; there is a lack of energy—whether it is mental, emotional, physical, or spiritual." Fatigue repeatedly has been shown to be prodromal to minor illness as well as major disease processes. It can also be a message to slow down. Nearly everyone has said at some point, "I just don't feel right. I feel like I'm coming down with something." Often, fatigue is the symptom of a major medical disorder that brings individuals to see a health care provider. They do not know what is wrong, but know *something* is wrong; they feel they are at the point where they cannot go on.

The relationship between the symptom or syndrome of fatigue and what it can tell us about the state of our body, mind, and spirit is fascinating. For most of my career, I have worked with postoperative patients who have had general and cardiovascular surgery; in addition, I teach registered nurses how to care for this population. I observed that patients who complained of fatigue did not progress as well in their treatment and recovery phase. They appeared to develop more frequent complications, ranging from changes in mental status, especially depression, to physical problems such as infections. This is of particular concern to people with cancer, since many are elderly and also have other significant clinical problems such as heart disease and heart failure, lung disease, rheumatoid arthritis, and diabetes that lead to rapid functional decline. In addition, many people receive a diagnosis of cancer prior to or immediately following surgery. When I began my research on postoperative fatigue over ten years ago, there was little interest in fatigue (Smeeding, 1987). When I tried to find information on clinically related fatigue, I found very few data-based studies in the medical literature. I found most of the research was conducted in the disciplines of aerospace and industry. Hence, most of that research focused on developing research measurement tools and objective measures relevant to unrelated tasks.

As we near the end of this century, clinical science—nursing, medicine, the therapies, nutrition—has just begun to realize the significance of this common, seemingly mundane syndrome of fatigue as an alert to imbalances in mind, body, and spirit.

References

American Psychiatric Association. (1980). *DSM III: Diagnostic and statistical manual of mental disorders.* 3rd ed. Washington, DC: American Psychiatric Association.

Appley, T., and Trumbull, A. (1967). *On the concept of psychological stress.* New York: Appleton-Century-Croft.

Austin, R. (1968). *Air crew fatigue in international jet transport operations.* Department of Supply, Australian Defense Scientific Service, Aeronatical Research Laboratories, Human Engineering.

Bartlett, T. (1943). Psychological criterion of fatigue. In W. F. Floyd and S. T. Welford (Eds.), *Fatigue.* London: H. K. Lewis.

Bartley, S. H. (1965). *Fatigue: Mechanisms and management.* Springfield: Charles C Thomas.

Bartley, S. H., and Chute, E. (1947). *Fatigue and impairment in man.* New York: McGraw-Hill.

Brown, J. R. (1967). Car driving and fatigue. *Triangle, 8,* 131–137.

Cameron, C. (1968). *A questionnaire study of fatigue in civil aircrew.* Department of Supply, Australian Defense Scientific Service, Aeronautical Research Laboratories, Human Engineering.

Cameron, C. (1969). Fatigue in a changing technological environment. In *Proceedings of the Australia and New Zealand Association for the Advancement of Science,* 41st Congress, Section 32.

Cameron, C. (1973). Theory of fatigue. *Ergonomics, 16,* 633–648.

Cannon, W. C. (1984). *The way of an investigator.* New York: W. W. Norton. (Originally published in 1945; rereleased posthumously.)

Christensen, T., Bendix, T., and Kehlet, H. (1982). Fatigue and cardiorespiratory function following abdominal surgery. *British Journal of Surgery, 69,* 417–419.

Davis, H. (1946). The disorganization of behavior in fatigue. *Journal of Neurology and Psychiatry, 9,* 23–29.

Davis, H. (1948). *Pilot error.* London: H.M.S.O.

Dill, B. (1967). The Harvard fatigue laboratory: Its development, contributions and demise. *Circulation Research, 20* (supplement I), 1–161.

Drew, G. C. (1940). An experimental study of mental fatigue. In E. J. Dearnoley and P. S. Warr (Eds.), *Aircrew stress in wartime aviation* (pp. 20–62). New York: Academic Press.

Edwards, T., and Kilpatrick, R. (1948). A technique for the construction of attitude scales. *Journal of Applied Psychology, 32,* 374.

Fehlig, P., and Wahren, J. (1975). Fuel homeostasis in exercise. *New England Journal of Medicine, 239,* 1078–1084.

Friedlander, H. S. (1962). Fatigue as a presenting symptom: Management in general practice. *Current Therapy Research, 4,* 443–449.

Grandjean, E. (1970). Fatigue: Yant Memorial Lecture. *American Industrial Hygiene Association Journal, 5,* 401–441.

Grandjean, E. (1979). Fatigue in industry. *British Journal of Industrial Medicine, 36,* 175–186.

Guyton, A. C. (1981). *Textbook of medical physiology.* 6th ed. Philadelphia: W. B. Saunders.

Hamilton, M. (1982). Symptoms and assessment of depression: 8 + 12. In E. S. Payhil (Ed.), *Handbook of affective disorders* (pp. 45–49). New York: Guilford Press.

Harms, H. E., and Soniat, T. L. L. (1952). The meaning of fatigue. *Nursing Clinics of North America, 36,* 311–317.

Hermansen, L., Hultman, E., and Salten, B. (1967). Muscle glycogen during prolonged severe exercise. *Acta Physiologica Scandinavica, 71,* 129–139.

Hess, W. R. (1948). *The functional organization of the diencephalon.* New York: Grune & Stratton.

Holsti, O. R., Loomba, J. K., and North, R. C. (1968). Content analysis. In G. Lindzey and E. Aronson (Eds.), *The handbook of social psychology* (vol. 11, pp. 562–692). Reading, MA: Addison-Wesley.

Jackson, R. (1958). *Problems in human assessment.* New York: McGraw-Hill.

Jasper, H. (1949). Diffusion projection systems: The integrative action of the thalamic reticular system. *Electroencephalography Clinics of Neurophysiology, 1,* 405.

Jerrett, W. A. (1981). Lethargy in general practice. *Practitioner, 225,* 731–737.

Jouvet, M. (1967). The states of sleep. *Scientific American, 216,* 62.

Kashiwagi, S. (1971). Psychological rating of human fatigue. *Ergonomics, 114,* 17–21.

Kaye, P. (1980). Fatigue: Pervasive problem. *New York State Journal of Medicine, 80,* 1225–1229.

Kinsman, R. A., and Philip, W. C. (Eds.). (1976). Subjective symptomatology during work and fatigue. In *Psychological aspects of work and fatigue* (pp. 336–401). Springfield, IL: Charles C Thomas.

McFarland, R. A. (1971). Fatigue in industry: Understanding fatigue in modern life. *Ergonomics, 14,*10.

McNelly, G. (1976). The development and laboratory validation of a subjective fatigue scale. In J. Jeffers and E. McCormick (Eds.), *Industrial psychology* (pp. 20–40). London: George Allen & Unwin.

Megued, M. A., and Egdahl, R. H. (1977). Neuroendocrine response to operation. In J. D. Harding (Ed.), *Rhoads textbook of surgery: Principles and practice.* 5th ed. Philadelphia: J. B. Lippincott.

Mogoun, H. W. (1946). An inhibitory mechanism in the bulbar reticular formulation. *Journal of Neurophysiology, 9,* 165.

Morrison, F. D. (1980). Fatigue as a presenting complaint in family practice. *Journal of Family Practice, 10,* 795–801.

Moruzzi, G. (1960). Synchronizing influences of the brainstem and the inhibitory mechanism underlying the reduction of sleep by sensory stimulation. *Electroencephalography Clinics of Neurophysiology. 13*(suppl.), 231.

Moruzzi, G., and Majoun, H. W. (1949). Brain stem reticular formation and activation of the EEG. *Electroencephalography Clinics of Neurophysiology 1,* 455.

National Ambulatory Medical Care Survey (1975). *Summary.* Hyattsville, MD: National Center for Health Statistics.

Newsholme, E. A. (1981). The glucose/fatty acid cycle and physical exhaustion in human muscle fatigue: Physiological mechanism. *Pittman Medical Ciba Foundation Symposium, 82,* 89–101.

Nussbaum, H. E. (1963). Chronic fatigue. *Journal of the Medical Society of New Jersey, 60,* 499–503.

Pearson, R. G., and Byars, G. E. (1956). The development and validation of a checklist for measuring subjective fatigue. (Report no. 56-115), School of Aviation, USAF: Randolph AFB, Texas.

Poffenberger, D. (1928). The effects of continuous work upon output and feelings. *Journal of Applied Psychology, 12,* 459.

Rhoten, D. (1982). Fatigue and the postsurgical patient. In C. M. Norris (Ed.), *Concept clarification in nursing* (pp. 277–300). Rockville, MD: Aspen.

Rose, E. A., and King, T. C. (1978). Understanding postoperative fatigue. *Surgery, Gynecology Obstetrics, 147,* 97–102.

Saito, Y., Kogi, R., and Kashiwagi, S. (1970). Factors underlying subjective feelings of fatigue. *Journal of Science and Labor, 46,* 205–224.

Selye, H. (1974). *Stress without distress.* Philadelphia: J.B. Lippincott.

Selye, H. (1976). *The stress of life.* 2nd ed. New York: McGraw-Hill.

Selye, H. (1978). *The stress of life* (revised edition). New York: McGraw-Hill.

Smeeding, S. (1987). "Fatigue concept clarification." Master's thesis, University of Utah College of Nursing, Salt Lake City, Utah.

Solsberg, L. (1984). Lassitude: A preliminary care evaluation. *Journal of the American Medical Association, 251*(24), 3272–3276.

Thurstone, L. L. (1929). *The measurement of attitudes.* Chicago: University of Chicago Press.

Tourney, G. (1970). The severely depressed patient in medical practice. In Merck, Sharp, and Dome (Corporate Eds.), *Depression in medical practice* (pp. 171–191). West Point, PA: West Point.

Vander, S. L. (1980). *Human physiology: The mechanism of body function.* 3rd ed. New York: McGraw-Hill.

Weiser, W., and Stampes, P. (1973). Task-specific symptomatology changes resulting from prolonged submaximal bicycle riding. *Medicine and Science in Sports, 5,* 79.

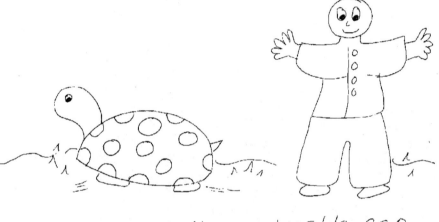

you feel like a turtle can
more faster than you can.

Brenda Heil, 33 years old, 9-year survivor

Psychoneuroimmunology: Foundations for Mind-Body Interaction

Kathryn Ann Caudell

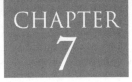

The first thing I'm going to try to do is stand up, if I'm able to. . . .
Astronaut Norman Thagard after nearly four months in orbit

Background

Psychoneuroimmunology (PNI) is a relatively new field of study in which relationships between the psyche, the neuroendocrine system, and the immune system are evaluated. Suggestions about the relationship between health and behavior go back over 2,000 years in Western religion and is a central theme in many world religions. Relationships between health, emotions, and stress have been studied empirically throughout this century by such well-known researchers as Walter B. Cannon (1910s through 1940s) and Hans Selye (1940s through 1970s), as well as many others. However, their attempts to identify mechanistic links were hampered by a lack of equipment and techniques that could measure the necessary neurohumoral-immunological factors and compare them with results of established psychological tests.

The first paper that attempted to theoretically integrate the relationships between stress, emotion, and immunological dysfunction with physical and mental disease was published in 1964 by Solomon and Moss. The authors discussed similarities that had been discovered between personality factors and the diseases of cancer and autoimmunity. At this point, researchers began to question the idea that cancer and autoimmunity might be linked to immune deficiency states and that certain diseases appeared to be the result of pathophysiology resulting from emotional disturbances.

The breakthrough in PNI occurred approximately 30 years ago when cell biologists and immunologists discovered the existence of similar cell surface receptors for a number of substances including hormones and white blood cells. Advancements in the field of neurophysiology led to discoveries that the central nervous system (CNS) actively innervates a number of lymphoid tissues throughout the body. This research excited scientists: Now there were highly controlled laboratory studies that provided strong evidence for a communication between the neuroendocrine system and the immune system. Further research found that several of the neuroendocrine hormones demonstrated immunomodulatory function.

Current PNI research investigates the influence of psychosocial factors on neuroendocrine and immune function, and the efficacy of various biobehavioral interventions in reducing maladaptive neuroendocrine and immune responses to stressful situations. Because of the broad scope of investigation that PNI encompasses, it is not surprising that other areas of study including psychology, behavioral medicine, neuroscience, endocrinology, and immunology are subsumed under the PNI umbrella. This chapter focuses on PNI, specifically stress, neuroendocrine responses to stressful external and internal stimuli, immune function, the bidirectional communication between the neuroendocrine and immune systems, the psychological factors that mediate the responses, and biobehavioral interventions that facilitate adaptation to stressful environments.

Stress

Stress is a popular and ubiquitous word in our society. It seems every ill is blamed on stress. Its alleged incidence is so high that stress-management programs are increasingly being offered and touted as a necessary component of preventive health. Bookstores carry a plethora of stress-reduction and self-help books, and several universities and private physicians publish newsletters focusing on ways to reduce stress and improve one's well-being. Historically, stress was characterized as part of basic survival needs, that is, getting enough food, safety from predators, and other more physical fundamentals of existence. Today, it appears to focus more on psychosocial issues, such as family and work relationships, and dealing with changes in technology.

One of the most significant reasons why the stress literature is confusing is that there have been so many inconsistencies in definitions associated with it. Definitions of *stress* have variously included (1) the generalized response of the organism to environmental demands (Selye, 1936), (2) a disturbance of homeostasis resulting from internal and/or external situations (Cannon, 1932), and (3) "an extraordinary demand on physiological or psychological defenses with concomitant responses of neuroendocrine systems to the external elicitor" (Solomon and Amkraut, 1981).

Despite the variations in definitions used to describe the phenomenon, it is hypothesized that the degree of physiological response to the initiating stimulus is mediated by vari-

About the Contributor

Kathryn Ann Caudell knew from the beginning that there were two things she didn't want to do: Be a nurse and teach. Working for several years as a nursing assistant on a high-risk obstetrics/gynecology unit peaked her interest in physiology. One day, she was temporarily assigned to the oncology unit. That was it: She was hooked. After graduating with a bachelor's of science in nursing from the University of Arizona, she moved to California where she worked in a bone marrow transplant unit and received her masters in 1987. The 35-mile-per-day round-trip commute on a California interstate "parking lot" in rush hour inspired an interest in how the body and mind respond to stress (psychoneuroimmunology). Combining

ables such as social support, coping style, mood, and personality factors (Lazarus and Folkman, 1984). In addition, how different individuals perceive the stressor can result in vastly different neuroendocrine responses (Frankenhaeuser, 1975). For the purpose of this chapter, the evoking stressful stimulus will be defined as a *stressor;* the response, as the *stress response;* and the factors that influence the response, as *mediators.*

Evaluation of the effects of stressors in humans is particularly challenging due to the numerous characterizations of stressors and their variability in duration. Stressors have been categorized according to their duration (acute or chronic) and type (daily hassles, major life events, psychological, and physiological). Furthermore, depending on the event, an initial acute stressor may become more long term. For example, the suspicion and subsequent diagnosis of cancer are initially devastating and frequently result in a myriad of immediate physical and emotional responses. After the cancer treatment is underway, the individual may begin to habituate to the treatment, but now is faced with learning to cope with symptom distress and changes in family and professional roles.

Effects of Stress on Psychophysiological Responses

A wide range of stressors can induce maladaptive psychoneuroimmune responses. The physiological responses differ depending on whether the stressor is acute or chronic in nature and the way in which the person copes or adapts to the stressor. This section first discusses the neuroendocrine system and the stress response, followed by specific responses that have been observed according to the temporal duration of the stressor.

Neuroendocrine System

The neuroendocrine system generally functions in a homeostatic manner that acts as an alarm system when individuals are exposed to real or perceived physical or mental stressors. The sympathetic nervous system (SNS) functions to assist individuals in improving alertness and physical prowess so they are able to effectively deal with the stressful event. When individuals are exposed to a stressor, a series of endocrine responses occurs as a result of SNS activation. These endocrine responses are mediated by specific cell populations

studies in the University of Washington's premiere nursing physiology program with work in the laboratory of a renowned immunology researcher led to Ann's dissertation research, which addressed natural killer cell activity (an immune indicator) with women's response to an acute stressor (1993). She is currently developing relaxation interventions using advanced technology. She is a person of many talents and interests. Her passion is dry-climate landscape gardening; in addition, she and her husband built the first "strawbale" construction home in New Mexico (R value of 2½ per square inch)!

located in the hypothalamus that exercise control over the two major SNS axes, the sympathetic-adrenal-medullary axis and the pituitary-adrenal-cortical axis. The hypothalamic efferent neurons stimulate the adrenal medulla to secrete both epinephrine and norepineprhine (in smaller amounts) and the sympathetic postganglionic neurons to secrete norepinephrine. Norepinephrine and epinephrine function to shunt peripherally pooled blood into the central circulation via vasoconstriction, increase heart rate and contractility, and through selective vasoconstriction, distribute blood to critical organs such as the heart, skeletal muscle, and brain.

Stressor = the evoking stressful stimulus (i.e., the thing that causes stress)

Stress response = how the person reacts (internally and externally)

Mediator = the factor(s) that influence the response and how it will be perceived

At the same time, specialized neurosecretory cells in the hypothalamus secrete neuropeptides such as corticotropin-releasing hormone into the hypophyseal portal system, a vascular network between the hypothalamus and the anterior pituitary. These neuropeptides then modulate the secretion of pituitary hormones such as adrenocorticotropic hormone (ACTH) into the circulation where they affect the activity of other organs. For example, ACTH modulates corticotrophs in the adrenal cortex to secrete cortisol and other related hormones (Madden and Felten, 1995) (see Figure 7-1). Cortisol functions to increase the

| Figure 7.1 | **Stress Response Pathways: The Hypothalamic–Pituitary–Adrenal (HPA) and the Sympathetic–Adrenal–Medullary (SAM) Axes** |

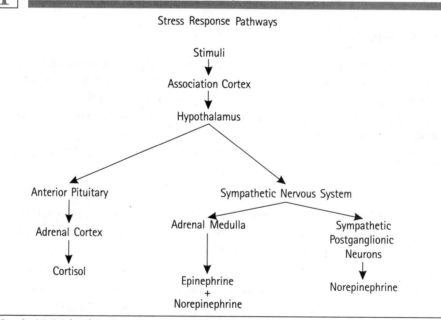

Source: From Caudell, K. A. (1996). Psychoneuroimmunology and innovative behavioral interventions in patients with leukemia. *Oncology Nursing Form, 23,* 494. Used with permission from Oncology Nursing Society.

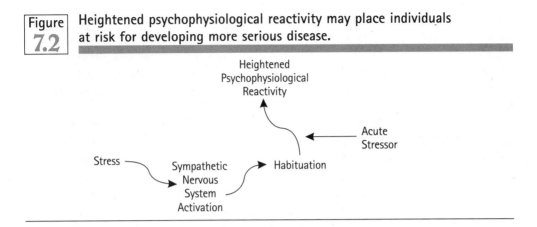

Figure 7.2 Heightened psychophysiological reactivity may place individuals at risk for developing more serious disease.

breakdown of glycogen and some tissue protein, while suppressing the activity of other hormones and organs such as growth hormone, insulin, the thyroid, and gonads, all of which assist in providing more energy to the individual.

If exposure to the stressor becomes more long term, the physiological responses change from the more acute response to one of habituation. Increased pulse and sweat rates may gradually resolve and be replaced by increased basal muscle tension. The problem occurs when individuals in this state are then exposed to an acute stressor: They may respond in an exaggerated way and have difficulty returning to the prestress state of relaxation. Often they will exhibit higher blood pressures, sweat rates, respiratory rates (Stoyva and Budzynski, 1993) and epinephrine levels (Pike et al, 1997) when compared to non-stressed individuals (see Figure 7-2). This physiological reactivity may place individuals at risk for developing more serious diseases such as high blood pressure or cancer.

Bidirectional Communication Between the Immune and Neuroendocrine Systems

How does stress cause alterations in immune function? A number of mechanisms support a bidirectional communication between the neuroendocrine and immune systems. Receptors for a variety of hormones such as cortisol, epinephrine, and norepinephrine are found on the cell surface of lymphocytes. The distribution and migration of monocytes tend to be influenced by hormones that are secreted in response to emotions. For example, monocyte and lymphocyte levels are inversely correlated with a person's anxiety and depression levels (Landmann et al, 1991).

ACTH as an Immunosuppressor

ACTH suppresses antibody and interferon-α synthesis. Many neuroendocrine peptides have immunoregulatory activities. Several peptides have suppressive actions on white blood cells, antibodies, and cytokines. For instance, ACTH causes suppression of immunoglobulin and interferon-γ synthesis. Others have beneficial actions such as the enhancement of cytotoxic T cells by growth hormone. In addition, various chemical mediators secreted by white blood cells possess hormonal functions. Interferon-α leads to elevated levels of plasma cortisol. This finding indicates that interferon-α may directly affect the adrenal cortex (Blalock, 1989).

Cells of the immune system produce some hormones. For example, lymphocytes synthesize ACTH, growth hormone, and prolactin. Helper T cells produce enkephalins and thyroid-stimulating hormone. Researchers characterized the molecular weights, cellular morphology, and function of these hormones and discovered that most were similar to the hormones produced by the endocrine system. Immunomodulatory substances such as cytokines are synthesized by certain hormones, and cells of the immune system exhibit hormone-type functions. For example, interferon-α and -γ induce steroid synthesis in the adrenal medulla whereas interleuken-1 and -2 can cause the pituitary gland to release ACTH and endorphins.

In summary, there is a bidirectional communication between the neuroendocrine and immune systems. Although there is a relationship between stressors and immune function that is mediated by neuroendocrine processes, these relationships are complex. It will be many years before the details of these relationships are elucidated. To complicate the picture, it seems these relationships can be influenced by psychosocial factors.

Acute Stressors

Space Flight

Numerous investigators have examined the influence of acute stress on human immune function in an attempt to understand the pathophysiology of human disease. The space programs in various countries have provided wonderful opportunities to study the effects of acute stressors on healthy individuals. During the Apollo spaceflight program, the National Aeronautics and Space Administration (NASA) included temporal examinations of immune function in their medical evaluation of the astronauts. Blood samples obtained before takeoff, during flight, and immediately after splashdown revealed decreased lymphocyte transformation in response to mitogens, elevated overall white blood cell counts, and increased absolute numbers of polymorphonuclear leukocytes on the day of splashdown (Kimzey, 1975). In addition, neuroendocrine measures also were elevated on the day of splashdown, indicating that the day of splashdown was apparently stressful for the astronauts (Leach and Rambaut, 1974). Immune function under conditions of space flight and microgravity is an ongoing area of study that promises to yield practical outcomes in understanding stress and disease.

Laboratory Stressors

Other clinical laboratory studies that involved exposing subjects to experimental stressors such as sleep deprivation and loud noise during various tasks discovered that interferon production increased, phagocytosis decreased transiently, and lymphoblast transformation was depressed following sleep deprivation. No changes were observed in granulocyte adherence and leukocyte alkaline phosphatase activity (Palmblad et al, 1979). The results indicate that *timing* and *duration* of exposure to stressors are important to consider when attempting to determine the nature of stress-induced immune dysfunction. In addition, various types of experimentally induced stressors most likely produce different neuroendocrine and immune responses.

Examination Stressors

A few studies investigated the relationships between neuroendocrine and immune responses to examination stress. Kiecolt-Glaser and colleagues (1984) examined the immunocompetence of medical students during final examinations. Specimens were drawn one month prior to and after the examinations. Natural killer cell (NKC) numbers were quantified by examining the number of larger granular lymphocytes and the number of cells expressing a NKC surface antigen. The total numbers of NKCs decreased from the sample taken before examinations to the postexamination sample. NKC cytotoxic activity, as examined in the chromium release assay, also declined significantly from the preexamination sample to the postexamination sample. These studies demonstrated that examinations produced decreases in total T-lymphocyte numbers, T4/T8 ratios, mitogen responsiveness, interferon-γ production, and the ability of the cellular immune system to maintain herpesviruses in a latent state.

McClelland, Ross, and Patel (1985) examined salivary immunoglobulin A (IgA) and norepinephrine levels in students experiencing examination stress. Salivary samples were taken immediately after the examination and 1¾ hours after the examination. The subjects gave an additional sample several days after the examination day that provided baseline data during a period in which they were relaxed. Increases in both norepinephrine and salivary IgA were observed in both of the postexamination samples. However, the correlation between the increase in norepinephrine and salivary IgA from baseline to examination time was very low ($r = .09$). On the other hand, the increase in norepinephrine from the immediate postexamination measurement to the 1¾-hour measurement was associated with a greater decline in salivary IgA at the same measurement times. It was postulated that another hormonal mechanism was responsible for the increase in salivary IgA levels. The investigators suggested that increased adrenergic output may lower immune function by stimulating adrenergic receptors on B lymphocytes, which subsequently depresses their functional capacity.

Cancer Diagnosis

The *diagnosis* of cancer is also sufficient to induce alterations in immune function. One hundred sixteen women diagnosed with stage II or III invasive breast cancer and who underwent surgery were invited to participate in a study examining the stress of diagnosis on immune function (Andersen et al, 1998). Prior to the beginning of chemotherapy, each subject completed a questionnaire designed to determine stress levels. Based on the scores, the women were categorized as either high stress or low stress. The investigators examined the extent of NKC demise and their response to interferon gamma in addition to T-lymphocyte responsiveness to the mitogens phytohemagglutinin and concanavalin A and to monoclonal antibodies. Women placed in the high-stress category exhibited 15.4% greater destruction of NKCs, a 20.1% lower response of NKCs to interferon gamma, and a 19.8% lower T-lymphocyte response to the mitogens and monoclonal antibodies. This study represents one of the largest stress and immunity studies to date that demonstrates the emotional and immunological threat posed by the diagnosis of cancer. This is a critical area that demands more investigation. Is there a way we can make this devastating experience less threatening? Is there a way we can provide a more supportive environment and buffer the stress? This obviously warrants further research.

Chronic Stressors

Many studies have used various paradigms to examine the meaning of physiological responses to acute stress. Several studies, however, were based on chronic stressors. *Chronic stress* has been defined as "demands, threats, perceived harm or loss, or responses that persist for long periods of time" (Baum, 1990). This definition suggests that the perceived loss or harm can continue to elicit responses in animals or humans long after the specific event has terminated. This is supported by studies that examined physiological responses to the loss of a loved one, to a nuclear power plant disaster, and to crowded living situations.

Bereavement

Bereavement, characterized as the psychological, physiological, and behavioral responses to the loss of someone or something that is valued, can be anticipatory, acute, or chronic. Several studies have exemplified the long-term effects of bereavement on immune function in grieving family members. For example, lymphocyte responsivity to mitogens declines significantly within a month or two after the death of a spouse, and, in some cases, these responses remain low for up to one year (Irwin et al, 1987; Schleifer et al, 1983).

Nuclear Plant Disaster

The destruction of a nuclear core at the Three Mile Island (TMI) nuclear plant in 1979 induced a variety of concerns in the residents living in the vicinity of the plant. The accident involved the release of radioactive gas and water, potentially exposing individuals living close to the plant. Exposure to radiation instills a great deal of fear and apprehension in people because of the known illness and death associated with radiation exposure at Hiroshima, Nagasaki, and Chernobyl. Furthermore, mismanagement of information given to residents during the incident, loss of privacy due to increased news media coverage, and the evacuation of pregnant women and small children added to the threat of the incident (Baum, 1990).

Individuals living within five miles of the plant exhibited higher urinary concentrations of epinephrine and fewer B lymphocytes, cytotoxic T cells, and NKCs (McKinnon et al, 1989). They also performed more poorly on tasks and reported more symptoms than did control subjects living 80 miles away during periods in which the trapped radioactive gases were released from the containment building (Baum, Gatchel, and Schaeffer, 1983). Data continued to be collected during the 1980s. A surprising finding was that the reporting of symptoms, poor task performance, and elevated catecholamine levels remained consistently elevated in the TMI residents through 1985. The same group also exhibited higher blood pressure, had more health complaints, and purchased more prescriptions.

Crowding

The effect of crowding has also been examined in both humans and animals. Individuals living for extended periods in crowded neighborhoods and those living in uncrowded neighborhoods were examined for symptoms of stress, urinary catecholamine levels, and cardiovascular reactivity. Subjects were given a task to perform in their home. Heart rate, blood pressure, and 24-hour urine samples were assessed as well. Crowded residents exhibited higher catecholamine levels, lower baseline heart rates, and greater increases in heart rate and blood pressure in response to the task. They also reported more bothersome symptoms than did the uncrowded control subjects. This dramatic study indicated that chronically stressed individuals exhibit a more heightened reactivity in response to novel stressors than do individuals who do not experience a high level of chronic stress (Fleming et al, 1987).

Our modern health care system, in its self-absorbed quest for high-technology treatments, has sacrificed the very thing that people have known for thousands of years as the key to recovery: quality rest and periodic privacy.

These findings about crowding may have significance for the hospital and outpatient treatment of people with cancer. The constant disturbance and noise, the invasion of privacy, and threats to intimacy during times of crisis should be considered and minimized as much as possible. Our modern health care system, in its self-absorbed quest for high-technology treatments, has sacrificed the very thing that people have known for thousands of years as the key to recovery: quality rest and periodic privacy. We need to examine what environments are optimal to promoting healing and give patients choices when they need to have protected quiet and uninterrupted time. Patients frequently comment they need to go home to get some rest!

Disease

Few studies have examined the effect of chronic disease symptomatology on neuroendocrine and immune function. One such study investigated individuals hospitalized for psychiatric illness. Kiecolt-Glaser, Ricker, and George (1984), in a study examining loneliness in psychiatric inpatients, found that patients who exhibited higher loneliness scores and described themselves as more distressed had significantly higher urinary cortisol levels, lower levels of NKC activity, and poorer T-lymphocyte responses to the mitogen phytohemagglutinin.

Another population experiencing a chronic and potentially fatal disorder are those infected with the human immunodeficiency virus (HIV). Individuals who perceive they are at a greater risk of developing acquired immunodeficiency syndrome (AIDS) as a result of previous sexual or drug use behaviors exhibit higher levels of psychological and social distress. Many of these individuals also have lost friends and partners because of AIDS and experience repeated bereavements.

As mentioned earlier, bereavement is commonly associated with immunosuppression. In addition to this, individuals with HIV infection also face active discrimination in employment, housing, insurance eligibility (Ostrow, Grant, and Atkinson, 1988), and rejection from family and friends. These changes in life events and health certainly constitute a chronic stressor.

A study by Kemeny and colleagues (1994) examined both HIV seropositive and seronegative males and grouped them according to whether they were bereaving the loss of loved ones or friends. No differences in immune parameters were observed between the bereaved and the nonbereaved subjects. However, a depressed mood in the HIV-seropositive nonbereaved males was strongly associated with lower lymphocyte proliferative responses, fewer CD4 (helper) T cells, and a greater number of CD8 (suppressor) T cells. Depressed mood in the seropositive bereaved group, however, was not associated with immune parameters. The investigators hypothesized that depression may be a cofactor in some HIV-positive men that contributes to the variable decline in CD4 cells and the progression to AIDS.

The suspicion of and subsequent diagnosis of cancer are usually very stressful for the person with cancer and family members. Treatment and changes in the person's professional as well as family roles add to this stress and often lead to a chronic stress response (Lazarus and Folkman, 1984; Post-White, 1998). Depression is one of the most frequently experienced effects during the course of cancer diagnosis and treatment and has also been associated with immune dysfunction. It is possible that the emotional, cognitive, and behavioral responses of an individual to a stressor may play a potential role in the development of cancer. An endocrine pathway may mediate the development of some cancers, such as breast cancer. Given this, it may be likely that psychophysiological responses that are hormonally mediated may be associated with certain cancer outcomes (Heiden and Levy,

1991). At present we must be cautious about making assumptions about individuals from studies on groups. There is still a strong social stigma as well as punitive treatment by many third-party payers associated with the diagnosis and treatment of psychiatric disorders such as depression.

Psychological Mediators

A number of psychological variables influence neuroendocrine and immune responses. The way in which a person responds depends on the perception or appraisal of the stressor, and the ability of the person to effectively cope with, adapt to, or completely eliminate the stressor (Lazarus and Folkman, 1984; Post-White, 1998).

Appraisal

According to Lazarus and Folkman (1984), when people are exposed to stressors, they immediately evaluate or appraise if and how the stressor affects their well-being. The appraisal of a stressor directly affects the neuroendocrine response. Frankenhaeuser (1975) found that individuals who performed a self-paced task secreted elevated amounts of catecholamines. Those who were instructed to perform the task within a time frame secreted higher amounts of cortisol. These findings demonstrate that those who felt time pressure and perhaps a loss of control exhibited different neuroendocrine responses than did those without time restrictions. Others also found significant correlations between helplessness and elevated cortisol levels (Breier, Albus, and Wolkowitz, 1991).

Norepinephrine is released from the sympathetic postganglionic neuron terminals in response to exercise and to certain stress tests in which expenditure of effort is required. Its release is not typically related to the emotional connotation of the challenge (Lovallo et al, 1990). In contrast, in response to mental stress tests where the competency of the individual is threatened or at stake, epinephrine, which is synthesized and released from the adrenal medulla, is more commonly released in higher amounts than norepinephrine. Therefore, a strong emotional component is associated with the stressor. For example, epinephrine levels were elevated in interns who gave lectures to experienced and critical audiences. The stressor in this situation was one in which the competency or adequacy of the physician was questioned (Dimsdale and Moss, 1980). Data from both animal and clinical human studies suggest that stressors that require physical effort result in the secretion of catecholamines such as epinephrine. In contrast, subjects who experience distress and loss of control demonstrate comparatively more cortisol excretion (Hennessy et al, 1979).

When an animal perceives a stimulus as *relevant*, contrasting types of responses occur and are associated with the concepts of challenge and defeat. It is suggested that the hippocampus, contained in the limbic system, functions as a cognitive mapping system. When a discontinuity occurs between the animal's current perception of its position or rank in the environment and its stored representation of the environment, ACTH is secreted. This occurs when the animal loses control of its position in its social hierarchy. ACTH enables the animal to rapidly learn new information, which will update the existing cognitive map into one that will be more suitable for the current situation (Henry, 1992).

If the animal, on the other hand, perceives the stimulus as a *threat* to its control, the amygdala is activated, resulting in defense response behaviors such as aggression. Amygdalar activation leads to activation of the sympathetic-adrenal-medullary system and is characterized by elevations in both norepinephrine and epinephrine levels with no change in corticosterone levels (Henry, 1992). Based on this collection of information, it appears that if an animal maintains control of its environment and social interrelationships, the pathophysiological impact of stress is minimized.

When developing patient, family, and health care provider education programs, facilitate an environment of contextual relevance and minimize threat and the learning environment will be optimized. When patients, family, or staff are embarrassed, exhausted, or having trouble focusing, it is not a good time for education. We often try to cram information about drugs, side effects, and schedules into patients who are already fatigued as a result of their clinic visit and treatment.

The appraisal of an event also affects several aspects of the individual stress response. For instance, Turner, Clancy, and Vitaliano (1987) observed that individuals' appraisals of their pain problems were significantly associated with the way in which they coped with the pain. If individuals accepted the pain and did not feel that the pain should restrict their activities, they were more likely to utilize problem-focused coping. These data may suggest that individuals' initial appraisal affects not only their physiological response but also the coping strategies they select to utilize. Unfortunately, as individuals experience increased and debilitating fatigue, it is common to hear clinical reports of how their customary coping strategies require too much energy and their pain becomes increasingly overwhelming. By maintaining patients' functional status and minimizing potential loss, we may contribute to keeping other symptoms under control.

After individuals determine the significance of an event on their well-being, the available resources or coping strategies to manage the event will be evaluated. *Coping* is an adaptive process that attempts to manage, reduce, or eliminate a stressful demand placed on an individual. Coping strategies are usually driven by context in that they are based on the type of stressor and the situations associated with them (Bush, 1998). According to Lazarus and Folkman (1984), coping strategies are primarily problem focused or emotion focused. *Problem-based strategies* are used if individuals want to direct their efforts at eliminating or managing the specific event. *Emotion-based strategies* are those used to manage emotional reactions to the event.

The type of coping style used also depends on the person's stable personality traits and the coping resources the person has. For example, a person's optimism and locus of control influence the type of coping style used (Somerfield and Curbow, 1992). Coping is also thought to be characterized as a trait in which the style becomes a pattern of coping for the person, or a process that is used to manage a specific stressful event (Bush, 1988). This process tends to vary according to the diverse adaptational significance and the associated demands or concerns (Heim, Valach, and Schaffner, 1997).

Impaired cognitive functioning, often described as "foggy thinking," and threats to emotion-based strategies such as the emotional lability (very much a type of very-rapid-cycling bipolar behavior) often experienced with treatment, disease progression, anemia, and fatigue seriously challenges functioning. Most individuals have limited prior experience applying practiced coping strategies and styles to the multiple problems related to the cancer experience. Even in individuals with multiple recurrences (such as with non-Hodgkin's lymphoma), the recurrence creates doubt about the effectiveness of prior coping strategies. Fatigue in the cancer experience leaves people with less free (cognitively and emotionally unencumbered) energy when they most need it.

Coping styles influence neuroendocrine and immune responses in both animals and humans. Depending on the coping style, individuals experiencing stress may practice poor health behaviors such as smoking, poor diets, or poor sleeping habits that can affect immunocompetence (Cohen, 1994). Conversely, they may become involved in activities that have known beneficial effects in reducing SNS arousal and that may subsequently have indirect effects on immune function such as relaxation (Holland et al, 1991) and imagery (Post-White, 1991).

Personality Variables

It has long been thought that personality characteristics moderate the relation between stress and the development of disease. Studies in which the probands (proband refers to a person with an illness or disorder who is part of a group, usually a family, who is the focus of a study of hereditary and genetic factors to determine if others of the family are carriers or have the disorder) were followed over a ten-year period found that personality variables were much more predictive of death from cancer or cardiovascular disease than was smoking. Furthermore, those susceptible to one of these two diseases were characterized by a certain personality type (Eysenck, 1988). *Personality type* was defined in terms of different ways of dealing with interpersonal stress. The study found that stress was a potent contributor to mortality in that the stressed probands had a 49% higher death rate than did the nonstressed probands.

Personality factors have also been associated with the onset of autoimmune disease. Individuals with rheumatoid arthritis, for instance, have been found to be restricted in expression of emotion, self-sacrificing, sensitive to criticism, and rigid. The onset of an autoimmune disease often followed either a period of psychological stress or interruption of the ability to maintain previous patterns of defense and adaptation (Solomon and Amkraut, 1981). Stress and failure of psychological defenses coupled with psychological distress are frequently observed in many diseases associated with dysfunction of the immune system.

Social Support

Kennedy, Kiecolt-Glaser, and Glaser (1988) suggested that interpersonal resources such as supportive interpersonal relationships may contribute to enhanced immune function and thus may have an impact on health. Persons maintaining satisfactory support networks may experience fewer health consequences when exposed to stressful events, in comparison with those who demonstrated limited or inadequate social networks.

Social support also strongly mediates the development of cancer in a number of populations. In an early review of 75 studies on psychological factors associated with the development of cancer, LeShan (1959) discovered that the most consistently documented, significant psychological factors present prior to the first noted symptoms of neoplasm were the loss of a major emotional relationship. The same investigator followed this report with a large epidemiological study that evaluated mortality rates among different groups of people (LeShan, 1966). Based on the results from this study, LeShan successfully predicted that cancer mortality rates would be higher for widowed and divorced people and lower for married and single people.

Two more recent studies corroborated the beneficial effects of social relationships on survival. A seminal study by Speigel and colleagues (1989) discovered that women with advanced breast cancer who had social support incorporated into a multicomponent intervention survived an average of 36 months, while women who did not participate in a support group lived for 18.9 months. Fawzy and Fawzy (1994) investigated the effects of a short-term group intervention for malignant melanoma patients that contained health education, stress management, coping instruction, and psychological support. They found that those who participated in the support-group component experienced a statistically significant higher survival rate than did those who did not.

What about patients who are too fatigued to participate? Many have no energy to participate in an additional activity, or they are limited by family responsibilities. Speigel and colleagues did not examine functional status or role demands that would limit social activity and be a confounding variable. Interventions for those who cannot participate in groups and who may have limited family support may include using electronic mail, Internet "chat" groups, or telephone support.

Mood

Disturbances in mood result from ineffective coping as well as alterations in neuroendocrine and immune function. For example, the relationship between loneliness, cortisol, and immune dysfunction was examined in hospitalized psychiatric inpatients (Kiecolt-Glaser, Ricker, and George, 1984). Patients who had high values on the University of

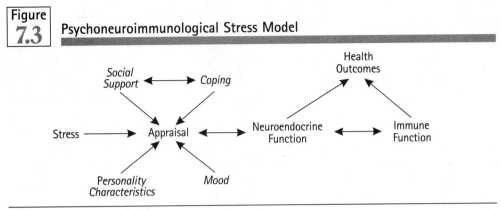

Figure 7.3 Psychoneuroimmunological Stress Model

California at Los Angeles Loneliness Scale exhibited significantly higher urine and plasma cortisol levels than did those who had lower loneliness values. The high-loneliness patients also had lower NKC cytotoxicity and poor T-lymphocyte responses to the mitogen phytohemagglutin in and reported higher amounts of distress than did the low-loneliness group.

Depression has also been correlated with several parameters of immune dysfunction. Schleifer and colleagues (1985) observed suppressed lymphocyte reactivity in depressed patients, and the degree of immune suppression was associated with the severity of depression. Irwin and colleagues (1987) discovered that NKC activity was significantly lower in patients hospitalized for major depression.

Social support, coping, personality factors, and mood are suggested to be major variables that influence how an individual perceives and responds to stressful events. The extent to which these variables influence a person's appraisal of an event and the subsequent psychophysiological responses is unknown. Nonetheless, relationships between these variables have been observed in a number of studies and should be considered as possible mediators between stress and physiological responses (Figure 7-3).

Measurement Issues

A number of variables affect both the function and the measurement of the neuroendocrine and immune systems. Some of these, such as gender, age, and genetics, are innate and unchangeable, whereas others are related to behavior.

Innate Variables

At birth, the immune system is immature and characterized by small levels of immunoglobulins that are able to confer resistance to bacteria and other harmful microbes.

Immunocompetence is acquired through continued exposure to a variety of antigens (Abbas, Lichtman, and Pober, 1995). Conversely, aging affects immunocompetence via the natural involution of the thymus gland, resulting in increasing suppression of cell-mediated immunity by the fifth decade of life. The immune system loses between 5% and 30% of its original capacity over an individual's lifetime (Haddy, 1987). Individuals over 50 years old tend to secrete higher levels of norepinephrine than do younger individuals (Aslan et al, 1981; Ziegler, Lake, and Kopin, 1976).

There appear to be differences in catecholamine levels between men and women and across the age span during resting and challenge states. Data from several studies indicate that women secrete lower levels of epinephrine than do men in response to cognitive laboratory testing (Aslan et al, 1981; Ziegler, 1989). Menstrual cycle also influences plasma and urine levels of norepinephrine, with higher levels occurring in the luteal phase compared to the follicular phase (Leibenluft, Fiero, and Rubinow, 1994).

Gender may play a role in the development of certain autoimmune diseases. The incidence of Graves' disease, autoimmune thyroiditis, rheumatoid arthritis, and systemic lupus erythematosus (SLE) is higher in women than men. Variations in gender-specific hormones may precipitate or exacerbate some diseases. For instance, the incidence of rheumatoid arthritis in women taking oral contraceptives may be half that in those who do not, and during pregnancy rheumatoid arthritis has been observed to go into remission (Turiel and Wingard, 1985). Although the mechanisms underlying these observations are unknown, the existence of a bidirectional communication between pituitary hormones, gonadal steroids, thymic hormones, and components of the immune system makes it feasible for these hormones to influence the development of various autoimmune disorders (Grossman, 1984).

Both genetics and a shared environment can place family members at risk for developing the same disease. Sørenson and colleagues (1988), in a prospective study, examined the deaths of adoptive children and their biological and adoptive parents. The adopted children who had at least one biological parent die before the age of 50 exhibited mortality rates 1.7 and 1.8 times higher than those whose two biological parents were alive. The death of an adoptive parent had no effect on the children's mortality rates. The most significant finding was that if the biological parent died from an infection before the age of 50, the mortality rate of the adoptee increased fivefold. This finding indicates that the strength of the immune system is likely genetically determined.

The secretion and activity of several neuroendocrine peptides and lymphocytes are influenced by circadian rhythms. For example, ACTH is secreted in irregular bursts throughout the 24-hour day and plasma cortisol levels tend to parallel these bursts. In humans the bursts occur more frequently during the night, and peak levels of both ACTH and cortisol normally occur in the morning between 5:00 and 9:00.

Two studies in human and murine models demonstrated rhythmic variations of the immune system (Cove-Smith et al, 1978; Lee et al, 1977). In rats, the maximum activity of a delayed hypersensitivity response occurred at the beginning of the light phase when corticosterone levels were the lowest.

Another study examined cortisol and lymphocyte subpopulation levels in peripheral blood samples taken from healthy males every three hours. The lowest total lymphocyte numbers occurred at 10:00 AM, three hours after cortisol values peaked at 7:00 AM. While the evening peak and trough levels did not neatly follow the precise three-hour lag as did the morning levels, the highest numbers of lymphocytes were observed between 7:00 PM and 10:00 PM while the lowest cortisol levels occurred at 10:00 PM. Nevertheless, it is conceivable that the redistribution of cortisol in various compartments and tissues in the body requires a certain time lag before effects on circulating lymphocytes are observed (Dammacco et al, 1984).

It has long been suggested that hospitals arrange to have patients undergo surgery at a time of day when their bodies would have the greatest neurohormonal advantage. Unfortunately, surgical schedules are set by quite different factors than the well-being of patients!

Age, gender, genetics, and circadian rhythms are all factors that introduce variability in the measurement of stress responses. While PNI investigators have little control over altering the effect of these factors on hormonal and immune measurement, they can control for their influence in research studies methodologically and statistically.

Influential Variables

A number of behaviors affect the immune system's function. For instance, sleep deprivation can cause depressed neutrophil function, decreased lymphocyte response to the mitogen phytohemagglutinin, and decreased phagocytosis by polymorphonuclear granulocytes (Palmblad et al, 1979). Deficits in both calorie and protein intake can also affect immunocompetence. For example, cell-mediated immune dysfunction commonly results from protein-calorie malnutrition. Thymic hormone synthesis is impaired, thereby potentially altering T-cell regulation and differentiation (Chandra, 1980). Prolonged fasting impairs the chemotactic activity of neutrophils (Turiel and Wingard, 1985). Inadequate vitamin and mineral intake can cause significant alterations in immune function. For instance, vitamin A and B_6 deficiencies alter T-cell and B-cell functions. Vitamin B_6 catalyzes the biosynthesis of nucleic acids, which may explain the reduction in the number and function of both T and B lymphocytes. T-lymphocyte and neutrophil functions are also greatly affected by iron deficiencies (Lahita et al, 1984).

Cigarette smoking also depresses lymphocyte responses to several mitogens and may increase the mitotic rate in cytotoxic T cells (Petersen, Steimel, and Callaghan, 1983; Holmen et al, 1995). While these findings indicate both suppressive and stimulating effects on the immune system, they support the notion that cigarette smoking induces alterations in cell-mediated immunity.

Exercise produces physiological responses very similar to those resulting from psychosocial stress. Exercise can either enhance or suppress immune function. For instance, ß-endorphin, catecholamine, and glucocorticoid levels increase with exercise (Howlett et al, 1984). Catecholamines influence lymphocyte migration, which may explain the observations that some long-distance runners have elevations in blood leukocyte levels (Shinkai et al, 1992). Granulocyte (Davidson et al, 1987) and NKC numbers and activity (Sevier, 1994) also increase during exercise. These responses are thought to be mediated by the increase in epinephrine released during exercise, which results in a release of lymphocytes from reserve pools located in the lungs, liver, and spleen (Eichner and Calabrese, 1994).

> *Smoking, exercise, sleep, and diet can potentially influence neuroendocrine and immune function. This is of particular importance for the person who is experiencing chronic stress, has a preexisting immune dysfunction from an autoimmune disease, or has a chronic infection such as with HIV.*

Hall and colleagues (1998) investigated the relationships among bereavement-related depression, intrusive thoughts, sleep disturbance, and immune function. The subjects who scored higher on intrusive thoughts exhibited lower numbers of NKCs and greater time awake during the first phase of non–rapid eye movement sleep. Although there was no significant association between intrusion scores and functional NKC measures, the data suggest that electroencephalographic sleep disruptions are associated with immune function in humans.

Assay Factors

Catecholamine measurement can be affected by a number of situations that may influence the degree to which they are secreted or that interfere with the laboratory assays. For example, a number of stimuli including rising from sleep, eating a meal, smoking, drinking coffee, and copulation trigger the secretion of catecholamines. Catecholamines are also released in response to emotional stimuli. For example, Baum, Grunberg, and Singer (1982) observed that the anticipation of having an intravenous catheter placed for drawing blood significantly increases norepinephrine and epinephrine levels. For this reason, investigators should incorporate a 30-minute stabilization period after catheter insertion to control for this naturally occurring response (Pike et al, 1997).

Several drugs are known to alter catecholamine levels or interfere with the measurement assay. For this reason, some protocols may limit inclusion of subjects who are taking certain drugs. For example, guanethidine, methyldopa, radiographic contrast agents, and reserpine decrease catecholamine levels, while nitroglycerin, prochlorperazine, desipramine, theophylline, and β-blockers increase catecholamine levels. Drugs that may cause catecholamine levels to appear higher than they are when measured with high-performance liquid chromatography (HPLC) include acetaminophen, methyldopa, and medazepam. High doses of vitamin B (riboflavin) can also cause a rise in catecholamine levels (Keiser, 1995; Koller, 1988).

A variety of factors influence the synthesis and release of hormones, the migration and functional ability of lymphocytes, and the reliability of laboratory assays to appropriately measure the hormone or lymphocyte of interest. The need to control these factors must be considered when attempting to measure the influence of stress on immune function.

Biobehavioral Interventions

While early PNI research focused on identifying mechanisms of communication between the neuroendocrine and immune systems, more recent research has involved testing the efficacy of various biobehavioral interventions in reducing maladaptive psychophysiological responses to stressful events or situations and perhaps in preventing poor health outcomes.

Relaxation techniques are quite effective in inducing a state of both physiological and mental rest. Individuals are instructed to focus on internal sensory processes such as breathing while relaxing various muscle groups. *Active relaxation* involves tightening specific muscle groups at varying degrees followed by relaxation of the muscles. This enables the individual to learn to recognize variations in muscle tension so that relaxation techniques may be instituted while the muscle tension is still at a manageable level (McGuigan, 1993). *Passive relaxation* involves passively relaxing muscle groups and requires no energy expenditure.

Relaxation training, alone or in combination with imagery or hypnosis, has produced beneficial results in cancer patients by decreasing anxiety, pain, emotional distress, nausea, vomiting, and general dysphoria (Burish et al, 1987; Burish, Snyder, and Jenkins, 1991; Carey and Burish, 1987; Holland et al, 1991). Although most investigators and clinicians report few, if any, adverse effects from relaxation training, several have been documented in the literature. (See Chapter 17.) It is not surprising that increased perception of physical sensations also relates to increased reports of discomfort in patients. Achieving a relax-

---

Patients are often accused of being able to "do much more when nobody is by." It is quite true that they can. . . . A very weak patient finds it really much less exertion to do things for himself than to ask for them. And he will, in order to do them . . . calculate the time his nurse is likely to be absent, from a fear of her "coming in upon" him or speaking to him, just at the moment when he finds it quite as much as he can do to crawl from his bed to his chair, or from one room to another. . . . Some extra call made upon his attention at that moment will quite upset him. . . . Remember that many patients can walk who cannot stand or even sit up. Standing is, of all positions, the most trying to a weak patient.

Florence Nightingale, *Notes on Nursing*

ation state also induces a feeling of floating in some people. As the person continues training and begins to master the relaxation techniques, the beneficial effects of relaxation may be experienced.

Another important consideration in relaxation training is choosing the appropriate type of relaxation technique based on the functional status of the individual. For example, persons who experience fatigue from either chronic stress, disease processes, or treatment should avoid active relaxation techniques that expend energy. In this case, passive relaxation with imagery might be the more appropriate technique.

Patients who are anemic often report a racing heart rate and agitation that are aggravated by the slightest exertion and excitement. They indicate it is almost impossible to achieve a state of passive relaxation, even if they have practiced it before. They may experience distress because relaxation techniques and restful sleep that formerly helped now seem frustratingly elusive. In this case, gentle distractions such as quiet music or a restful picture (e. g., cut-up, old, large calendars of nature scenes) may help.

In addition, individuals who are dying and who are suffering from cachexia and profound fatigue are not able to engage in even passive relaxation. Some patients who are agitated may actually be engaging in a personal or spiritual struggle and may require time to work things through. On the other hand, they may welcome the offer for someone to pray for them or ask about their need for a spiritual support person of their choice such as a minister, a rabbi, or a priest. In Chapter 21, Kelly talks about resisting the temptation to engage in "premature rescuing." We must be sensitive to which intervention is appropriate on an individual basis.

Cognitive or attentional distraction is another biobehavioral strategy frequently used in oncology patients to reduce symptom distress during procedures or treatments. The use of video games during chemotherapy for pediatric patients has produced beneficial results in decreasing nausea (Kolko and Rickard-Figueroa, 1985; Redd, Andresen, and Minagawa, 1982). Although the distraction was successful in reducing nausea, physiological arousal increased, suggesting that nausea reduction occurred independently of relaxation.

Mental imagery has also had positive results in improving immune function in adult oncology patients (Post-White, 1991, 1998). Solid-tumor patients attended a four-month mental imagery training program. Levels of β-endorphins, NKC cytotoxicity, lymphokine-activated killer activity, and monocyte cytotoxicity were examined before, immediately, and 6 and 12 months after the completion of the program. Although no association between imagery and immune function was identified, mortality rates were lower in the imagery group than in the control group.

Other interventions such as therapeutic or healing touch, massage, acupuncture, prayer, and exercise are currently being evaluated for their effectiveness in reducing physiological arousal and reducing symptom distress (see Table 7-I). Before selecting a biobehavioral intervention, clinicians and researchers should determine the individual's motivation, interest, functional status, and philosophical or religious perspective. Inclusion

Table 7.1	Behavorial Interventions for Patients with Cancer		
Intervention	Description	Advantages	Disadvantages
Active relaxation	Differential contraction and relaxation of specific muscle groups	Teaches recognition of varying degrees of muscle tension Decreases muscle tension Decreases emotionality Improves psychosomatic disorders	Increases awareness of sensations in body Causes a floating sensation May increase fatigue in patients with advanced disease or compromised functional status
Guided imagery plus relaxation	Concentration on specific relaxing images using all senses	Evokes relaxation response Decreases pain, anxiety, emotional distress, depression, and nausea and vomiting	Inability to relax in response to image Difficulty obtaining image in people with nonvisual orientation
Hypnosis plus relaxation	A passive state in which perception and memory are altered, leading to increased responsiveness to the suggestion of relaxation	Decreases anticipatory nausea Elicits deep muscle relaxation Decreases blood pressure and pulse rate Provides cognitive distraction Provides sense of control	Inability to obtain hypnotic state Reappearance of anticipatory nausea in absence of therapist-induced hypnosis
Cognitive/attentional distraction (e.g., music, video games)	Cognitive techniques that block sensory stimuli by directing a portion of attention away from the stimulus	Decreases behavioral distress Decreases side effects of chemotherapy Decreases anxiety	Increases physiological arousal Decreases ability of the intervention to affect a person's response over time
Therapeutic touch	Attempts by a practitioner to discriminate and adjust energy-flow imbalances between individual and environment	Decreases anxiety and stress Decreases pain Evokes relaxation response Requires no energy expenditure or cognitive effort by recipient	Efficacy in reducing symptom distress in patients with cancer not determined Requires skilled practitioner

Source: From Caudell, K. A. (1996). Psychoneuroimmunology and innovative behavioral interventions in patients with leukemia. *Oncology Nursing Form, 23,* 497. Used with permission from Oncology Nursing Society.

of the individual or patient in all treatment decisions is critical in the success of biobehavioral programs.

Where Do We Go From Here?

The promising field of PNI represents a paradigm shift in our thinking about the mind-body relationship. As continued basic science research increases our knowledge base regarding mechanisms of communication between the neuroendocrine and immune systems, more health care clinicians and researchers may begin to appreciate the importance of this new field.

A number of studies have illustrated how stress affects psychophysiological responses in terms of acute responses, habituated responses to chronic stressors, and the hyper-reactive responses by those experiencing chronic stress when exposed to acute stressors. Evidence strongly suggests that continued exposure to stress with subsequent maladaptive responses leads to unfavorable health outcomes such as the development of infections and, more seriously, autoimmune diseases and cancer. Owing to the enormous number of variables that also influence the development of these diseases, at present it is difficult to determine more than the correlation between stress and disease.

Increasingly, insurance plans are beginning to offer stress-management and complementary therapy programs that help individuals learn to manage stress and respond in more adaptive ways. Integrative medicine groups that include allopathic physicians along with alternative practitioners such as acupuncturists, herbalists, Reiki and healing touch therapists, yoga and Feldenkrais practitioners, and chiropractors are developing across the country. Persons with diseases historically difficult to treat with allopathic techniques, such as fibromyalgia, are slowly beginning to respond favorably to treatment team approaches that consider the mind and body. Indeed, the emerging field of PNI may represent a paradigm shift in the way health care providers and consumers approach the entire health and illness continuum.

References

Abbas, A. K., Lichtman, A. H., and Pober, J. S. (Eds.) (1995). *Cellular and molecular immunology.* Philadelphia: W.B. Saunders.

Andersen, B. L., Farrar, W. B., Golden-Kreutz, D., Kutz, L. A., MacCallum, R., Courtney, M. E., and Glaser, R. (1998). Stress and immune responses after surgical treatment for regional breast cancer. *Journal of the National Cancer Institute, 90,* 30–36.

Aslan, S., Nelson, L., Carruthers, M., and Lader, M. (1981). Stress and age effects on catecholamines in normal subjects. *Journal of Psychosomatic Research, 25,* 33–41.

Baum, A. (1990). Stress, intrusive imagery, and chronic distress. *Health Psychology, 9,* 653–675.

Baum, A., Gatchel, R. J., and Schaeffer, M. A. (1983). Emotional, behavioral, and physiological effects of chronic stress at Three Mile Island. *Journal of Consulting and Clinical Psychology, 51,* 565–572.

Baum, A., Grunberg, N. E., and Singer, J. E. (1982). The use of psychological and neuroendocrinological measurements in the study of stress. *Health Psychology, 1,* 217–236.

Blalock, J. E. (1989). A molecular basis for bidirectional communication between the immune and neuroendocrine systems. *Physiology Reviews, 69,* 1–32.

Breier, A., Albus, M., and Wolkowitz, O. M. (1991). The effects of psychological and physical stress in humans. In N. Plotnikoff, A. Murgo, R. Faith, and J. Wybran (Eds.), *Stress and immunity* (pp. 47–60). Boca Raton, FL: CRC Press.

Burish, T. G., Snyder, S. L., and Jenkins, R. A. (1991). Preparing patients for cancer chemotherapy: Effect of coping preparation and relaxation interventions. *Journal of Consulting and Clinical Psychology, 59,* 518–525.

Burish, T. G., Snyder, S. L., Krozely, M. G., and Greco, F. A. (1987). Conditioned side effects induced by cancer chemotherapy: Prevention through behavioral treatment. *Journal of Consulting and Clinical Psychology, 55,* 42–48.

Bush, N. J. (1998). Coping and adaptation. In R. M. Carroll-Johnson, L. M. Horman, and N. J. Bush (Eds.), *Psychosocial nursing care. Along the cancer continuum* (pp. 35–52). Pittsburgh: Oncology Nursing Press.

Cannon, W. B. (1932). *The wisdom of the body.* New York: W.W. Norton.

Carey, M. P., and Burish, T. G. (1987). Providing relaxation training to cancer chemotherapy patients: A comparison of three delivery techniques. *Journal of Consulting and Clinical Psychology, 55,* 732–737.

Caudell, K. A. (1996). Psychoneuroimmunology and innovative behavioral interventions in patients with leukemia. *Oncology Nursing Form, 23,* 493–502.

Chandra, R. (1980). Cell-mediated immunity in nutritional imbalance. *Federal Proceedings, 39,* 3088–3092.

Cohen, S. (1994). Psychosocial influences on immunity and infectious disease in humans. In R. Glaser and J. Kiecolt-Glaser (Eds.), *Human stress and immunity* (pp. 301–319). San Diego: Academic Press.

Cove-Smith, M. S., Kabler, P. A., Pownall, R., and Knapp, M. S. (1978). Circadian variation in an immune response in man. *British Medical Journal, 2,* 253.

Dammacco, F., Campobasso, N., Altomare, E., and Iodice, G. (1984). Analogues in immunology. *LaRicerca Clinical Lab, 14,* 137–147.

Davidson R. J. L., Robertson J. D., Galea G., and Maughn, R. J. (1987). Hematological changes associated with marathon running. *International Journal of Sports Medicine, 8,* 19–25.

Dimsdale, J. E., and Moss, J. (1980). Short-term catecholamine response to psychological stress. *Psychosomatic Medicine, 42,* 493–497.

Eichner, E. R., and Calabrese, L. H. (1994). Immunology and exercise. Physiology, pathophysiology, and implications for HIV infection. *Medical Clinics of North America, 78,* 377–388.

Eysenck, H. J. (1988). Personality, stress and cancer. Prediction and prophylaxis. *British Journal of Medical Psychology, 61,* 57–75.

Fawzy, F., and Fawzy, N. W. (1994). Psychoeducational interventions and health outcomes. In R. Glaser and J. Kiecolt-Glaser (Eds.), *Handbook of human stress and immunity* (pp. 365–402). San Diego: Academic Press.

Fleming, I., Baum, A., Davidson, L. M., Rectanus, E., and McArdle, S. (1987). Chronic stress as a factor in physiologic reactivity to challenge. *Health Psychology, 6,* 221–237.

Frankenhaeuser, M. (1975). Experimental approaches to the study of catecholamines and emotion. In L. Levi (Ed.), *Emotions and their parameters and measurement.* New York: Raven Press.

Grossman, C. J. (1984). Regulation of the immune system by sex steroids. *Endocrine Reviews, 5,* 435–455.

Haddy, R. I. (1987). Aging, infections and the immune system. *Journal of Family Practice, 27,* 409–413.

Hall, M., Baum, A., Buysse, D. J., Prigerson, H. G., Kupfer, D. J., and Reynolds, C. F. (1998). Sleep as a mediator of the stress-immune relationship. *Psychosomatic Medicine, 60,* 48–51.

Heiden, L. A., and Levy, S. M. (1991). Behavior as a biological response modifier. In N. Plotnikoff, A. Murgo, R. Faith, and J. Wybran (Eds.), *Stress and immunity* (pp. 3–28). Boca Raton, FL: CRC Press.

Heim, E., Valach, L., and Schaffner, L. (1997). Coping and psychological adaptation: Longitudinal effects over time and stages in breast cancer. *Psychosomatic Medicine, 59,* 408–418.

Hennessy, M. B., Kaplan, J. N., Mendoza, S. P., Lowe E. L., and Levine, S. (1979). Separation distress and attachment in surrogate-reared squirrel monkeys. *Physiology and Behavior, 23,* 1017–1023.

Henry, J. P. (1992). Biological basis of the stress response. *Integrative Physiological and Behavioral Science, 27,* 66–83.

Holland, J. D., Morrow, G. R., Schmale, A., Derogatis, L., Stefanek, M., Berenson, S., Carpenter, P. J., Breitbart, W., and Feldstein, M. (1991). A randomized clinical trial of alprazolam versus progressive muscle relaxation in cancer patients with anxiety and depressive symptoms. *Journal of Clinical Oncology, 9,* 1004–1011.

Holmen A., Karlsson, A., Bratt, I., and Hogstedt, B. (1995). Increased frequencies of micronuclei in T8 lymphocytes of smokers. *Mutation Research, 334,* 205–208.

Howlett T. A., Tomlin S., Ngahfoong, L., Rees, L. H., Bullen, B. A., Skrinar, O. S., and McArthur, J. W. (1984). Release of ß-endorphin and Met-enkephalin during exercise in normal women: Response to training. *British Medical Journal, 288,* 1950–1952.

Irwin, M., Daniels, M., Bloom, E. T., Smith, T. L., and Weiner, H. (1987). Life events, depressive symptoms, and immune function. *American Journal of Psychiatry, 144,* 437–441.

Keiser, H. R. (1995). Pheochromocytoma and related tumors. In L. J. Degroot (Ed.), *Endocrinology* (vol. 2, pp. 1853–1877). 3rd ed. Philadelphia: W.B. Saunders.

Kemeny, M. E., Weiner, H., Taylor, S. E., Schneider, S., Visscher, B., and Fahey, J. L. (1994). Repeated bereavement, depressed mood and immune response in HIV seropositive and seronegative homosexual men. *Health Psychology, 13,* 14–24.

Kennedy, S., Kiecolt-Glaser, J. K., and Glaser, R. (1988). Immunological consequences of acute and chronic stressors: Mediating role of interpersonal relationships. *British Journal of Medical Psychology; 61,* 77–85.

Kiecolt-Glaser, J. K., Garner, W., Speicher C., Penn, G. M., Holliday, J., and Glaser, R. (1984). Psychosocial modifiers of immunocompetence in medical students. *Psychosomatic Medicine, 46,* 7–14.

Kiecolt-Glaser, J. K., Ricker, D., and George, J. (1984). Urinary cortisol levels, cellular immunocompetence, and loneliness in psychiatric inpatients. *Psychosomatic Medicine, 46,* 15–21.

Kimzey, S. L. (1975). The effects of extended spaceflight on hematologic and immunologic systems. *Journal of the American Medical Womens Association, 30,* 218–232.

Kolko, D. J., and Rickard-Figueroa, J. L. (1985). Effects of video games on the adverse corollaries of chemotherapy in pediatric oncology patients: A single case analysis. *Journal of Consulting and Clinical Psychology, 53,* 223–228.

Koller, M. (1988). Results for 74 substances tested for interference with determination of plasma catecholamines by "high performance" liquid chromatography with electrochemical detection. *Clinical Chemistry, 34,* 947–949.

Lahita, R., Levy, J., Weksler, M., et al. (1984). Effects of sex hormones, nutrition, and aging on the immune response. In C. Stites, J. Stobo, H. Fudenbery, and J. Wells (Eds.), *Basic and clinical immunology* (pp. 288–311). 5th ed. Los Altos, CA: Lange Medical.

Landmann, R. M. A., Perini, C., Müller, F. B., and Bühler, F. R. (1991). Catecholamine and leukocyte phenotype responses to mental stress in subjects with anxiety or suppressed aggression. In N. Plotnikoff, A. Murgo, R. Faith, and J. Wybran (Eds.), *Stress and immunity* (pp. 235–246). Boca Raton, FL: CRC Press.

Lazarus, R. S., and Folkman, S. (Eds.) (1984). The stress concept in the life sciences. In *Stress, appraisal, and coping* (p. 19). New York: Springer.

Leach, C. S., and Rambaut, P. C. (1974). Biochemical responses of the Skylab crewmen. *Proceedings of the Skylab Life Sciences Symposium, 2,* 427–454.

Lee, R. E., Smolensky, M. H. L., Leach, C., and McGovern, J. P. (1977). Circadian rhythms in the cutaneous sensitivity to histamine and selected antigens including phase relationships to urinary cortisol excretion. *American Allergy, 38,* 231–236.

Leibenluft, E., Fiero, P. L., and Rubinow, D. R. (1994). Effects of menstrual cycle dependent variables in mood disorder research. *Archives of General Psychiatry, 51,* 761–781.

LeShan, S. (1959). Psychological states as factors in the development of malignant disease. A critical review. *Journal of the National Cancer Institute, 22,* 1–18.

LeShan, S. (1966). An emotional life-history pattern associated with neoplastic disease. *Annals of the New York Academy of Sciences, 125,* 780–793.

Lovallo, W. R., Pincomb, G. A., Brackett, D. J., and Wilson, M. F. (1990). Heart rate reactivity as a predictor of neuroendocrine responses to aversive and appetitive challenges. *Psychosomatic Medicine, 52,* 17–26.

Madden, K. S., and Felten, D. L. (1995). Experimental basis for neural-immune interactions. *Physiology Reviews, 75,* 77–106.

McClelland, D. C., Ross, G., and Patel, V. (1985). The effect of an academic examination on salivary norepinephrine and immunoglobulin level. *Journal of Human Stress, 11,* 52–99.

McGuigan, F. J. (1993). Progressive relaxation: Origins, principles, and clinical applications. In P. Lehrer and R. L. Woolfolk (Eds.), *Principles and practice of stress management* (pp. 17–52). 2nd ed. New York: Guilford Press.

McKinnon, W., Weisse, C. S., Reynolds, C. P., Bowles, C. A., and Baum, A. (1989). Chronic stress, leukocyte subpopulations, and humoral response to latent viruses. *Health Psychology, 8,* 389–402.

Ostrow, D., Grant, I., and Atkinson, H. (1988). Assessment and management of the AIDS patient with neuropsychiatric disturbances. *Journal of Clinical Psychiatry, 49* (suppl), 14–22.

Palmblad, J., Petrini, B., Wasserman, J., and Akerstedt, T. (1979). Lymphocyte and granulocyte reactions during sleep deprivation. *Psychosomatic Medicine, 41,* 273–278.

Petersen, B. H., Steimel, L. F., and Callaghan, J. T. (1983). Suppression of mitogen-induced lymphocyte transformation in cigarette smokers. *Clinical Immunology and Immunopathology, 27,* 135–140.

Pike, J. L., Smith, T. L., Hauger, R. L., Nicassio, P. M., Patterson, T. L., McClintick, J., Costlow, C., and Irwin, M. (1997). Chronic life stress alters sympathetic, neuroendocrine, and immune responsivity to an acute psychological stressor in humans. *Psychosomatic Medicine, 59,* 447–457.

Post-White, J. (1991). "The effects of mental imagery on emotions, immune function, and cancer outcome." Doctoral dissertation, University of Minnesota, Minneapolis, MN. Dissertation Abstracts International, 52, 12B (University Microfilms No. 92-5462).

Post-White, J. (1998). Psychoneuroimmunology: The mind-body connection. In R. M. Carroll-Johnson, L. M. Horman, and N. J. Bush (Eds.), *Psychosocial nursing care. Along the cancer continuum,* (pp. 349–364). Pittsburgh: Oncology Nursing Press.

Redd, W. H., Andresen, G. V., and Minagawa, R. I. (1982). Hypnotic control of anticipatory emesis in patients receiving cancer chemotherapy. *Journal of Consulting and Clinical Psychology, 50,* 14–19.

Schleifer, S. J., Keller, S. E., Camerino, M., Thornton, J. C., and Stein, M. (1983). Suppression of lymphocyte stimulation following bereavement. *Journal of the American Medical Association, 250,* 347–377.

Schleifer, S. J., Keller, S. E., Siris, S. B., Davis, K. L., and Stein, M. (1985). Depression and immunity. Lymphocyte function in ambulatory depressed patients, hospitalized schizophrenic patients, and patients hospitalized for herniorrhaphy. *Archives of General Psychiatry, 42,* 129–133.

Selye, H. (1936). Thymus and adrenals in the response of the organism to injuries and intoxications. *British Journal of Experimental Pathology, 17,* 234–248.

Sevier, R. L. (1994). Infectious disease in athletes. *Sports Medicine, 78,* 389–397.

Shinkai, S., Shore, S., Shek, P. N., and Shephard, R. J. (1992). Acute exercise and immune function. *International Journal of Sports Medicine, 13,* 452.

Solomon, G. F., and Amkraut, A. A. (1981). Psychoneuroendocrinological effects of the immune response. *Annual Reviews of Microbiology, 35,* 155–184.

Solomon, G. F., and Moss, R. H. (1964). Emotions, immunity and disease: A speculative theoretical integration. *Archives of General Psychiatry, 11,* 657–674.

Somerfield, M., and Curbow, B. (1992). Methodological issues and research strategies in the study of coping with cancer. *Social Science Medicine, 34,* 1203–1216.

Sørensen, T. I. A., Nielsen, G. G., Anderson, P. K., and Teasdale, T. W. (1988). Genetic and environmental influences on premature death in adult adoptees. *New England Journal of Medicine, 318,* 727–732.

Spiegel, D., Bloom, J. R., Kraemer, H. C., and Gottheil, E. (1989). Effect of psychosocial treatment on survival of patients with metastatic breast cancer. *Lancet, 2,* 888–891.

Stoyva, J. M., and Budzynski, T. H. (1993). Biofeedback methods in the treatment of anxiety and stress disorders. In P. Lehrer and R. L. Woolfolk (Eds.), *Principles and practice of stress management* (pp. 263–300). 2nd ed. New York: Guilford Press.

Turiel J., and Wingard, D. (1985). *Estrogens and cancer: A multi-disciplinary focus on diethylstilbestrol (DES).* Berkeley: University of California Press.

Turner, J. A., Clancy, S., and Vitaliano, P. P. (1987). Relationships of stress, appraisal and coping to chronic low lack pain. *Behavior Research and Therapy, 25,* 281–288.

Ziegler, B. G. (1989). Catecholamine measurement in behavioral research. In N. Schneiderman, S. M. Weiss, and P. B. Kaufmann (Eds.), *Handbook of research methods in cardiovascular behavioral medicine* (pp. 167–183). New York: Plenum Press.

Ziegler, M. G., Lake, C. R., and Kopin, I. J. (1976). Plasma noradrenaline increases with age. *Nature, 261,* 33.

Resources

This is an exciting field of study. Frequently, various biochemical components of the psychoneuroimmunological system are identified by inference. They may go through several name changes as their function is elucidated. The *Cytokine Online Pathfinder Encyclopedia* lists the etymology of these various biochemicals, making it easier to keep current on newer developments in the literature. For those who are curious about the biochemical discoveries relevant to psychoneuroimmunology on a daily basis, here are some interesting Internet sites. Many of these sites have excellent links:

National Center for Biotechnology Information: http://www3.ncbi.nlm.nih.gov/

Johns Hopkins Genome Database: http://gdbwww.gdb.org/

BodyMap: Anatomical Expression Database of Human Genes:
    http://www.imcb.osaka-u.ac.jp/bodymap/

Cytokine Family cDNA Database: http://cytokine.medic.kumamoto-u.ac.jp/

COPE V 2.1 Cytokines Online Pathfinder Encyclopedia:
    http://bioinfo.weizmann.ac.il/cgi-bin/cope/cope.pl

The Cytokines Web at Oxford UK: http://www.psynix.co.uk/cytweb/index.html

Cytokines Web 3-D Structures of Cytokines: http://www.psynix.co.uk/cytweb/cyt_strucs/index.html

Cytokines Web Clinical Significance Table: http://www.psynix.co.uk/cytweb/roles/index.html

PART
II

Clinical Issues

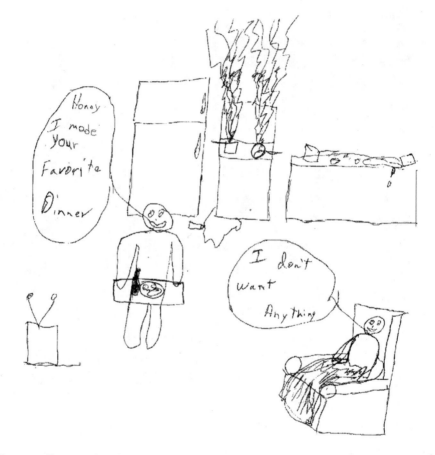

When my wife was undergoing her chemotherapy treatments, nothing seemed to cheer her up too much.

Robert Heil, spouse of breast cancer survivor

CHAPTER 8

Treatment:
An Overview

Patricia C. Buchsel
Margaret Barton-Burke
Maryl L. Winningham

Getting out of bed is all you can do somedays.
Brenda Heil, 33 years old, 9-year survivor

Background

Fatigue is an experience common to all life. Among healthy individuals, it is usually followed by rest and, with the appropriate fluid and nutrition, leads to regeneration. Under normal circumstances, it is considered to be protective and short term. However, the fatigue often experienced by cancer patients as a result of disease or treatment can be enormously debilitating. Patients report that it is not equivalent to anything they have experienced before the advent of their cancer. This symptom is the most common complaint experienced by oncology patients prior to, during, and after treatment. It is also the longest-lasting symptom, interfering with every aspect of life (Fatigue Coalition, 1998; Winningham et al, 1994).

In a recent article, Vogelzang and colleagues (1997) reported that only 31% of randomly surveyed cancer patients mentioned fatigue to their doctors on every visit, while three-fourths (74%) of these patients reported that fatigue is an untreatable condition. Significantly, only 5% of surveyed oncologists reported that their patients mention fatigue at every visit. It is puzzling that this symptom, while so destructive, is the source of so much miscommunication.

Cancer-related fatigue (CRF) results in significant disability and adversely affects quality of life. Despite the ubiquitous presence of CRF, it is a condition that is poorly understood, inadequately studied, often overlooked, and certainly undertreated. Current research is aimed at identifying the incidence, severity, and causative factors of fatigue; its impact on other symptoms such as pain, nausea, and vomiting; and supportive care measures to lessen the effects of CRF.

A study by Pater and colleagues (1997) examined factors affecting the level of fatigue among cancer patients participating in clinical trials. Patients reporting the greatest amount of fatigue were females with ovarian or lung cancer who had metastatic disease and poor performance status. This corroborates empirical observations and the scientific literature in which the population reported to be most at risk for fatigue is younger women, that is, women with breast or ovarian cancers (Jamar, 1989; Vogelzang et al, 1997). Another important finding of the study by Pater and colleagues (1997) was that patients treated with prophylactic antiemetics experienced significantly less fatigue than did those not receiving this treatment. This finding supports the propositions presented by Winningham (see Table 8-1, page 156) that efficient symptom management can decrease the experience of fatigue (Barnett, 1997; Winningham, 1995, 1999). In a recent clinical research project, Buchsel found that patients randomized to a clinical intervention that involved use of a pain-control algorithm (protocol or recipe) reported less pain and generally improved well-being compared to the control group. The control group received standard pain management. These findings suggest that optimal and organized management of one symptom may reduce the intensity of another symptom.

This chapter presents the general problem of fatigue and then discusses how the broad variety of treatments may influence it. This can be a review for health care professionals or an introduction for patients, families, and nonmedical support providers such as social workers, pastoral counselors, or massage therapists who do not understand the confusing world into which their patients, friends, family members, or cancer survivors have been thrust.

The Etiology of Cancer-Related Fatigue

The etiology of fatigue in cancer patients is complex, multifactorial, and multidimensional, encompassing the physiological, psychological, and situational aspects of a patient's life. Some of the physiological factors that exacerbate fatigability in cancer, in addition to specific aspects of cancer itself, include diabetes and cardiac, renal, or respiratory conditions. In addition, the side effects of cancer therapy—anemia, infection, fever, pain, anorexia, nausea, vomiting, diarrhea, dehydration, fluid and electrolyte imbalances, and malnutrition—contribute to CRF (Barton-Burke, 1998; Piper, Lindsay, and Dodd, 1987; Portenoy and Miasakowski, 1998; Winningham et al, 1994).

Fatigue precedes, accompanies, and follows most malignancies and treatments. Since tumors can produce abnormal chemicals that are toxic to the body, CRF may be a direct

About the Contributor

Patricia Buchsel has been a nurse for 25 years; 15 of those years have been in oncology. She describes her career path as "traditional," starting with work on a medical surgical unit in a community hospital. She spent over ten years at the Fred Hutchinson Cancer Research Center as nursing director of ambulatory care. Consequently, her specialty area has been in bone marrow and stem cell transplantation. She has edited or coedited a number of books on cancer nursing. Patricia has been actively involved in the Oncology Nursing Society at the local and national levels, and has generously given of herself to her community in a diverse number of cancer causes.

result of those chemical changes. It is often the primary concern that causes individuals to see a physician. Most notably, patients with leukemia or lung cancer complain of unusual fatigue; if a patient has a concomitant illness such as cardiac, respiratory, or renal disease, the fatigue that is experienced may be distorted and exacerbated (Barton-Burke, 1998).

Side effects of therapy, including anemia and infection, cause or potentiate the CRF experienced by the patient. Cancer-related anemia arises either as a result of direct kidney damage or from myelosuppression (depression of cells normally produced in the bone marrow) secondary to chemotherapy or irradiation, blood loss, iron or vitamin deficiency, hemolysis (destruction of red blood cells), tumor impinging on marrow function, or the anemia that develops with chronic illness. Cancer patients are often susceptible to infections, which cause fever and can contribute to anorexia, diarrhea, nausea, and vomiting. In addition, patients often report infections as contributing to feelings of depression. These things, in turn, contribute to dehydration, fluid and electrolyte imbalances, and malnutrition.

Symptoms such as pain further compound the incidence and severity of CRF. Pain causes interrupted sleep and anorexia; it also contributes to decreased activity, which results in decreased strength and endurance and increased exhaustibility. As clinical interest in fatigue increases and there is an increased demand for research-based interventions, attention to these other correlates will have to be considered.

Surgery

Surgery is experienced by most cancer patients as a diagnostic tool or first-line approach to treatment. Fatigue following surgery can persist for as long as six months and may be due to increased cardiac output, metabolism of anesthetics, pain medication, alterations in nutrition, and decreased physical activity (Barnett, 1997; Piper, Lindsay, and Dodd, 1987; Winningham et al, 1994). Patients requiring major invasive surgery are at risk for CRF as a result of the previously mentioned side effects of surgical intervention and for anemia resulting from blood loss sustained during the surgical procedure. In Chapter 22, McDade details CRF from the perspective of both the surgeon and the patient.

Patricia has an educational background in nursing and business administration (bachelor of science in nursing from Seattle University, a degree from the University of Washington in integrated business administration), and a master of science in nursing administration from Seattle Pacific University.

Her "human being" time is spent gardening, playing tennis and bridge, and reading. A few years ago, she also started running marathons. She rates time with her family, especially with her husband and grandchildren, as her greatest treasure.

Table 8.1	Winningham's Ten Propositions Relating Fatigue, Symptom Management, Functioning, and Quality of Life

The relationships among activity, energy, fatigue, symptom management, and functional status in people with cancer can be summarized in the following propositions:

1. Too much rest as well as too little rest contributes to increased feelings of fatigue.

2. Too little activity as well as too much activity contributes to increased feelings of fatigue.

3. A relative balance between activity and rest promotes restoration; an imbalance promotes fatigue and deconditioning.

4. Deconditioning is the adaptive energetic response whereby an organism's biological work potential is decreased over time.

5. Everyday energy expenditure in activity is the most potent known regulator of the body's energy systems. ("Use it or lose it.")

6. Any symptom/condition that contributes to decreased activity will lead to deconditioning, increased fatigue, and decreased functional status.

7. Any intervention that provides relief of a symptom/condition that contributes to decreased activity may simultaneously serve to mitigate fatigue and promote functioning, provided that intervention does not have a sedating or catabolic effect.

8. The experience of fatigue potentiates distress associated with other symptoms/conditions.

9. The experience of other symptoms/conditions potentiates feelings of fatigue.

10. Deconditioning and perceived fatigue interact to make every aspect of life more stressful and to negatively influence quality of life, thus contributing to increased suffering.

Chemotherapy

A majority of CRF studies have been conducted on patients receiving chemotherapy. It is suggested that the prevalence of fatigue related to the administration of chemotherapy may occur at rates approximating 75% to 100% (Smets et al, 1993). Chemotherapy may cause CRF either directly or indirectly. It may contribute directly to CRF by suppressing bone marrow or kidney function, thus causing a hypoproliferative anemia. Indirectly, chemotherapy may have an effect on cytokines either directly or indirectly at the cellular level, peripheral neuromuscular junction, or central nervous system.

Berger (1998) described the pattern of fatigue, activity, and rest, and the relationship between these three variables during adjuvant chemotherapy for breast cancer. Women with stage I or II breast cancer were treated with one of three cycles of either (1) cyclophosphamide, methotrexate, and fluorouracil or (2) cyclophosphamide, doxorubicin, and fluorouracil. Total and subscale fatigue scores were significantly different over time, with scores higher at treatment times and lower at cycle midpoints. Clearly, activity levels were lower when perceived fatigue was greater. This study substantiated what clinicians and patients reported, that fatigue in patients receiving chemotherapy occurred in predictable *patterns*.

In 1995, Richardson used patient diaries to document the onset, pattern, duration, intensity, and distress associated with fatigue for 109 patients receiving different cancer chemotherapy protocols. Data indicated that although fatigue may be essentially similar among groups receiving different chemotherapy regimens, there is significant individual variation in its severity and the amount of associated perceived distress.

Radiation Therapy

Patients receiving radiation either alone or in multimodal therapy (in combination with chemotherapy or some other kind of therapy) are at risk for considerable treatment-related fatigue that can last months or years after treatment (Blesch et al, 1991). Several plausible explanations exist to describe the fatigue mechanism that is operational with radiation therapy. However, these mechanisms are not well understood and still require considerable guesswork; for instance, (1) CRF may be the direct result of cellular death as a result of radiation therapy, or (2) CRF may be the result of a specific tumor lysis syndrome secondary to radiation therapy. In either case, toxic intracellular materials are released into the bloodstream and may affect many of the major organs of the body such as the kidneys, lungs, or brain and central nervous system. (3) An alternative theory may be that radiation therapy causes an increased basal metabolic rate, which rapidly depletes energy stores. Finally, it is well established that radiation therapy has a direct effect on a patient's bone marrow metabolism.

One recent study by Irvine and colleagues (1998) reported on patterns and duration of fatigue in women with breast cancer who were receiving radiation therapy. Fatigue significantly increased over the course of treatment, peaked from the second to the last week of therapy, and returned to pretreatment levels three months after therapy. The strength of this study lay in the identification of peak times of fatigue and it confirmed fatigue patterns similar to those identified in the pioneering study by Haylock and Hart (1979).

The most frequent self-reported strategies used to ease the fatigue symptoms were to "take it easy" or to "get plenty of rest" (Irvine et al, 1998; Winningham, 1983, 1992). In the study by Irvine and colleagues (1998), fatigue was not influenced by patient age, stage of disease, time since surgery, body weight, or length of time since diagnosis. The authors reported a strong relationship between fatigue and symptom distress, psychological distress, and select physiological variables. This, again, supported predictions made in Winningham's ten propositions (see Table 8-1) and her psychobiological entropy model (see Figure 2-4), that efficient symptom management can decrease the experience of fatigue (Barnett, 1997; Winningham, 1995). (See Chapter 2 for details.)

Biotherapy

An overwhelming, flu-like fatigue is the dose-limiting toxicity of this cancer treatment and it has been suggested that the fatigue of biotherapy may be more intense, protracted, and debilitating, with mechanisms that differ completely from those of the other three major treatment interventions. As someone described it, "It's like having flu all the time, only ten times worse!" Biological response modifiers (BRMs) include white cell colony-stimulating factors such as granulocyte colony-stimulating factor (G-CSF) and granulocyte macrophage colony-stimulating factor (GM-CSF), interferon, interleukin-2, monoclonal antibodies, and tumor necrosis factor (TNF). Each BRM causes fatigue that is dependent on the dose, duration, and route of administration (Jassak, 1995).

Often fatigue is manifested in a constellation of symptoms known as *flu-like syndrome,* which includes fever, chills, myalgia, headache, and fatigue. Flu-like syndromes are usually well tolerated and managed with acetaminophen and rest (Shelton and Turnbough, 1996). Interferon, however, presents dose-limiting hurdles requiring dose reductions, treatment delays, or termination of treatment.

Treatment compliance related to fatigue intolerance becomes a major hurdle to successful disease management. Support groups for patients self-administering interferon therapy and their family members are routinely organized to assist with issues of managing fatigue.

Marrow and Stem Cell Transplantation

Bone marrow transplantation (BMT) represents one of the most intense treatment therapies for thousands of patients with leukemia, lymphoma, solid-organ disease, and immunological disorders. Most BMT recipients have received prior treatment with chemotherapy and irradiation followed by ablative (intended to wipe out the body's normal immune system) conditioning regimens for BMT. Intense symptom management until trilineage engraftment and clinical stability is one of the mainstays of supportive care. Effective new therapies for nausea, vomiting, diarrhea, and pain management have greatly reduced fatigue, yet this symptom remains an understudied phenomenon in the BMT population. Given the intensity of symptoms arising from ablative therapy (designed to wipe out the patient's diseased bone marrow cells), patient fatigue is profound.

Buchsel (1993) studied the presence, duration, and intensity of symptoms of BMT recipients enrolled in a randomized, controlled clinical trial testing the safety and cost of early hospital discharge. Fatigue, along with symptoms related to gastrointestinal, liver, and renal systems, was found to be present, enduring, and intense for all groups being studied. In a study comparing quality of life in unrelated allogeneic bone marrow recipients to that in a normal population, Sutherland and colleagues (1997) determined that recipients less than three years after marrow grafting had diminished scores on physical activity, vitality, and general health compared to scores for the general population. In contrast, the group who survived longer than three years after BMT scored significantly higher than the three-year group and not significantly different than a normal population. Interestingly, 20% of the subjects reported moderate to severe fatigue, sleep disturbances, and pain (Sutherland et al, 1997). This paper represents one of the rare quality-of-life studies that compares long-term sequelae in unrelated marrow recipients to normal populations (Syrjala et al, 1993).

Research by Molassiotis and Morris (1998) supported the findings by Sutherland and colleagues. Molassiotis and Morris reported on the correlates of fatigue in the BMT population. In the group receiving marrow from a related donor, lack of energy showed high correlations with tiredness, depression, overall psychosocial adjustment, psychological symptom distress, difficulty concentrating, and shortness of breath. In the group receiving marrow from an unrelated donor, fatigue was associated with general pain, depression, overall psychosocial adjustment, weight loss, and anorexia.

Donor Fatigue

One type of fatigue that is not often discussed or identified when considering CRF in the BMT population is that of donor fatigue. Allogeneic marrow donors undergo general or spinal anesthesia for marrow harvest with minimal postoperative morbidity and mortality (Buckner et al, 1984). The incidence of fatigue manifested by related donors is reported to be similar, but published studies do not indicate causes. It is likely that causal factors for donor fatigue in this population mirror those of unrelated donors.

Most donors receive autologous or allogeneic red blood cell transfusions as a supportive measure after bone marrow harvest. York and colleagues (1992) examined the benefit of administering exogenous erythropoietin prior to harvest in order to decrease the risk of anemia and the need for subsequent transfusions. The investigators concluded that exogenous erythropoietin could be given safely to normal marrow donors, with a significant increase in hematocrit occurring in the two to three weeks prior to marrow harvesting. Unfortunately, there are no published studies in the literature to advance this premise.

Medications

Cancer patients require numerous medications for treatment as well as supportive care. Many of these medications, such as antiemetics and anxiolytics, may cause or exacerbate fatigue. These are discussed in more detail in Chapter 10.

Depression

Psychological correlates such as depression, anxiety, anticipatory nausea and vomiting, and pain can exhaust patients and overwhelm coping mechanisms. Symptoms of depression and fatigue mimic or exacerbate each other, making diagnosis and treatment difficult. Assessment includes evaluation of the impact of fatigue on the patient. Proper care focuses on psychotherapeutic and psychopharmacological treatment of psychological or psychiatric diagnoses and introduction of behavioral and cognitive strategies for reducing the negative effects of fatigue in all areas of the patient's life (Portenoy and Miaskowski, 1998).

Assessment of Fatigue

Because fatigue is a subjective condition, assessment is at times difficult. Clinical assessment and diagnosis are accomplished by performing hematological studies, monitoring for underlying bleeding, hemolysis, and possible marrow involvement of tumor. Assessment for symptoms and problems that compound fatigue–such as pain, infection, fever, and poor nutritional status–is imperative. Evaluation for psychological and situational stressors such as depression, anxiety, and sleep disturbances can assist in the diagnosis of the causative

Hospital Standard Time

As a patient who has endured two lengthy hospital confinements, I can tell you all, as health care providers, that I have some serious complaints. Does that mean I am gearing up to vent without measure all my petty frustrations, and fears built on emotional distress and physical discomfort? No, it doesn't. I am asking that you assume a cool and nondefensive posture and rationally evaluate my direct experience.

After 36 hours of serious puking, I was admitted, exhausted, through the emergency room at 7:30 PM, diagnosed by an attending internist with a critical bowel blockage, and scheduled for surgery in the first suite available. Seven hours later, at about 3:00 AM, the surgeons removed a 2.5- to 3-centimeter tumor that was growing through my cecal valve from a bowel that had not been mechanically prepared. I "third-spaced" most of the fluid administered by the anesthesiologist, and on my way to the recovery room, my blood pressure dropped to 60 systolic. After 48 hours in ICU, my blood pressure stabilized; I was sent to the floor.

By now I was worse than exhausted; I was drained, emotionally and physically. I had a seemingly endless supply of tubes in my nose and throat, a Foley catheter, one IV pump, one IV tree with two or three bags hanging on it, and very limited capacity to either address on my own, or communicate to others, any of my distress. Because my bowel was not clean, the wound became infected. You are no doubt aware of the additional treatments that problem entails! Other complications followed: severe postop cholecystitis, more IV drugs, old IV sites collapsed, IVs started in new sites, inability to hold down any food or any liquid other than water, malnutrition, . . . for 24 days.

Over and above all this, twice a day (4:30 AM and 4:30 PM) someone was waking me up to draw blood. At 10:00 PM, midnight, 2:00 AM, 4:00 AM, and 6:00 AM, someone was waking me up to do blood pressure, pulse, and oxygen saturation. At times other than these, someone was changing IV bags. For the first seven or eight days on the floor, the surgeons would wander in at some ridiculous hour in the morning to take off the bandages and poke and prod.

As soon as I got the tubes out of my nose and mouth, aides began showing up three or four times a day to tell me it was time for "us" to take a walk. I am 1.9 meters tall and weigh 160 kilograms. The aides averaged about 1.65 meters in height and weighed 60 to 65 kilograms. Malnourished, exhausted,

problems leading to fatigue (Piper et al, 1998). Chapter 14 discusses the clinical assessment of fatigue.

When one is discussing fatigue, the terms *assessment, evaluation,* and *measurement* are used interchangeably or synonymously. However, these are distinctly different ways of identifying the subjective phenomena composing CRF. Clinicians *assess* or *evaluate* cancer patients in the hospital, in the clinic, or at home about the general impact that a symptom has on their life and health. *Measurement* is a term used in empirical or quality-control studies, when it is essential to determine differences for treatment or research. The word *measurement* implies a more rigorous determination than is used in everyday clinical settings.

dehydrated, and shaking, I questioned the wisdom of these walks with so little support. I was told by several aides, "That's all right, we are trained to handle it." On the one occasion when "we" actually did fall, the "training" didn't live up to its billing.

They were giving me care, perhaps the best they could, as they understood it. And very expensive care, from the bill. But the "delivery of medical care" was at their convenience, for their purposes, to meet their schedules. It had nothing to do with health. I was just another problem to be "solved." I was pronounced cured and sent home, 24 days postop. I had lost nearly 30 kilograms. I was sleep deprived and so physically debilitated that I couldn't walk unaided more than 40 feet.

Do I know and understand why hospitals work to certain schedules? Yes, I do. I know what aide rounds are and nursing rounds. I understand doctors' rounds and why they make them when they do.

However, I was sick, literally in jeopardy of my life! Did I need to sleep? Yes! Was there any provision for protected time when I didn't have to fear being pounced upon and attacked? NO! Any time when I could really rest? NO!

Did the lab need the blood? Yes! Did they have to bang the bedside table into the radiator everytime they came in to get it? NO! Did they have to talk to one another over me, every time, about their personal interests, regardless of the hour? NO!

Did the nurse need to change the IV bags? Yes! Did she have to stand right outside the door to my room at 3:15 AM and yell down the hall to have an aide bring her a new line setup? NO!

Vital signs are "things" aides monitor. The things that are most "vital" are relegated to the least trained of the hospital clinical staff. Do they ever consider that the patient lying in the bed is not a thing?

People cannot be taught to care. Either they care or they don't. Being professionals, they can however, one presumes, be trained in the simple processes of courtesy and consideration. I can't imagine that the patient's experience of it all is taken into consideration.

And whatever happened to the idea that rest is necessary to getting better? I'm not sure what took longer: (1) time to recover from my cancer or (2) time to recover from the hospital? I don't understand. If we can schedule surgeries and airplanes, why can't we schedule patient care so patients can also get rest?

Clinical interventions usually grow out of clinical observations and trial and error. They are followed by more detailed study through patient-researcher interaction, are studied using empirical techniques, and then are quantified. Afterward, they are tested again on the clinical population. Hence, in this case, *measurement* is a term used by scientists and researchers to quantify the variable CRF. Scientific, theoretically based interventions used in research are applied to the subject in an attempt to measure and manipulate the variable and find the most effective intervention(s). (See Chapter 3 about measurement issues and Chapter 14 on clinical assessment.)

Treatment of Fatigue

The treatment of fatigue is often hampered by misperceptions and myths. Often clinicians and patients believe this problem is inherent to cancer and its treatment, that it must be endured and few interventions are available. Most of the chapters in this book present how different medical specialists could approach this problem. For example, Chapter 9 discusses how a medical oncologist views the diagnosis and treatment of fatigue-related issues; Chapter 11 presents a psychiatrist's perspective; Chapter 12, an immunologist's perspective; Chapter 15, a physiatrist's perspective; and Chapter 22, a surgeon's perspective. Many chapters also present how advanced practice nurses and various therapists view and treat the problem. Each chapter is an adventure into the minds of specialists from different disciplines.

Management of Cancer-Related Anemia

Anemia is the most common hematological abnormality in cancer patients. Management of cancer-related anemia results in red blood cell administration in up to 18% of patients with solid tumors, with lung cancer patients accounting for the highest percentage. Up to 75% of leukemia patients and 25% of lymphoma patients also require red blood cell administration arising from either the disease or the treatment (Skillings et al, 1993).

Historically, the management of cancer-associated anemia has depended on the transfusion of packed red blood cells; under these circumstances, this was generally implemented only when symptoms were severe enough to significantly compromise the patient. The advantage of a red blood cell transfusion is rapid red blood cell recovery, resulting in alleviating distressing symptoms and improving the patient's functional status.

Graft-versus-host disease, usually limited to BMT recipients, can occur, albeit rarely, as an immunological reaction of blood donor lymphocytes–recognizing the patient as foreign and mounting a defense resulting in this problem (Spector, 1995). Infectious agents not detected by standard enzyme immunoassay techniques and inadvertently administered place patients at risk for hepatitis, cytomegalovirus (CMV), acquired immunodeficiency syndrome, and a host of other bacterial, viral, and parasitic infections. Another possible disadvantage of blood product transfusion is depressed immune function such as lowered levels of cytokines and helper T lymphocytes, increased T-cell function, and decreased natural killer cell activity.

Of interest, Miller and colleagues (1990) noted that patients with cancer-related anemia due to chronic disease experience insufficient endogenous erythropoietin levels (levels produced by their own body to stimulate red blood cell production) for their degree of anemia. Since the recognition of this blunted erythropoietin response, numerous investigations supporting the use of exogenous erythropoietin have occurred.

Recombinant human erythropoietin (r-HuEPO) has become a recognized and effective approach to treating cancer treatment–related anemia. (See Chapter 10 by Meadows on the pharmacological use of r-HuEPO.) Answers to the many questions, however, concerning the best and most appropriate use of this medication (classified as a colony-stimulating factor) require additional research. Most studies to date were performed in patients with non-myeloid malignancies, and it is not known if anemia in patients with other diseases can be treated as effectively. Similarly, clinical trials have focused on patients receiving chemotherapy, and studies are needed to test the efficacy of r-HuEPO in patients receiving radiation treatment for various kinds of cancer.

Psychostimulants

Some clinicians are suggesting the use of psychostimulants such as methylphenidate (Ritalin), pemoline (Cylert), and dextroamphetamine, administered in low dosages, to promote a sense of well-being, decrease fatigue, and increase appetite. These drugs have potential for great benefit; they also have a long list of adverse effects including insomnia, euphoria, and mood lability. Long-term use may produce anorexia, nightmares, insomnia, paranoia, and possible complications. The National Cancer Institute has posted suggested dosages of these drugs on its Physician's Data Query (PDQ) fatigue management page (see Resources at end of this chapter); however, it is significant that only one clinical study to date has supported the use of methylphenidate in cancer patients. This study was on brain cancer patients (Meyers et al, 1998; see Chapter 17). At present, other uses of these drugs are considered "off label," which means the U.S. Food and Drug Administration has not approved their use for treatment of fatigue in cancer patients. However, the severity of distress associated with fatigue in cancer, as well as the potential benefits, demands that the evaluation of pharmacological interventions be treated as seriously as medication for pain has been addressed. Well-designed clinical trials are needed to confirm risks as well as benefits, especially in elderly cancer patients who may exhibit paradoxical reactions. Currently, the optimal approach for treatment is to take a preliminary psychiatric history (as presented in Chapter 11) and refer patients to a staff psychiatrist for evaluation.

Promoting Sleep and Rest

Oddly enough, few studies exist on the relationship of sleep disorders to fatigue. Of these studies, most addressed the effects of hospital noise on sleep. A few scattered abstracts and letters to editors addressed insomnia and cancer, but they depended on self-report (most studies examining sleep disturbances rely on subjective self-report). Studies on sleep disturbances in healthy individuals as well as people with cancer need to address actual versus perceived amount and quality of sleep. Understanding the discrepancy between the two may make a valuable contribution to research. Research is needed to document sleep patterns in cancer patients and institute therapeutic sleep measures. Such studies should include a comparative group of "normal, healthy" patients with similar everyday socioeconomic stressors (i.e., work, social obligations, family needs).

Numerous symptoms associated with cancer, its treatment, and recovery have the potential to dramatically disrupt sleep cycles. Urinary frequency, hot flashes, pain, nausea, muscle cramps, cough, and diarrhea are symptoms that can be managed so that patients can benefit from optimal night sleep. Effective symptom management may decrease sleep interruptions and possibly reduce daytime fatigue. Other measures include decreasing noise levels, avoiding caffeine late in the day, taking *appropriate* naps (see Chapter 11), implementing reasonable physical exercise, and using relaxation techniques or guided imagery.

Nutritional Support

When energy requirements exceed nutritional intake, fatigue can ensue. Three potential mechanisms may be (1) alterations in the body's ability to process nutrients efficiently, (2) an increase in the body's energy requirements, and (3) a decrease in intake of energy sources. Many studies indicated that early nutritional intervention improves or preserves self-image, sense of control, appetite, and ability to continue daily activities. In addition, well-nourished individuals generally have more rapid recovery times and are better able to tolerate therapy, thereby enhancing quality of life (Splett, 1996).

Fatigued individuals often neglect to maintain an adequate fluid intake as well as nutritional intake. National Aeronautics and Space Administration (NASA) studies, over a period of more than a decade, demonstrated that dehydration was a consequence of bed rest and prolonged exposure to microgravity. This contributes to actual muscle weakness and a sensation of mental confusion (Greenleaf and Kozlowski, 1982). In addition, symptoms such as pain, dyspnea, and nausea, as well as treatment-related diarrhea, aggravate the state of dehydration.

Alternative Therapies

Alternative measures such as relaxation techniques, biofeedback, and massage therapy are frequently suggested to counter stress-related fatigue. No large controlled studies have evaluated these nonpharmacological techniques, and scientific investigation using multidisciplinary approaches is required to validate their use. The expertise of physicians, pharmacists, nurses, physical therapists, social workers, and other health care providers is needed to address these alternative therapies (Aistars, 1987).

Energy Conservation and Body Mechanics

Energy conservation is perhaps the most simple, sensible, and economic approach to fatigue management, but is often overlooked. In Chapters 15 and 16, the roles of physical medicine and occupational and physical therapy are explored in relation to fatigue.

Exercise

Moderate, prescriptive exercise may be an effective means of minimizing fatigue (MacVicar and Winningham, 1986; Winningham, 1983, 1991). It was initially used in 1982–83 by Maryl L. Winningham at Ohio State University as a means of counteracting the known energetic deterioration due to decreased activity and bed rest. This deterioration was well established in the 1950s through 1970s in NASA aerospace medicine studies. These studies demonstrated that even healthy, young athletes became depressed, weakened, and deconditioned (generalized organ system deterioration) when placed on bed rest. NASA studies also established that select types of exercise could minimize this deterioration. Exercise recommendations for cancer patients should adhere to safety guidelines established by the American Heart Association and the American College of Sports Medicine as a minimal standard of care. In 1983, Winningham and MacVicar reported on a survey of cancer patients who were physically active. Results indicated that cancer survivors found exercise particularly useful in helping them control the stress associated with their cancer. Their symptom reports also led to the development of a clinical, symptom activity survey to ensure the safety of exercise in people with cancer. See Chapter 18 for more details.

A Posttreatment Athletic Program

The University of Washington Cancer Center sponsors a program for women with cancer called Team Survivors Northwest. Women cancer survivors of various ages participate in weekly walks, runs, and exercise sessions as well as monthly hikes, swims, and bike rides. Each year, the members of Team Survivors Northwest participate in the Danskin Women's Triathlon, consisting of a 0.5-mile swim, 10-mile bike ride, and a 3-mile run. The team has coaches who train women for this event. In addition, the Team Survivor Northwest program incorporates regular exercise, diet, positive thinking, and team spirit. Major athletic challenges, such as the annual triathlon, encourage women to set goals and participate in adventures as a means of celebrating life and their achievements, despite their cancer diagnosis. Treatments related to cancer can have long-term toxic effects. This program combines appropriate medical supervision with the satisfaction of athletic challenges. For those who find it to be an important component of their quality of life, it is an example of how recreational sports and athletics can celebrate life in cancer survivors.

Moderate, noncompetitive exercise is all that is necessary to optimize fitness and health in most individuals. For nonathletic patients, it may be a preferred strategy to encourage long-term compliance because the commitment is not as demanding. Guidelines and recommendations for exercising cancer survivors published by Winningham (1994) and Winningham, MacVicar, and Burke (1986) are intended for use by coaches and therapists, as well as clinicians, to provide safe parameters for training.

Caregiver Fatigue

Family and caregiver fatigue is a well noted but rarely studied phenomenon. The economic mandates of managed care organizations have shifted care from the hospital to the outpatient and home setting, placing a greater burden and responsibility for the cancer patient's care on family members. Unfortunately, the costs of time lost from work and increased fatigue on the part of the caregiver are rarely considered. For a rare and personal account of an experience caring for a loved one, the reader is referred to an article by an oncology nurse and wife of a stem cell transplant recipient (Rivera, 1997). Chapter 20 examines caregiver fatigue in greater detail.

Fatigue as a Long-Term Consequence

Little is known about the presence, duration, and intensity of fatigue as a long-term consequence of cancer and its therapy. The BMT research literature serves as a model in identifying those most at risk for acute fatigue related to deconditioning and has wide implications for cancer patients in general. More than any patient population, BMT recipients are followed by teams worldwide to monitor long-term engraftment, disease, cure, and complications arising from this treatment.

For example, cataracts are a known consequence of total body irradiation. However, patients receiving single-dose chemotherapy regimens are not likely to manifest this problem. Researchers studying the effects of BMT are fortunate in working with a group of patients that is in a large database and tends to be responsive to contributing to the knowledge of long-term outcomes.

Many recipients and their families return to transplant centers annually for up to five years after treatment and data collected at that time have contributed further to the known consequences of high-dose chemotherapy, total body irradiation, graft-versus-host disease, and treatment failure.

Where Do We Go From Here?

One area of research that is just beginning to expand is that of fatigue in the pediatric cancer population. Two researchers, Hockenberry-Eaton and Hinds, have begun to investigate fatigue in this population. As discussed in Chapter 4, the ability of children to speak in metaphors with honesty and dignity serves as an excellent model for communicating with adults.

Researchers must be sensitive to the fact that the clinical and personal management of fatigue has not considered the importance of fatigue as a family and personal role problem. Future studies need to be directed toward identification and interventions for this problem. Furthermore, economic investigations need to examine the broader picture of costs to caregivers, the workplace, and the community. Only with the fullest elaboration of the experience of fatigue, not just the identification of fatigue symptoms, can clinical interventions and supportive management of fatigue be addressed adequately. The most effective treatment for fatigue may be models of intervention rather than one treatment per se. Realistic expectations from the patient's point of view may reduce the distress experienced, thus enabling the use of self-care and coping strategies. Strategies that may be useful in developing empirically based interventions for cancer patients include exercise and attention-restoring activities. The safety, content, and timing of these interventions require considerable research that can be modeled and replicated in multiple settings.

In brief, fatigue is a multidimensional subjective symptom that encumbers thousands of cancer patients before, during, and after treatment. Only recently have health care providers, patients, caregivers, and advocacy groups come together to attempt to solve or resolve this universal symptom.

References

Aistars, J. (1987). Fatigue in the cancer patient: A conceptual approach to a clinical problem. *Oncology Nursing Forum, 14*, 25–30.

Barnett, M. (1997). Fatigue. In S. Otto (Ed.), *Cancer Nursing* (pp. 669–678). St. Louis, MO: Mosby.

Barton-Burke, M. (1998). Fatigue and quality of life. In C. R. King and P. S. Hinds (Eds.), *Quality of life: From nursing and patient perspectives* (pp. 255–283). Sudbury, MA: Jones and Bartlett.

Berger, A. M. (1998). Patterns of fatigue and activity and rest during adjuvant breast cancer chemotherapy. *Oncology Nursing Forum, 25*, 51–61.

Blesch, K. S., Paice, J. A., Wickham, R., Harte, N., Schnoor, D. K., and Purl, S. (1991). Correlates of fatigue in people with breast or lung cancer. *Oncology Nursing Forum, 18*, 81–87.

Buchsel, P. (1993). "Patterns of symptoms experienced by bone marrow transplant recipients during an early discharge trial." Master's thesis, Seattle Pacific University, Seattle, WA.

Buckner, C. D., Clift, J. E., Sanders, J. E., Stewart P., Bensinger, W. I., and Doney, K. C. (1984). Marrow harvesting from normal donors. *Blood, 64*, 630–634.

Fatigue Coalition (September 22, 1998). Fatigue most prevalent, longest-lasting cancer-related side effect. <http://www.plsgroup.com/dg/b090c.htm>

Greenleaf, J., and Kozlowski, S. (1982). Physiological consequences of reduced physical activity during bed rest. *Exercise and Sports Science Review, 10*, 84.

Haylock, P. J., and Hart, L. (1979). Fatigue in patients receiving localized radiation. *Cancer Nursing, 2*(6), 461–467.

Irvine, D. M., Vincent, L., Graydon, J. E., and Bubela, N. (1998). Fatigue in women with breast cancer receiving radiation therapy. *Cancer Nursing, 21*, 127–135.

Jamar, S. (1989). Fatigue in women receiving chemotherapy for ovarian cancer. In S. Funk, E. Tournquist, M. Champagne, L. Archer-Cobb, and R. Wiese (Eds.), *Key aspects of comfort: Management of pain, fatigue and nausea.* New York: Springer.

Jassak, P. (1995). An overview of biotherapy. In P. T. Rieger (Ed.), *Biotherapy. A comprehensive overview* (pp. 3–13). Sudbury, MA: Jones and Bartlett.

MacVicar, M. G., and Winningham, M. L. (1986). Promoting the functional capacity of cancer patients. *Cancer Bulletin, 38,* 235–239

Meyers, C. A., Weitzner, M. A., Valentine, A. D., and Levin, V. A. (1998). Methylphenidate improves cognition, mood, and function of brain tumor patients. *Journal of Clinical Oncology, 16,* 2522–2527.

Miller, C. B., Jones, R. J., Piantodosi, S., Abeloff, M. D., and Spival, J. L. (1990). Decreased erythropoietin response in patients with the anemia of cancer. *New England Journal of Medicine, 322,* 1698–1692.

Molassiotis, A., and Morris, J. (1998). Fatigue after bone marrow transplantation: 5 years of experience. *Bone Marrow Transplantation, 21,* S250 (Abstract N937).

Pater, J. L., Zee, B., Palmer, M., Johnston, D., and Osoba, D. (1997). Fatigue in patients with cancer: Results with National Cancer Institute of Canada Clinical Trials Group studies employing the EORTC QOL-C30. *Supportive Care in Cancer, 5,* 410–413.

Piper, B. F., Dibble, S. L., Dodd, M. J., Weiss, M. C., Slaughter, R. E., and Paul, S. M. (1998). The revised Piper Fatigue Scale: Psychometric evaluation in women with breast cancer. *Oncology Nursing Forum, 25,* 677–684.

Piper, B. F., Lindsay, A. M., and Dodd, M. J. (1987). Fatigue mechanisms in cancer patients: Developing nursing theory. *Oncology Nursing Forum, 14,* 17–23.

Portenoy, R. K., and Miaskowski, C. (1998). Assessment and management of cancer-related fatigue. In A. M. Berger, R. K. Portenoy, and D. E Weissman (Eds.), *Principles and practice of supportive oncology* (pp. 109–119). Philadelphia: Lippincott–Raven.

Richardson, A. (1995). Patterns of fatigue in patients receiving chemotherapy (abstract). In *Fatigue: The impact and scope of the problem.* Amsterdam: Excerpta Medica.

Rivera, L. M. (1997). Blood cell transplantation: Its impact on one family. *Seminars in Oncology Nursing, 13,* 194–199.

Shelton, B. K., and Turnbough, L. (1996). Flu-like syndrome. In S. L. Groenwald, M. H. Frogge, M. Goodman, and C. H. Yarbro (Eds.), *Cancer symptom management* (pp. 59–76). Sudbury, MA: Jones and Bartlett.

Skillings, J. R., Sridhar, F. G., Wong, C., and Paddock, L. (1993). The frequency of red cell transfusions for anemia in patients receiving chemotherapy: A retrospective cohort study. *American Journal of Clinical Oncology, 16,* 22–25.

Smets, E. M. A., Garssen, B., Schuster-Uitterhoeve, A. L., and de Haes, J. C. J. M. (1993). Fatigue in cancer patients. *British Journal of Cancer, 68,* 220–223.

Spector, D. (1995). Transfusion-associated graft-versus-host disease: An overview and two case reports. *Oncology Nursing Forum, 22,* 97–101.

Splett, P. L. (1996). *Costs outcomes of nutrition intervention* (part 1 of a 3-part monograph). Evansville, IN: Mead Johnson.

Sutherland, H. J., Fyles, G. M., Adams, G., Hao, Y., Lipton, J. H., and Minden, M. D. (1997). Quality of life following bone marrow transplantation: A comparison of patients' reports with population norms. *Bone Marrow Transplantation, 19*, 1129–1136.

Syrjala, K. L., Chapko, M. K., Vitaliano, P. P., Cummings, C., and Sullivan, K. M. (1993). Recovery after allogeneic marrow transplantation: Prospective study of predictors of long-term physician and psychosocial functioning. *Bone Marrow Transplantation, 11*, 319–327.

Vogelzang, N. J., Breitbart, W., Cella, D., Curt, G. A., Groopman, J. E., and Horning, S. J. (1997). Patient, caregiver, and oncologist perceptions of cancer-related fatigue: Results of a tripart assessment survey. *Seminars in Hematology, 34*, 4–12.

Winningham, M. L. (1983). "Effects of bicycle ergometry on functional capacity and feelings of control in women with breast cancer." Doctoral dissertation, Ohio State University, Columbus, OH.

Winningham, M. L. (1991). Walking program for people with cancer: Getting started. *Cancer Nursing, 14*, 270–276.

Winningham, M. L. (1992). How exercise mitigates fatigue: Implications for people receiving cancer therapy [Monograph]. *Oncology Nursing Forum: The Biotherapy of Cancer-V*(Suppl.), 16–21.

Winningham, M. L. (1994). Cancer and exercise. In Goldberg, L., and Elliot, D. L. (Eds.), *Exercise for prevention and treatment of illness* (pp. 301–315). Philadelphia: F. A. Davis.

Winningham, M. L. (1995). Fatigue: The missing link to quality of life. *Quality of Life Research 4*, 2.

Winningham, M. L. (1999). Fatigue. In C. Yarbro, M. Frogge, and M. Goodman (Eds.), *Cancer symptom management* (pp. 58–76). 2nd ed. Sudbury, MA: Jones and Bartlett.

Winningham, M. L., and MacVicar, M. G. (1983). Exercise as a tension reduction mechanism in cancer patients. *Ohio Journal of Science, 83*, 75 (Abstract).

Winningham, M. L., MacVicar, M. G., and Burke, C. (1986). Exercise for cancer patients: Guidelines and precautions. *Physician Sportsmedicine, 14*, 125.

Winningham, M., Nail, L., Barton-Burke, M., Brophy, L., Cimprich, B., Jones, L., Pickard-Holly, S., Rhodes, V., St. Pierre, B., Beck, S., Glass, E. C., Mock, V. L., Mooney, K. H., and Piper, B. (1994). Fatigue and the cancer experience: The state of the knowledge. *Oncology Nursing Forum, 21*, 23–36.

York, A., Clift, R., Sanders, J., and Buckner, C. D. (1992). Recombinant human erythropoietin (rHu-Epo) administration to normal marrow donors. *Bone Marrow Transplantation, 10*, 412–417.

Resources

Consumers are urged to call 1-800-4CANCER or contact their local chapter of the American Cancer Society for further information. Many of the large comprehensive cancer centers around the United States have Web sites for local referrals. Quality information is also available at the following Web sites:

The National Cancer Institute's CancerNet: http://cancernet.nci.nih.gov/

The University of Pennsylvania's Oncolink covers people as well as information about cancer in domestic animals: http://cancer.med.upenn.edu/

The American Cancer Society: http://www.cancer.org/

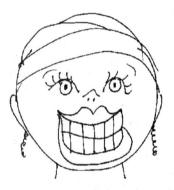

In my doctor's
office....

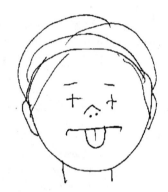

Later, at home....

A Medical Oncologist's View

Brian T. Pruitt

You know, when I was feeling so sick after treatment, I didn't want anyone around. Just having to talk with them and try to explain things to them was more than I could even imagine. I seemed to be too tired to sleep. My mind fought to concentrate, but I couldn't. I kept coming back to my cancer. What was this monster inside? Was the therapy doing any good? Did my doctor even know what was going on? Somehow, I seem to look so good in the clinic. She runs in the room: "How are you doing, Marge?" "Fine!" I chirp. They can't fool me—before she even comes in the room, she pushes the button to signal the cleaning staff to get the room ready for the next patient. You know, I even get charged extra if I have questions? And anyway, at that very moment I can't think of anything else to say. I even forget about the wilted list of questions I wanted to ask that is forgotten, right there, in my perspiring hand.

All this comes back when I go home and lie down. I can't even remember what it was they were telling me about my drugs. The questions are coming back now to haunt me. Fear stalks me, and I can't escape it. My mind is too tired to do the things I used to do to escape or to relax, and no one seems to understand. I don't even have the energy to explain, and my thoughts just buzz around and around in circles. I want to escape, but I am bound in the prison of gravity and my bed.

Long-term breast cancer survivor, 56 years old, with recent metastases

Background

I hesitated to address the problem of fatigue. I encountered fatigue every day in my clinic patients, but like most physicians, I had no special knowledge about it. My medical education included almost nothing about fatigue as experienced by cancer patients, and when I tried to read more about it, I did not find it listed in the indexes of standard oncology textbooks. In addition, there are no standard medical tests that give a "fatigue count" or an "exhaustion level." Further, in cancer patients, the underlying causes of fatigue are not always treatable. In view of traditional medical practice, which tends to emphasize objective clinical measures such as diagnostic tests and laboratory values, this is particularly frustrating. How can I do something about a problem that I cannot see or touch, for which there is no direct and objective evidence? I have learned most of what I know in the past few years by listening to my patients and asking about their fatigue.

In this chapter, I present a more traditional medical approach to evaluating patients with fatigue by looking for treatable disorders that can cause the problem. To help others understand the medical approach, I describe some of the common medical disorders that are known to cause fatigue in people with cancer. These disorders usually fall under one of the following categories: (1) depression, (2) anemia (low red blood cell count), (3) cancer chemotherapy, (4) hypoxemia (low levels of oxygen), (5) hyponatremia (low sodium), (6) hypercalcemia (high calcium levels in the blood), and (7) advanced cancer. I also present a few of my observations about long-term fatigue after cancer chemotherapy is completed.

Depression

When patients complain of fatigue, I think initially of depression. Although estimates vary widely, about 30% or more of cancer outpatients experience a reactive depression at some point in their illness, and fatigue is one of the common symptoms presenting with depression. A diagnosis of depression by *Diagnostic and Statistical Manual of Mental Disorders,* fourth edition (DSM-IV) criteria (American Psychiatric Association, 1994) requires that a patient have at least five of the following symptoms almost every day for the preceding two weeks, and either dysphoria or anhedonia must be one of the five symptoms.

- Dysphoria (pervasive, depressed mood, feeling sad).
- Anhedonia (diminished interest or pleasure in daily activities)—not just dread of vigorous activity (which often accompanies long-term anemia).
- Significant weight loss (without intentional dieting) or weight gain (at least 5%).
- Insomnia (trouble sleeping) or hypersomnia (too much sleep). Insomnia may include trouble falling asleep, staying asleep (keep waking up), or waking up too early.
- Psychomotor retardation (slowing down) or agitation (nervous activity or restlessness) observable by others and not just felt by the individual. This may be observed by others before the individual feels it.

About the Contributor

Prior to engaging in the practice of oncology, Brian Pruitt's background included the three M's: mathematics, medical school, and the military. He is currently actively involved in both research and clinical practice. He also teaches, is part of many cancer-associated committees, keeps up-to-date through his participation in several general medical and oncology professional organizations, publishes, and contributes to his community. Brian has great clinical knowledge, balanced by compassion and intuitive clinical insight.

- Feelings of fatigue or loss of energy on a daily basis that are not relieved by rest. (People with cancer-related fatigue may feel better in the morning or feel a little better after rest. In people with depression, awakening in the morning may be accompanied by feelings of dread or exhaustion.)
- Feelings of worthlessness and excessive or inappropriate guilt (not just related to feeling of guilt over what the person cannot do because of the illness).
- Trouble concentrating; diminished ability to focus or make decisions.
- Recurrent thoughts of death or suicide (in contrast to fear of dying).

Some of these symptoms may occur with fatigue from other causes, potentially mimicking depression.

I find that patients may deny feeling "depressed" but readily admit to easy tearfulness, fatigue, sleeplessness (especially waking up after sleeping a short time), and trouble concentrating. These patients often feel much better with effective antidepressant therapy, and fatigue is one of the first symptoms to be relieved. The newer selective serotonin reuptake inhibitor (SSRI) antidepressants have an energizing effect that can relieve the fatigue from depression even when the other contributors to fatigue persist. It is important to emphasize to cancer patients that receiving treatment for depression is entirely appropriate. It is not a sign of moral or spiritual weakness, nor is it cheating.

Anemia

Anemia is defined as a blood hemoglobin concentration below 12 grams per deciliter (g/dL) for women or below 13 g/dL for men. These normal values may vary somewhat between individuals and depend on altitude; that is, hemoglobin levels adjust to living at higher altitude (i.e., Denver, Mexico City, Salt Lake City). Mild anemia may lead to few symptoms other than fatigue with exertion. Patients with more severe anemia (e.g., hemoglobin levels of ≤ 8 g/dL) will usually experience more continual fatigue, dizziness, headache, irritability, and trouble concentrating. However, the hemoglobin level associated with these symptoms is quite variable. Patients who rapidly become anemic may have significant symptoms at a hemoglobin level of 10 g/dL, while those who become anemic more slowly may be asymptomatic at a hemoglobin level of 5 or 6 g/dL. Also, patients with

One coworker described him as a "Renaissance man." When he modestly expressed doubt about his worthiness to write this chapter, we told him, "There are no real experts. This is too new. Write it from a traditional oncology background, as someone who is in the process of learning about fatigue." He is learning in the best way a physician can: He is listening to his patients.

other medical problems (such as pulmonary disease) may experience more symptoms than expected from a relatively mild degree of anemia.

Whenever possible, the best treatment for anemia is to correct the underlying cause. Problems like iron deficiency, for example, are often readily correctable. However, the most frequent causes of anemia in cancer patients are (1) chronic disease, (2) bone marrow invasion by tumor, and (3) chemotherapy or radiotherapy. These underlying problems are not always correctable, and it is often necessary to use blood transfusions, a synthetic form of erythropoietin (r-HuEPO), or both. Erythropoietin is a natural product of the body that stimulates red blood cell production. The recombinant pharmaceutical erythropoietin equivalent (epoetin alfa), approved for use by the U.S. Food and Drug Administration, is marketed under the name Procrit and Epogen.

Transfused red blood cells carry a risk of viral and bacterial infections as well as allergic reactions. For patients with early malignancies, there is also some concern that blood transfusions may exert an immunosuppressive effect and may worsen the prognosis from the cancer. At the least, this can be stressful on the body.

If started early enough, r-HuEPO therapy can sometimes help avoid transfusions. After a dose of 10,000 units of r-HuEPO is given parenterally three times per week, the hemoglobin concentration may not increase significantly for several weeks. Recent evidence suggests that the entire week's r-HuEPO dose of 30,000 units may be administered in one weekly injection. When 30,000 units is ineffective, the dose may be increased to 45,000 units, 60,000 units, and even up to 90,000 units per week as needed. (Readers are referred to the latest U.S. Food and Drug Administration–approved guidelines for the use of this drug.)

Cancer Chemotherapy

Fatigue is almost always one of the side effects of chemotherapy. The severity of the fatigue varies considerably. The neurotoxicity of some chemotherapeutic agents such as cisplatin and vinblastine produces a great deal of fatigue, while other agents have milder effects. Chemotherapy-related fatigue is often so mild that it is not reported to the oncologist. (One must also consider the individual and cultural influences that affect how people express their fatigue.)

In preparation for writing this chapter, I reviewed the charts of 40 breast cancer patients whom I had treated recently with doxorubicin and cyclophosphamide as adjuvant treatment (after mastectomy or lumpectomy). Of these patients, 17 had no fatigue (or more likely, I had not documented any information about their fatigue) during or after their chemotherapy. Fifteen patients complained of mild fatigue that did not interfere with everyday activities. Eight patients complained of moderate fatigue that limited activities but was not described as severe. Of the patients having mild or moderate fatigue, about half were depressed. Which came first, the fatigue or the depression? Although chemotherapy-associated fatigue could surely predispose to depression, I had automatically considered the fatigue to be a symptom of depression.

I resolved that I would more carefully ask the patients in my clinic about their fatigue. The first patient I questioned was a woman being treated with the regimen mentioned above. She said initially that she had no fatigue. After further inquiry, she told me that she had experienced fatigue during the first two weeks of each three-week chemotherapy cycle. Because of the fatigue, she had reduced the number of hours she worked each day and had taken a daily nap. However, she had expected to be tired during the chemotherapy, and she did not find the symptom significant enough to report. I wonder if she even would have mentioned it to me if I had not asked.

Hypoxemia

Hypoxemia, an abnormally low blood oxygen concentration, often presents with fatigue rather than shortness of breath. The problem has many possible causes in cancer patients, including pleural effusions, tumor infiltration of the lungs, pulmonary emboli, chemotherapy-induced lung toxicities, and heart failure. The easiest method for documenting hypoxemia is pulse oximetry, in which a portable, noninvasive device is attached to a patient's finger to estimate the percent oxygen saturation of hemoglobin. The normal result is 95% or greater. A value less than 90% is an indication for supplemental oxygen therapy. For most patients with hypoxemia, supplemental oxygen will relieve the fatigue almost immediately. A more precise method for assessing a patient's oxygenation is arterial blood gas (ABG) analysis, which requires an arterial puncture. ABG parameters include the percent oxygen saturation, the partial pressures of oxygen and carbon dioxide, the pH, the bicarbonate concentration, and the oxygen content of the blood. The oxygen content is abnormally low in the presence of either hypoxemia or anemia, or a combination of the two. Although it is not widely used, measurement of oxygen content is potentially helpful in assessing patients with fatigue.

Hyponatremia

Hyponatremia may be defined as a serum sodium concentration less than 135 milliequivalents per liter (mEq/L). However, symptoms are unusual with sodium concentrations above 125 mEq/L unless the fall in sodium concentration has been rapid. The symptoms of hyponatremia include fatigue, headache, loss of appetite, and confusion. With severe or sudden hyponatremia, the symptoms may progress to seizures or coma.

Some of the causes of hyponatremia (e.g., diuretics) are associated with dehydration, while others (e.g., congestive heart failure, cirrhosis) are associated with edema. Patients with small-cell lung cancer may have hyponatremia without either dehydration or edema. In these patients, the cancer produces *antidiuretic hormone,* a factor that prevents the kidneys from excreting water. The retained water dilutes the serum sodium concentration. Patients with this disorder need to restrict their fluid intake to avoid becoming hyponatremic. Demeclocycline, a tetracycline derivative, can help these patients by temporarily decreasing the sensitivity of their kidneys to antidiuretic hormone, allowing them to excrete water.

Hypercalcemia

Hypercalcemia, a serum calcium concentration of more than 10.5 milligrams per deciliter (mg/dL), may cause fatigue, confusion, loss of appetite, constipation, renal insufficiency, and cardiac arrhythmias. Some patients develop these problems at calcium concentrations of 11.5 to 12.0 mg/dL, while others remain asymptomatic at higher concentrations. The calcium level must be interpreted carefully when the serum albumin concentration is lower than 4 g/dL. When the albumin level is low (as it often is in poorly nourished cancer patients), the calcium measurement is falsely low. To avoid missing significant hypercalcemia when the albumin level is low, a simple formula should be used to correct the serum calcium:

$$\text{Corrected calcium} = \text{The measured calcium} + (4 - \text{Serum albumin})$$

I have developed the habit of haunting garage sales, yard sales, and bookstores, pestering my neighbors for copies of large, outdated calendars with beautiful and pleasing pictures. I cut them up so someone doesn't have to hold or balance anything heavy to look at them. I made a file of them with major categories— outdoor scenes of mountains and seas, religious pictures, pictures of cute little animals—things people tell me they find pleasurable and places their minds can escape to in times of emotional darkness and distress and exhaustion. The pictures have to be big, so they can be seen without glasses, or when people's eyes don't focus well, and when taped to the wall, and I often put them in a clear plastic folder so the picture can be easily changed or wiped off with disinfectant without damaging the wall or the picture.

You don't know how many patients have held on to my hand to thank me, or even cried, because it gave them something to think about besides their cancer, or their pain. And if they need to escape from it, all they have to do is close their eyes and rest. If they want to take the picture with them in their minds, they can do that, too. I have seen people in pain finally drift off to sleep with a peaceful, weary smile, thinking about playing puppies, or the wind through the trees on a mountain.

Hospice volunteer

Advanced Cancer

Patients with advanced malignancy may experience fatigue in the absence of the problems just discussed. This fatigue is often accompanied by anorexia, weight loss, and other constitutional symptoms. Some cancers (lung cancer, for example) characteristically cause severe fatigue and anorexia, while others (breast cancer is the best example) cause relatively little fatigue and almost no anorexia. The causes of these symptoms are not clearly understood. It would be valuable to know whether the fatigue results from excessive energy utilization by the cancer or whether the fatigue is a neurological effect of a tumor-secreted factor.

Long-Term Fatigue

I find that almost every patient experiences some degree of fatigue during combination chemotherapy. Generally the fatigue lasts just a few months, resolving gradually but completely after the chemotherapy is completed. For a few patients, however, the fatigue is more persistent and more severe. For example, I recently saw a young woman who has had continual fatigue since her chemotherapy and mediastinal radiotherapy for Hodgkin's disease six years ago. By the time she gets her children up and off to school every morning,

---

The effect in sickness of beautiful objects, of variety of objects, and especially of brilliance of colour is hardly at all appreciated. . . . I have seen, in fevers (and felt, when I was a fever patient myself), the most acute suffering produced from the patient not being able to see out of [the] window and having [only one] view. I shall never forget the rapture of fever patients over a bunch of bright-coloured flowers. I remember (in my own case) a nosegay of wild flowers being sent me, and from that moment recovery becoming more rapid.

People say the effect is only on the mind. It is no such thing. The effect is on the body, too. Little as we know about the way in which we are affected by form, by colour and light, we do know this, that they have an actual physical effect.

Variety of form and brilliancy of colour in the objects presented to patients are actual means of recovery.

But it must be slow variety, e.g., if you show a patient ten or twelve [pictures] successively, ten-to-one that he does not become cold and faint, or feverish, or even sick; but hang one up opposite him, one on each successive day, or week, or month, and he will revel in the variety.

The folly and ignorance which reign too often supreme over the sick-room cannot be better exemplified than by this. . . .

Volumes are now written and spoken upon the effect of the mind upon the body. Much of it is true. But I wish a little more was thought of the effect of the body on the mind.

Florence Nightingale, *Notes on Nursing*

she has significant fatigue. At work in her job as a schoolteacher, she is exhausted by noon. She has found that she can function all day only if she goes to bed in the early evening every night. Although she experiences guilt about the limited time she spends with her children, she is not depressed. Most of the patients I have seen with this degree of fatigue cannot work a full day.

Here is a rule of thumb I have found useful: *Patients with chemotherapy-associated fatigue generally feel better at the beginning of the day and increasingly tire after some activity. Patients who are depressed wake up tired and find it difficult to initiate any activity.*

Where Do We Go From Here?

Fatigue, as it afflicts people with cancer, is variable in its causes, severity, and duration. When the fatigue is secondary to depression or medical problems such as anemia or hypoxemia, it may improve when the underlying problem is corrected. The fatigue from advanced cancer is usually unrelenting. While the palliative management of pain and nausea has improved immensely in recent years, we lack effective methods to treat fatigue in patients with advanced malignancies.

Fatigue may also be caused by chemotherapy. The fatigue that occurs with chemotherapy is usually mild and self-limited, but some patients are permanently disabled by fatigue. Many of these patients are long-term survivors who are considered "cured" of their cancers. Because they no longer have cancer, they are no longer considered ill, but they certainly are not well. There seems to be no place for them in the health care system. Newer chemotherapy agents and combinations with reduced neurotoxicity may help to avoid the problem.

I have also found it helpful to discuss fatigue with my patients before starting their chemotherapy. I advise them to get plenty of sleep at night, maybe an hour more than usual, and I encourage them to maintain their physical fitness by exercising during the day, perhaps walking four or five times per week. (See Chapter 18 for more information.) These recommendations need more research before they can be formalized, but they do seem to help patients avoid fatigue during chemotherapy.

For the patients who are already fatigued after chemotherapy, we are sorely limited in what we can offer. I have found that simply asking about my patients' fatigue, listening, and taking the problem seriously helps them to cope and adjust to the problem. It helps legitimize that their fatigue is a real phenomenon. To be able to offer more than that, we need to understand more about the nature and mechanisms of cancer-related fatigue.

References

American Psychiatric Association (1994): *Diagnostic and statistical manual of mental disorders.* 4th ed. Washington, DC: American Psychiatric Association.

Resources

The American Cancer Society publishes and/or distributes a series of authoritative references and texts for both physicians and nurses that are updated on a regular basis. These include the following:

American Cancer Society, Massachusetts Division (1990). *Cancer manual.* 9th ed. Boston: American Cancer Society.

Murphy, G. P., Lawrence, W., Jr., and Lenhard, R. E., Jr. (1995). *American Cancer Society textbook of clinical oncology.* 2nd ed. Atlanta: American Cancer Society.

Varricchio, C., Pierce, M., Walker, C. L., and Ades, T. B. (1997). *A cancer source book for nurses.* 7th ed. Sudbury, MA: Jones and Bartlett.

Most nursing references are attuned to symptom management as part of integrative nursing care. The following can be used as good resources on both disease and treatment in oncology:

Barton-Burke, M. (1996). *Cancer chemotherapy: A nursing process approach.* 2nd ed. Sudbury, MA: Jones and Bartlett.

Buchsel, P. (1993). *Oncology nursing in the ambulatory setting: Issues and models of care.* 1st ed. Sudbury, MA: Jones and Bartlett.

Groenwald, S. (1996). *Cancer symptom management.* 1st ed. Sudbury, MA: Jones and Bartlett.

Groenwald, S. L., Frogge, M. H., Goodman, M., and Henke Yarbro, C. (1998). *Cancer nursing: Principles and practice.* 4th ed. Sudbury, MA: Jones and Bartlett. (Available on CD-ROM.)

Otto, S. (1997). *Oncology nursing.* 3rd ed. St. Louis: Mosby Year-Book.

Internet Resources

Although there is much cancer-related information of a questionable nature on the Internet, the following Web sites are well-developed, trustworthy resources with large amounts of information useful for patients, health care professionals, and researchers:

The National Cancer Institute has a Web site called CancerNet with a broad variety of resources including those sponsored by the U.S. Government: http://cancernet.nci.nih.gov/. This site has public as well as professional information. It includes information on clinical trials and access to the Physician's Data Query (PDQ). In addition, patients may obtain information by calling 1-800-4CANCER.

OncoLink is an impressive resource hosted by the University of Pennsylvania Cancer Center: http://cancer.med.upenn.edu/.

The American Cancer Society also has a Web site: http://www.cancer.org/.

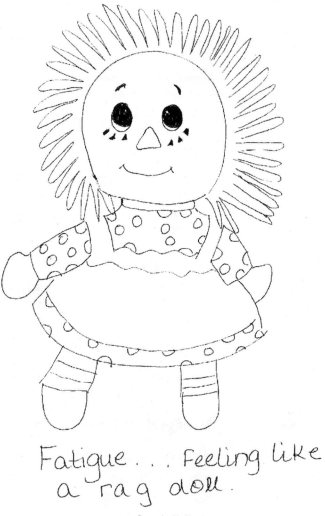

Fatigue ... Feeling like a rag doll.

Brenda Heil, 33 years old, 9-year survivor

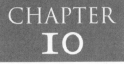

CHAPTER 10

The Pharmacist's Perspective

Lisa N. Meadows

All hurry or bustle is peculiarly painful to the sick. . . . Always sit down when a sick person is talking business to you, show no sign of hurry, give complete attention and full consideration if your advice is wanted, and go away the moment the subject is ended.

Florence Nightingale, *Notes on Nursing*

Background

Debilitating fatigue is now known to be the most frequently reported symptom related to cancer (Magnusson et al, 1997; Vogelzang et al, 1997; Winningham et al, 1994). Causes probably include not only the disease process, but also various cancer treatments, supportive therapies, changes in activity, and associated stressors of multiple origins. Fatigue has serious detrimental effects on quality of life (QOL) and may even interrupt or delay cancer therapy by altering nutrition, mood states, energy level, and the ability to contend with adverse treatment effects. All members of the health care team can take part in evaluating and managing fatigue. Fatigue no longer has to be an accepted component of the disease process for patients because options are available for controlling its impact. Pharmacists can advise other health care professionals and cancer patients on how to balance pharmaceutical treatment alternatives and drug doses with individual patient needs to secure optimal symptom—and fatigue—responses without sacrificing successful outcomes.

It is essential to determine whether patients are taking other medications or even over-the-counter drugs outside of their normal treatment regimen. Some highly promoted herbal or "natural" remedies may actually cause health problems, affect laboratory tests, or interfere with treatment. Ultra-high vitamin dosages may do the same. Health food stores feature many products that advertise an increase in energy or vigor. It is essential to gain the patient's confidence and determine whether any of these are being taken, whether they could pose a health threat, and whether they could interfere with treatment. Pharmacists can play a significant role by alerting other members of the health care team to nontraditional remedies that could present a problem to the patient's health and well-being.

Symptom management in cancer patients has focused mainly on pain and nausea. Little effort has been applied to assessing and treating fatigue, although it is considered by patients to exceed pain and nausea as a distressing phenomenon. This is possibly because fatigue was not viewed as a sign of pathophysiological danger or risk. For instance, pain may indicate disease progression or inhibit postsurgical ambulation, which could prevent such serious complications as atelectasis, pneumonia, or blood clots. Nausea and vomiting have been associated with electrolyte imbalances and dehydration. In comparison, fatigue appears to be relatively innocuous: Its effects are much more global and far-reaching rather than acutely obvious and threatening.

In a national study by Vogelzang and colleagues (1997) at the University of Chicago, 80% of oncologists surveyed believed fatigue to be overlooked and undertreated. Seventy-eight percent of their patients surveyed had experienced fatigue during the course of disease and treatment. Moreover, 74% of these patients believed fatigue to be a symptom they simply had to endure. The same study showed fatigue to be a symptom that was rarely discussed and even more rarely viewed as treatable.

At a recent international conference of professional oncology pharmacists, fatigue was identified as a unique therapeutic entity in the symptom management of the oncology patient. It is particularly important because it may reduce a patient's ability to cope with other symptoms like pain and nausea. In 1992 and 1995, Winningham proposed an interactive relationship between fatigue, other symptoms, and suffering wherein fatigue potentiated the distress associated with other symptoms, and other symptoms intensified the perception of fatigue (propositions 8 and 9 of the 10 propositions in Table 8-1). In recent validation of these propositions, a National Cancer Institute of Canada clinical trial examined factors affecting fatigue level. Patients in whom emesis was better controlled showed significantly less perceived fatigue after chemotherapy than in those in whom it was not controlled (Pater et al 1997). Figure 10-1 features a model that demonstrates the relationship between fatigue and two of the most clinically treated symptoms, pain and nausea. It suggests a relationship between symptom impact on patient's activities of daily living and the multiple dimensions of their QOL. This model includes critical elements such as nutrition, relationships, and emotional state to QOL. Successful interventions by an informed health care team can slow or break the symptom relationships demonstrated in this model.

Assessing Fatigue

Fatigue should be monitored on a regular basis. All health care providers can work with patients in monitoring these distressing cancer symptoms. Families should be included in these assessments as they often see changes in activity before the patient notices them. To

About the Contributor

After graduating from the University of Richmond (Virginia) in 1990 with a bachelor of arts in biology, Lisa Neurohr Meadows attended the Virginia Commonwealth University–Medical College of Virginia School of Pharmacy. Graduation in 1993 was followed by a wedding ceremony, honeymoon, and the National Board exams. She then moved across the Atlantic to join her husband and work for the U.S. military hospital in Landstuhl, Germany. During this time she was part of a team that established an outpatient pharmacy clinic in the largest European military community and supported the Bosnian relief

<table>
<tr><td>Figure
10.1</td><td>The Cancer Symptom Interrelational Model</td></tr>
</table>

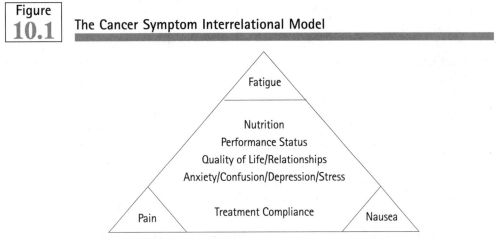

monitor symptoms in general, and fatigue specifically, a multidisciplinary approach utilizing standardized evaluation tools and clinical guidelines should be established as a standard of practice in every oncology setting. For example, a simple linear analogue scale such as is commonly used for pain or was proposed by Rhoton for fatigue can be utilized. This type of scale allows patients to assign a number from 0 to 10 (0 = none, 10 = the most) to represent the intensity of the three symptoms as they are experienced (Rhoton, 1982). Recording scale results along with daily activities in a journal permits comparisons as changes occur in patients' perceived energy levels and their difficulty with the other symptoms. Consistent evaluation of these diaries by the health care team provides necessary information on trends that can aid in symptom management.

Many options exist for treating cancer: chemotherapy, immunotherapy, hormone therapy, surgery, and radiation. One of the most common treatment-related sources of fatigue experienced by oncology patients is anemia. This phenomenon is usually cyclic in nature, depending on phases of treatment cycles. Suppression of erythropoiesis from bone marrow

effort with on-site pharmacy services for evacuated refugees. Her oncology experience began in Germany with exposure to European pharmaceuticals and pharmacognosy (pharmacology of natural drugs) in addition to the current U.S. therapies. Her former position as the oncology pharmacy specialist at the New England Veterans Affairs Medical Center and her current position at the Dana Farber Cancer Center in Boston have provided continued experience with oncology issues facing an aging population. She may occasionally still be heard to say "y'all."

or blood loss due to invasive procedures reduces levels of healthy red blood cells. Other adverse effects of these treatments contributing to fatigue include electrolyte imbalances from vomiting and diarrhea, painful mobility from neuropathy, combating infection from neutropenia, and damage to large organs such as the heart, resulting in reduced cardiac output. Adjunctive medications used to manage these toxicities of anticancer therapies may cause sedation and compound fatigue. Increased blood levels of drugs due to altered metabolism from liver or kidney impairment and inappropriate use of medications increase the potential for any side effects. Because high-dose therapies are utilized as treatment for many tumor types, aggressive supportive care strategies to address toxicities and ameliorate myelosuppression are necessary (Henry, 1997).

A frequent treatment strategy involves the use of several chemotherapeutic agents, each drug with a different mechanism of action, at once. The synergistic effect from a combination of drugs is more powerful than the effect of a single drug because each drug targets a different phase of the tumor cell's growth cycle. Chemotherapy may also be used concomitantly with surgery or radiation for some tumor types like head and neck (squamous cell) cancer, to aid in shrinking the tumor by sensitizing tumor cells and increasing the response to treatment (Jacobs and Pinto, 1995). All classes of chemotherapy have the potential for causing myelosuppression, though bleomycin (an antibiotic) and vincristine (a plant alkaloid) have a reported incidence of less than 1%. Tamoxifen, an oral antiestrogen agent used to treat breast cancer, may contribute to myelosuppression and reports of fatigue. Other biological drug alternatives exist for some tumor types. Interferon used in treating malignant melanoma and multiple myeloma is notorious for causing fatigue associated with a flu-like syndrome accompanied by myelosuppression (Quesadactal, 1986). Although combined treatment modalities can increase tumor response and survival rates for many cancers, they may also increase the impact of overlapping side effects like myelosuppression and fatigue. Examples of dose-limiting toxicities in various chemotherapeutic agents are listed in Table 10-1.

Anemia

Anemia is the most common hematological abnormality in oncology patients (Koeller, 1998). As red blood cell count diminishes, so does the body's ability to supply oxygen to working tissues. This contributes to metabolic exhaustion, or true energetic fatigue. Symptoms related to anemia that can also be documented in patient journals include dyspnea on exertion, tachycardia, edema, palpitations, dizziness, skin pallor, and hypersensitivity to cold. All these phenomena can be clarified through the associated pathophysiological mechanisms.

Anemia may be caused by bleeding, decreased red blood cell production (hypoproliferation) from nutritional insufficiency, myelosuppression, hemolysis from autoimmune disorders, and certain drug reactions. With some cancers, tumor infiltration of bone replaces healthy marrow and leads to the impaired production of blood cells.

Table 10.1 Myelosuppressive Cytotoxic Agents	
Drug	**Reported Incidence of Myelosuppression**
Alkylating drugs—agents that interrupt DNA replication by cross-linking	
Carboplatin	>10% (dose-limiting toxicity)
Carmustine	>10% (delayed, dose dependent)
Cisplatin	>10% (dose dependent)
Cyclophosphamide	1%–10%
Ifosfamide	1%–10%
Antibiotics—agents that intercalate base pairs of DNA, interrupting replication, and have no antibacterial properties	
Doxorubicin	>10% (dose-limiting toxicity)
Mitomycin	>10% (dose dependent)
Topotecan	>10% (dose-limiting toxicity)
Antimetabolites—agents that inhibit DNA synthesis	
Fludarabine	>10% (dose-limiting toxicity)
Fluorouracil (5FU)	>10%
Methotrexate	1%–10% (dose dependent)
Plant alkyloids/derivatives that feature varied mechanisms of action	
Docetaxel	>10%
Etoposide	>10% (dose-limiting toxicity)
Paclitaxel	>10%
Vinblastine	>10% (dose-limiting toxicity)

Source: Adapted from Lacy et al., 1997–98.

Evaluation

Laboratory findings most commonly associated with anemia include decreasing or subnormal hemoglobin (Hgb) and hematocrit (Hct) levels. Normal Hgb is generally considered to be 14 to 18 grams per deciliter (g/dL) in men and 12 to 16 g/dL in women (Chernecky and Berger, 1997). In a study at Rush-Presbyterian-St. Luke's Medical Center in Chicago, patients with Hgb levels greater than 12 g/dL reported significantly less fatigue, fewer nonfatigue anemia-related symptoms, better physical and functional well-being, and better QOL (Cella, 1997). Other laboratory measures used to determine the presence of anemia included red blood cell indices (e.g., total red blood cell count, mean corpuscular volume, red blood cell size, distribution, and width) and reticulocyte count (Chernecky and Berger, 1997). Vitamin deficiencies and low nutritional cofactors may also play a role in the development of anemia. These are evaluated by measurement of, for example, serum iron, ferritin, folate, and cyanocobalamin (B_{12}) levels, as erythropoiesis requires adequate levels of these cofactors. Nutritional deficiency of cyanocobalamin or folic acid results in failure of erythrocyte nuclear formation. Iron is necessary for development of the heme component of hemoglobin and myoglobin. An inadequate supply of iron results in reduced ability of red blood cells to carry oxygen. Since anemia is often multifactorial in cancer patients (Koeller, 1998), the combination of objective clinical data with subjective reporting of fatigue and concurrent symptoms provides practitioners with a picture of the relationship between anemia and how it affects patients.

Treatment

The diagnosis and treatment of anemia require careful assessment. It may resolve with successful management and the elimination of contributing factors, or it may reflect more serious underlying conditions. For acute treatment of symptomatic anemia, such as may result from blood loss, transfusions replenish the circulating volume to control symptoms and prevent oxygen-deficiency damage to body tissues. Recombinant human erythropoietin (r-HuEPO) stimulates the production of red blood cells from the bone marrow in the nonacute setting.

Nutritional Deficits

For nutritional deficits, various oral forms of iron, including ferrous sulfate or ferrous gluconate, are available. A polysaccharide formulation that is available may be better tolerated by some patients. Iron should be administered on an empty stomach to maximize absorption but may be given with meals to reduce stomach upset. Calcium, antacids, and some antibiotics interact with iron and reduce absorption; two to three hours should be allowed between dosing of each medication. Patients should be advised that iron can cause constipation and discoloration of stools. If symptoms occur, the addition of a stool softener such as docusate sodium to the treatment regimen may be required.

For treatment of folate deficiency, a 1-milligram (mg) tablet of folic acid is available by prescription. Folic acid has been associated with decreased levels of phenytoin and increased seizure activity, especially when given in high doses (i.e., > 5 mg/day). Caution should be used with the concomitant use of these drugs. Patients should be warned not to self-treat with over-the-counter versions of these drugs.

Cyanocobalamin (vitamin B_{12}) is given intramuscularly every month for maintenance therapy. Vials of cyanocobalamin contain 100 or 1,000 micrograms per milliliter (μg/mL). The physiological maintenance dose required is 100 to 200 micrograms per month.

With any drug therapy, full prescribing information should be *reviewed prior to treatment and periodically during treatment.* It is important to note that patients often do not remember instructions, particularly when they are stressed and exhausted. Written instructions and making an appointment for telephone follow-up can be effective in reinforcing prescribing information. Further, responses should be monitored regularly by evaluating both subjective and objective data.

Recombinant Human Erythropoietin

Erythropoietin, a glycoprotein secreted mainly by interstitial cells of the kidneys, causes proliferation and differentiation of erythroid precursor cells in bone marrow. Cancer patients have been shown to have a blunted production of endogenous erthropoietin relative to their degree of anemia (Miller, 1990). The r-HuEPO is indicated for the treatment of anemia in patients with nonmyeloid malignancies whose anemia is due to the effect of concomitantly administered chemotherapy. The r-HuEPO is also indicated to reduce the need for blood transfusions in these patients (Medical Economics Company, 1997).

Many providers are already familiar with r-HuEPO because of its success in treating anemia and improving the QOL in patients with chronic renal failure (Macdougall, 1998). Oncology dosing differs significantly from the dosages given to chronic renal failure patients. In the oncology setting, r-HuEPO is dosed at 150 units per kilogram (U/kg) via subcutaneous injection three times weekly and increased to 300 U/kg if a 1.0 g/dL increase in Hgb is not achieved after four weeks (see treatment algorithm in Figure 10-2). A once-weekly dosing schedule, based on the r-HuEPO indication for surgery, offers a more convenient method of administration and is currently being studied in the oncology population. Because response usually takes four weeks, r-HuEPO is not an option for the acute management of anemia; however, with appropriate patient monitoring, r-HuEPO can reduce the severity of anemia before fatigue and related symptoms have a significant impact on QOL.

A number of clinical trials have evaluated the impact of r-HuEPO therapy on the QOL of cancer patients. In a series of double-blind, placebo-controlled trials, QOL measures (i.e., perceived energy level, activity level, overall QOL) were assessed by a 10 0-millimeter visual analogue scale in 413 anemic cancer patients either receiving or not receiving concomitant chemotherapy (Abels et al, 1991). The r-HuEPO–treated patients received doses of 100 to 150 U/kg subcutaneously three times a week for 8 to 12 weeks, or until a target Hct of 38% to 40% not related to transfusion was achieved. The dose of r-HuEPO was then titrated to maintain the Hct in the target range. Patients treated with r-HuEPO that achieved a 6% increase in Hct or higher unrelated to transfusion exhibited a significantly greater improvement in all three indicators of QOL as compared to the placebo group ($p < 0.05$).

An open-label, community-based study assessed clinically relevant outcomes to r-HuEPO therapy, including QOL measures, in more than 2,000 anemic cancer chemotherapy patients (Glaspy et al, 1997). The r-HuEPO was given at a dose of 150 U/mg subcutaneously three times a week for up to four months, with a dose increase to 300 U/kg if a satisfactory response as determined by the physician was not seen after eight weeks. As in the placebo-controlled trials, patients were asked to rate their energy levels, ability to perform daily activities, and overall QOL on a visual analogue scale. Prestudy scores were compared to poststudy scores to determine improvement in functional status associated with r-HuEPO therapy. By the completion of the study, statistically significant improvements over baseline values were observed in energy level, activity level, and overall QOL with

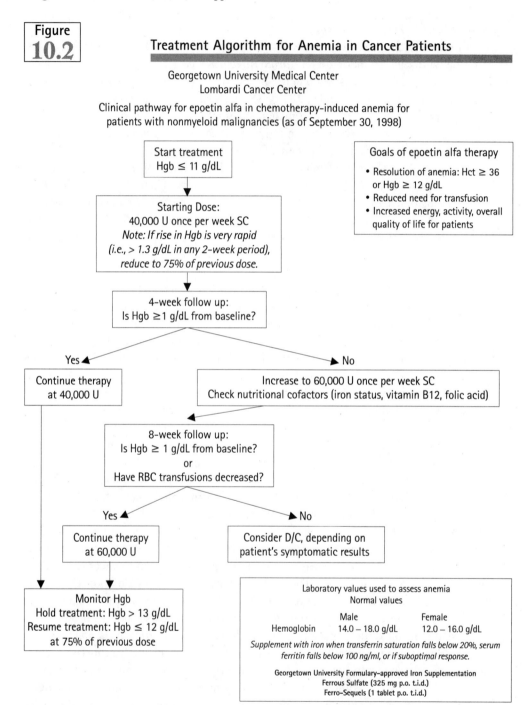

Figure 10.2

Treatment Algorithm for Anemia in Cancer Patients

Georgetown University Medical Center
Lombardi Cancer Center

Clinical pathway for epoetin alfa in chemotherapy-induced anemia for
patients with nonmyeloid malignancies (as of September 30, 1998)

Start treatment
Hgb ≤ 11 g/dL

Goals of epoetin alfa therapy

• Resolution of anemia: Hct ≥ 36
  or Hgb ≥ 12 g/dL
• Reduced need for transfusion
• Increased energy, activity, overall
  quality of life for patients

Starting Dose:
40,000 U once per week SC
*Note: If rise in Hgb is very rapid
(i.e., > 1.3 g/dL in any 2-week period),
reduce to 75% of previous dose.*

4-week follow up:
Is Hgb ≥1 g/dL from baseline?

Yes

Continue therapy
at 40,000 U

No

Increase to 60,000 U once per week SC
Check nutritional cofactors (iron status, vitamin B12, folic acid)

8-week follow up:
Is Hgb ≥ 1 g/dL from baseline?
or
Have RBC transfusions decreased?

Yes

Continue therapy
at 60,000 U

No

Consider D/C, depending on
patient's symptomatic results

Monitor Hgb
Hold treatment: Hgb > 13 g/dL
Resume treatment: Hgb ≤ 12 g/dL
at 75% of previous dose

Laboratory values used to assess anemia
Normal values

	Male	Female
Hemoglobin	14.0 – 18.0 g/dL	12.0 – 16.0 g/dL

*Supplement with iron when transferrin saturation falls below 20%, serum
ferritin falls below 100 ng/ml, or if suboptimal response.*

Georgetown University Formulary-approved Iron Supplementation
Ferrous Sulfate (325 mg p.o. t.i.d.)
Ferro-Sequels (1 tablet p.o. t.i.d.)

r-HuEPO therapy (p <0.001). The degree of improvement for each QOL parameter was directly correlated to the degree of increase in Hgb level (p <0.001).

Another large, open-label, community-based study was recently completed in anemic (Hgb <11 g/dL) cancer patients receiving chemotherapy. The tumor response was evaluated prospectively with the collection of Hgb values and QOL scores (Demetri et al, 1997). In this study, r-HuEPO was administered at an initial dose of 10,000 units subcutaneously three times a week. After four weeks of therapy, if the Hgb level did not increase by at least 1 g/dL, the subcutaneous dose was increased to 20,000 units, three times a week. The results of the study confirm the findings of the previous community-based study: Hgb level is an important factor involved in patient QOL and is independent of tumor response to chemotherapy.

Patients who are self-administering r-HuEPO should be counseled on proper injection technique and disposal of sharp instruments. Reimbursement for self-administration of r-HuEPO and other injectable drugs in the oncology setting is now universal. Iron supplemention may be necessary to support increased erythropoiesis. Patient counseling on a follow-up plan is important to promote compliance. Patients should be encouraged to keep "fatigue journals" to monitor daily activities, perceived energy level, and overall sense of well-being. Journals should be brought to clinic visits to document subjective responses to treatment and support objective findings. It is often striking what patients with cancer can accomplish when they have the energy for everyday living!

Fatigue Caused by Medications Used to Manage Symptoms

Side effects of medications often used to manage symptoms and toxicities of cancer treatments include fatigue and sedation. Drugs used to manage pain, nausea, mucositis/stomatitis, diarrhea, depression, and anxiety can compound fatigue from other causes. For example, morphine and adjunctive medications such as amitriptyline used to treat pain cause sedation in most patients. Likewise, agents used for treating nausea such as metoclopramide and prochlorperazine can cause drowsiness. Proper patient education is important to avoid confusing disease progression with a controllable drug side effect. A list of medications that may have sedating effects is in Table 10-2.

Abrupt cessation of corticosteroid treatment also is associated with emotional depression and feelings of exhaustion. It is not uncommon to hear patients report, "As long as I was on the prednisone, I was crawling the walls. I was up at midnight looking for laundry to do." However, when they are taken off the medication abruptly, the change in perceived energy levels is profound and they frequently report depression.

Drugs Used to Control Fatigue

It is not always easy to differentiate between fatigue and depression in cancer. Patients with depression should be treated appropriately with antidepressants and psychotherapy.

Table **10.2**	Medications Common to Cancer Patients That May Cause Sedation or Fatigue
Therapeutic Classes	**Generic Examples**
Antianxiety agents	Lorazepam, diazepam
Anticonvulsants	Carbamazepine, phenytoin
Antidepressants	Amitriptyline, imipramine
Antidiarrheals	Loperamide, diphenoxylate/atropine
Antiemetics	Prochlorperazine, trimethobenzamide
Antihistamines	Diphenhydramine, hydroxyzine
Antihypertensives	Clonidine, propranolol
Antipsychotics	Haloperidol
Gastrointestinal motility agents	Metoclopramide
Hormone therapy	Tamoxifen
Immunotherapy	Interferon
Muscle relaxants	Cyclobenzaprine
Opiates and derivatives	Morphine, oxycodone, codeine
Phenothiazines	Perphenazine

Recently, there has been some experimentation with using methylphenidate (Ritalin) to treat fatigue in cancer. It is important to emphasize that this is an off-label (not yet approved for this use by the U.S. Food and Drug Administration) use of the drug and is controversial. A recent review (Micromedix, 1997, see Chapter 1) of the use of methylphenidate in depression examined issues that should be evaluated in clinical trials before this drug can be recommended for use in fatigued cancer patients. Studies going back as early as 1958 have consistently showed no improvement in depressed patients as a result of methylphenidate treatment; however, studies showed rapid symptom improvement in medically ill, depressed patients. This was attributed to lessened fatigue and increased motor activity. Several cancer centers are currently evaluating methylphenidate in clinical trials as a possible treatment for cancer-related fatigue. (See further discussions in Chapters 11 and 17).

It is critical, when using psychotropic medications of any kind, to get a careful personal and family mental health history. For instance, patients who have a personal or family history of bipolar disorder (manic depression) have been known to have a full-fledged manic episode precipitated by prednisone. The use of methylphenidate in bipolar or schizophrenic disorders can lead to increased agitation, anxiety, mania, psychosis, or depression. Patients requiring psychotropic medications during cancer treatment should be referred to a psychiatrist affiliated with a cancer center for appropriate evaluation and individualized management. Paradoxical reactions to methylphenidate similar to those found in children have

Figure 10.3	Checklist for Taking Medications

❑ Your name: _____ Telephone number: _____

❑ Name of pharmacy/pharmacist: _____

❑ Telephone number of pharmacy: _____

   ❑ Less busy hours at pharmacy: _____

❑ Number for your pharmacy reimbursement card: _____

❑ Emergency telephone number for clinic/physician/nurse: _____

   ❑ During hours clinic/office is closed: _____

❑ Vitamins, minerals, or herbal (natural) products you are taking:

   ❑ _____

   ❑ _____

❑ Allergies to foods, medications, dental products, or environment (to what, when, what kind of reaction):

   ❑ _____

   ❑ _____

❑ Current medications (name, dose, how to take it, when, instructions, refills, etc.):

   ❑ _____

   ❑ _____

   ❑ _____

   ❑ _____

❑ Safe storage place   ❑ Journal of symptoms and responses

Source: From Winningham and Barton-Burke (2000). *Fatigue in Cancer: A Multidimensional Approach.* Sudbury, MA: Jones and Bartlett. Permission granted to copy and distribute this checklist for not-for-profit use.

also been reported in the elderly, with a potential sedating effect and increase in fatigue rather than an increase in psychomotor activity. It is clear that this treatment requires much more study before recommendations can be made.

Minimizing Potential Drug Interactions and Side Effects

Smaller doses of some medications may achieve the same therapeutic effect in special populations of patients. Pharmaceutical effects, including toxicities, are often magnified in the elderly, women, and children and may be due to decreased lean body mass. Patients with impaired renal or liver function due to disease or drug-induced toxicity cannot metabolize some drugs efficiently, resulting in higher serum drug levels. Drug-drug interactions may be more likely to occur in the elderly and in oncology patients for whom multiple-drug regimens are required. Toxic or subtherapeutic serum drug levels may be the result of these interactions.

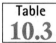

Table 10.3 | How Patients Can Get the Most Benefit From Medications

1. *Pharmacists are medication managers.* The pharmacist has the latest drug information and is trained to teach patients how to best manage medications. If possible, visit the pharmacy during slower work hours to have the pharmacist's undivided attention. Thoroughness takes time. If you find yourself too tired when you pick up your prescription, *ask about a telephone appointment* during off hours when you do not feel as stressed.

2. *Utilize only one pharmacy.* Computer profiles of allergies and adverse reactions as well as prescription history are maintained. Interactions between drugs may be avoided if the profile is complete.

3. *Request to be counseled about every medication,* including over-the-counter drugs, vitamins, and herbal remedies that do not require a prescription. *Natural* does not automatically mean "good." *Natural* can include uranium, arsenic, water, lead, and a host of other unhealthy things! Be honest with your pharmacist. Include, for instance, bad reactions you have had to certain foods or to treatments at the dentist. The pharmacist can offer valuable information on the potential for drug-drug, food-drug, drug-environment, and other interactions. Most states require an offer of counseling be made to patients, but it is up to you to accept. Get information in writing, if possible.

4. *Understand the basics*:*
   What is the medication for and what does it look like?
   How do you take it (i.e., time of day, with or without food, route of administration)?
   How often do you take it (or is it just "as needed")?
   What should you expect in terms of intended and potential side effects?
      What side effects require contacting the nurse or physician?
      What side effects may be the sign of a medical emergency?
   What should you do in case of a missed dose?
   Where should you store it (e.g., in the refrigerator or at room temperature)?
   How long will it have to be taken?
   Are there any refills?
   Are there other foods, drugs, environmental exposures (such as sunlight), or dietary supplements to be avoided during therapy?
   What is the expiration date of the medication?

5. *Read all the information provided with each prescription.* Make sure you get answers to your questions before you leave the pharmacy or hospital. Make sure all prescription labels are legible. Some patients may have changes in vision during drug treatments. Print on labels may have to be made larger, or bottle caps color-coded to aid with identification of medications.

6. *Obtain a new prescription at the next doctor's appointment if no refills remain.* Do not rely on the pharmacist to call for authorization. (The time spent on the phone could be better spent talking about medications.) One good way to remember this is to look at the label. When you go to refill a prescription and the bottle label reads "1 refill left," call your clinic about a refill or put your reminder for a refill at the top of your list for your next appointment. If the label reads "0 refills left," call immediately.

7. *Set up a "pill box" or an administration chart that is well labeled* with days and times when multiple medications are required. If a family member is helping, ensure that he or she is educated on all aspects of each drug given. Keep an up-to-date list of all medications and doses including over-the-counter vitamins, herbal, and natural products.

8. *With each hospital admission, bring the current medication list (including exact doses) and all medications for review.* This will save a lot of questions when you come in. It will also help the staff stay current

on what you are taking. Discard all discontinued drugs as directed by your pharmacist. Clarify any changes or additions to therapy by asking both the doctor and the pharmacist. Double-check to make sure the label on each bottle has current directions and that the refill and expiration information is current.

9. *Do not let others handle oral chemotherapy,* especially children or pregnant women. Keep all drugs in a locked cabinet if possible, and out of children's reach. Use child-proof caps whenever possible. Some drugs are toxic to children even in small doses.

10. *Keep a daily journal of signs or symptoms related to the disease or condition to be treated.* Monitor effects and outcomes of each treatment. (Communicate with members of the health care team regarding successes as well as failures!)

---

*Adapted from Federal Omnibus Budget Reconciliation Act of 1990 patient counseling guidelines.

Over-the-counter drugs, vitamin supplements, and herbal ("natural") medications are widely used and are important to include when evaluating a patient's medication and progress profile. Patients should be warned to avoid alcohol with any medication that causes fatigue or drowsiness due to central nervous system depression. Each patient's medication profile should be routinely reviewed and updated as changes take place (see Figure 10-3). Intended effects of drugs are always accompanied by unintended side effects. It is worth repeating that in addition to prescribed medications, pharmacists and other health care providers should also carefully ask questions about allergic or hypersensitive reactions, vitamin and mineral supplements the person may be taking, teas, nutritional natural supplements, and anything else related to self-treatment. It is not infrequent to find patients who do not acknowledge taking such products because they do not think of them as drugs. In addition, some patients are afraid that if they tell their pharmacist or health care provider they are using nontraditional treatments, they will be told not to use them.

Cancer patients, in particular, have many medications to manage, with frequent changes in dosing. These may be difficult to track, especially when they are already tremendously fatigued. The word *noncompliant* has often been used in a negative and accusatory manner toward patients. It is important for health care providers to ask whether alleged noncompliance is (1) the fault of health care providers who do not clearly communicate instructions; (2) the fault of health care providers who have failed to understand the patient's financial status, culture, and educational/literacy level; or (3) the fault of the patient because he or she really does not want to cooperate. We usually assume option 3 without thinking through options 1 and 2. Those who are noncompliant because of side effects or lack of appropriate counseling do not benefit from the intended goals of therapy (i.e., slowing of disease progression and symptom management).

With patients taking on more responsibilities for their care, good communication is vital to good health. Patients must know what to expect from their therapy, including the intended and unintended effects. The more informed patients are, the more compliant they will be, and the better they are able to make a difference in their own health care (see Table 10-3).

References

Abels, R. I., Larholt, K. M., Krantz, K. D., and Bryant, E. C. (1991). Recombinant human erythropoietin (r-HuEPO) for the treatment of the anemia of cancer. In *Blood cell growth factors: Their present and future use in hematology and oncology.* Dayton, OH: AlphaMed Press.

Barnett, M. L. (1997). Fatigue (pp. 669–678). In S.E. Otto (Ed.) *Oncology nursing.* 3rd ed. St. Louis: Mosby.

Cella, D. (1997). The Functional Assessment of Cancer Therapy–anemia (FACT-An) scale; a new tool for the assessment of outcomes in cancer anemia and fatigue. *Seminars in Hematology, 34*(3 suppl 2), 13–19.

Chernecky, C. C., and Berger, B. J. (1997). *Laboratory tests and diagnostic procedures.* 2nd ed. Philadelphia: W. B. Saunders.

Demetri, G., Wade, J., and Cella, D. (1997). Epoetin alfa improves quality of life in cancer patients receiving cytotoxic treatment independent of disease response: Prospective clinical trials results. *Blood, 90*(10 suppl 1), 175A.

Glaspy, J., Bukowski, R., Steinberg, D., Taylor, C., Tchekmedyian, S., and Vadhan-Raj, S. (1997). Impact of therapy with epoetin alfa on clinical outcomes in patients with nonmyeloid malignancies during cancer chemotherapy in community oncology practice. *Journal of Clinical Oncology, 15,* 1218–1234.

Henry, D. (1997). Haematological toxicities associated with dose-intensive chemotherapy, the role for and use of recombinant growth factors. *Annals of Oncology, 8* (suppl 3), s7–10.

Jacobs, C., and Pinto, H. (1995). Adjuvant and neoadjuvant treatment of head and neck cancers: The next chapter. *Seminars in Oncology, 22,* 540–552.

Koeller, J. M. (1998). Clinical guidelines for the treatment of cancer-related anemia. *Pharmacotherapy, 18,* 156–169.

Lacy, C., et al. (1997–98). *American Pharmaceutical Association drug information handbook.* 5th ed. Hudson, OH: Lexi-comp.

Macdougall, I. (1998). Quality of life and anemia: The nephrology experience. *Seminars in Oncology, 25*(3 suppl 7), 39–42.

Magnusson, K., Karlsson, E., Palmbad, C., Leitner, C., and Paulson, A. (1997). Swedish nurses' estimation of fatigue as a symptom in cancer patients–report of a questionnaire. *European Journal of Cancer Care, 6,* 186–191.

Medical Economics Company (1997). Procrit prescribing information (pp. 1212–1214). In *Physicians' desk reference.* 51st ed. Montvale, NJ: Medical Economics Company.

Micromedix. (1997). Topic: methylphenidate–therapy of depression. In *Drug consults, 97.* (Produced and distributed by Micromedix.)

Miller, C. (1990). Decreased erythropoietin response in patients with the anemia of cancer. *New England Journal of Medicine, 322,* 1689–1692.

Ortho Biotech (1998). Treatment algorithm for anemia in cancer patients. Raritan, NJ: Ortho Biotech.

Pater, J. L., Zee, B., Palmer, M., Johnson, D., and Osoba, D. (1997). Fatigue in patients with cancer: Results with National Cancer Institute of Canada Clinical Trials Group studies employing the EORTC QOL-C30. *Supportive Care in Cancer, 5,* 410–413.

Quesada, J., Talpaz, M., Rios, A., Kwizrock, R. and Gutterman, J. (1986). Clinical toxicity of interferons in cancer patients: A review. *Journal of Clinical Oncology, 4*(2), 234–243.

Rhoton, D. (1982). Fatigue and the postsurgical patient (pp. 277–300). In C.M. Norris (Ed.), *Concept clarification in nursing.* Rockville, MD: Aspen.

Vogelzang, N. J., Breitbart, W., Cella, D., Curt, G. A., Groopman, J. E., and Horning, S. J. (1997). Patient, caregiver and oncologist perceptions of cancer-related fatigue: Results of a tripart assessment survey. The Fatigue Coalition. *Seminars in Hematology, 34*(3 suppl 2), 4–12.

Winningham, M. L. (1992). How exercise mitigates fatigue: Implications for people receiving cancer therapy [Monograph]. *Oncolgy Nursing Forum: The Biotherapy of Cancer-V* (Suppl.), 16–21.

Winningham M. L. (1995). Fatigue: The missing link to quality of life. *Quality of Life Research,* 4, 2–6.

Winningham, M. L., Nail, L., Barton-Burke, M., Brophy, L., Cimprich, B., Jones, L., Pickard-Holly, S., Rhodes, V., St. Pierre, B., Beck, S., Glass, E. C., Mock, V. L., Mooney, K. H., and Piper, B. (1994). Fatigue and the cancer experience: The state of the knowledge. *Oncology Nursing Forum, 21,* 23–26.

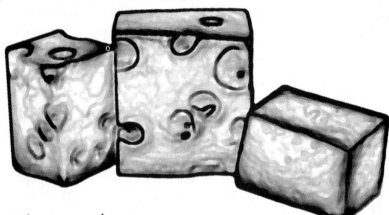

Like Swiss Cheese Memory . . .

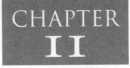

Select Psychiatric and Psychological Considerations

Henry Olders
Maryl L. Winningham

Introduction

The behavioral implications of this chapter fly into the face of tradition. If we are to make progress in the cancer-related fatigue syndrome, we have to be willing to examine the facts and think radically. Dr. Henry Olders' pioneering work in fatigue, sleep, and depression in cancer patients makes this chapter rich in new and challenging insights. In this presentation, Dr. Olders uses the "thought experiment" technique presented in Chapter 2.[1] Furthermore, his logic exemplifies the type of scientific inquiry proposed in the *Principia* (as related in Chapter 1) by Isaac Newton.

Among the disease- and treatment-specific conditions involved in the cancer-related fatigue syndrome (CRFS) are some that present a special opportunity in the field of oncological psychiatry. Complex metabolic, nutritional, pharmacological, lifestyle, genetic, and psychosocial issues challenge the clinician's ability to assess and appropriately intervene. The potential for psychiatry's contribution to the understanding and treatment of some aspects of the CRFS is only beginning to be appreciated.

A number of psychiatric conditions are of special concern in the context of the CRFS. On one hand, they may relate directly to the enigma of fatigue in cancer, such as the problem of differentiating and treating depression from fatigue. On the other hand, they may relate indirectly to the problem of the CRFS when the diagnosis and treatment of cancer threaten and overwhelm homeostatic coping mechanisms in vulnerable individuals. These threats, added to other compromises in patients, contribute to emotional exhaustion or counterproductive health belief practices. Examples include the effects of cognitive changes, depression, anxiety, prior trauma, and alterations in sleep patterns that frequently occur with the CRFS.

There are some excellent resources available on psychiatric conditions in cancer. Rather than reviewing what has already been well covered elsewhere, readers would better be served by a referral to other articles and books listed in the Resources section (Breitbart, 1995; Breitbart and Holland, 1988; Breitbart and Holland, 1993; Breitbart and Passik, 1993; Holland and Rowland, 1989; Kazak et al, 1996; Razavi and Stiefel, 1994). The present chapter focuses on topics that are less well known, but specifically significant to some components of the CRFS. Relatively little is mentioned in the literature about screening in oncology clinics, sleep disturbances, sleep-activity relationships, cognitive deficits resulting from cancer and its treatments, and the effect of traumatic life experiences on patients' responses to cancer. There are also new possibilities in pharmacological as well as behavioral interventions.

There are frequent questions about how much rest people with cancer should get, activity-rest issues, and how long people should nap. This chapter presents surprising insights on the traditional "get more rest" advice. Lay readers will find the comments surprising, clinicians will discover pearls of wisdom to pass along to their patients, and researchers should find the comments a stimulating basis for work in these areas.

—*M. L. W.*

Dr. Winningham: Dr. Olders, it is clear that cancer fatigue, or the CRFS, is different from tiredness experienced by healthy people or even the fatigue resulting from vigorous activity. Could you explain how cancer fatigue differs from other forms of fatigue?

Dr. Olders: The fact that a whole book can be devoted to the topic of fatigue in cancer testifies to its importance. Not only is it the most distressing symptom experienced by many cancer patients, but also it may interfere with self-care more than any other symptom.

I would like to make something clear: Fatigue is clearly not limited to cancer. It is also a significant issue in other medical illnesses and is often the chief reason why patients are unable to work. Here are some examples: Fatigue affects nearly 80% of patients with rheumatoid arthritis (Mahowald et al, 1989) and 68% with primary biliary cirrhosis (Cauch-Dudek et al, 1998). In the chronic fatigue syndrome, 28% of patients described their fatigue as being so severe that they became bedridden, able to do virtually nothing (Buchwald, Sullivan, and Komaroff, 1987). Complaints of tiredness and fatigue are universal during the initial weeks of Epstein-Barr viral infection (Guilleminault and Mondinir, 1986). Twenty percent of unemployed patients with acquired immunodeficiency syndrome (AIDS) or AIDS-related complex (ARC) reported that fatigue was largely responsible for the need to stop working (Darko et al, 1992). Most patients with chronic fatigue syndrome are unable

About the Contributor

When Henry Olders's service chief in consultation-liaison psychiatry at the Sir Mortimer B. Davis–Jewish General Hospital in Montreal asked him in 1995 if he were interested in being the liaison psychiatrist with the oncology department, he was unable to answer right away. Having lost his wife to colorectal cancer only three years earlier, he knew that daily contact with cancer patients would be sure to stir up painful feelings. But he felt also that what he had learned as witness to her courageous battle with her illness, her success at warding off depression, and the indomitable spirit that made it possible to accept her pain and fatigue while seeking (and finding!) something positive in every trial and setback, was something that he wanted to communicate to others. He finally concluded that fear of his own feelings should not stand in the way of helping relieve suffering by setting up a psycho-oncology clinic at the "Jewish."

to continue with full-time work, and many receive some form of disability payments for an extended period (Abbey and Garfinkel, 1991).

The fact that fatigue is so prominent in so many illnesses suggests that much of the fatigue experienced by cancer patients may be the result of having a serious illness. Certainly we need to consider those common elements when we address cancer fatigue.

Dr. Winningham: I'm glad to hear you say that. Chapter 1 in this book also suggests this approach. It is interesting that many of the individuals who initially present with one of the illnesses you mentioned are told they are depressed. I have had patients who told me they were *relieved* to have a diagnosis of cancer because they had been told they were crazy!

Dr. Olders: Fatigue is common and distressing in many medical conditions. It also figures prominently in the complex of symptoms of psychiatric affective disorders, whether major depression, dysthymic disorder, or bipolar depression.

The *Diagnostic and Statistical Manual of Mental Disorders*, fourth edition (DSM-IV) of the American Psychiatric Association (1994) includes the criterion "fatigue or loss of energy nearly every day" in its criteria for major depressive episode, and "low energy or fatigue" as a criterion for dysthymic disorder. The World Health Organization (1992) in its International Diagnostic Classification (ICD-10) includes the following in its description of a depressive episode: "In typical depressive episodes of all three varieties described below (mild, moderate, and severe), the individual usually suffers from depressed mood, loss of interest and enjoyment, and reduced energy leading to increased fatigability and diminished activity. Marked tiredness after only slight effort is common."

One of the problems is that various instruments used to aid in diagnosing depression consider fatigue an important component. For example, the Zung Self-rating Depression Scale (SDS) assesses the symptom "increased and unexplained fatigue" with the question "I get tired for no reason," which can contribute up to 4 points out of a total of 80 points.

A degree in electrical engineering (University of Waterloo, Ontario, 1970) and several years working as a computer systems engineer prior to studying medicine and then psychiatry at McGill University in Montreal comprise the backdrop to Henry's fascination with the biology of brain functioning. This background is particularly useful in his practice and research on interventions for treating cancer fatigue and depression by modulating rapid eye movement (REM) sleep.

Father of four and grandfather to three, Henry is happily remarried and fully occupied with family, work, singing in a community choir, lessons in ballroom dancing, and running with the "Wolf Pack." He nevertheless tries to find time for computer programming an artificial neural network to help diagnose psychiatric and neurological disorders.

The Beck Depression Inventory (BDI) includes 2 questions out of 21 that address fatigue: one about tiredness; the other about ability and motivation to work. The Hamilton Depression Scale permits a clinician to assess a patient's degree of depression; 2 questions, worth up to 6 points out of a possible 64, tap decrease in work and activities due to fatigue, as well as loss of energy and fatigability.

Dr. Winningham: For years, cancer fatigue was ignored because we didn't seem to realize how devastating it was, we thought it was depression, or thought it was an unavoidable part of cancer and cancer treatment. Could you address this?

Dr. Olders: Given that the fatigue associated with cancer and other serious illnesses may be indistinguishable from the fatigue of depression, it would be reasonable to explore whether illness-related fatigue may actually be a mild form of depression, perhaps a partial depressive syndrome that might occur in individuals who are *not predisposed* to develop a full-blown depression. If this is a reasonable hypothesis, then one might attempt to determine whether there are factors or circumstances associated both with depression and with fatigue in cancer and other illnesses.

Dr. Winningham: Wait a minute! For years we've been saying, "It's depression." More recently, we've been saying, "It's fatigue," and trying to get people to understand cancer fatigue. Now you're suggesting it may, indeed, be depression? You have defined your premises by alluding to the difficulty we have in discriminating fatigue from depression based on the DSM-IV diagnoses and the depression inventories. But what about the sleep disturbances, particularly insomnia, reported in cancer patients? Couldn't the fatigue experience in cancer be linked to insomnia?

Dr. Olders: Insomnia, defined as difficulty falling asleep or staying asleep, as well as hypersomnia, sleeping excessively, are common in patients with cancer, in other illnesses, and in depression. Fatigue and insomnia are reported to be closely linked in cancer (Grayden, 1994; Nail et al, 1991; Sarna, 1993) and during cancer treatment (Irvine et al, 1994). Fatigue and insomnia are also linked in people who have had heart attacks (McCorkle and Quint-Benoliel, 1983), who are receiving hemodialysis (Brunier and Graydon, 1993), and who suffer from rheumatoid arthritis (Mahowald et al, 1989). They are also linked in chronic fatigue syndrome patients, of whom 81% had at least one sleep disorder, most frequently sleep apnea (44%) and idiopathic hypersomnia (12%) according to one study (Buchwald et al, 1994). It may even be that you don't need cancer or another serious illness to experience crippling fatigue: Insomnia may be enough. Spielman, Saskin, and Thorpy (1987) found that insomnia patients have the same levels of fatigue as fibrositis syndrome patients.

On the surface, this connection between fatigue and insomnia seems self-explanatory. After all, if you don't get enough sleep, *of course* you'll be tired. As my teenage daughter says, "Duh!" But many people with fatigue seem to get lots of sleep: Bipolar depressed patients often have hypersomnia, yet complain of fatigue; chronic fatigue syndrome patients spend more time in bed and nap more than normal, healthy people (Sharpley et al, 1997). Insomnia also is closely linked to depression. Insomniacs had four times the rate of affective disorder and double the rate of anxiety disorder compared to the general population (Schramm et al, 1995).

Part of the problem may be terminology. Although the dictionary definitions for *tiredness* and *fatigue* are similar, and bear no relationship to drowsiness or sleepiness, these terms are frequently used interchangeably, by lay people (Carskadon, Brown, and Dement, 1982) as well as by researchers (Moldofsky, 1992; Nofzinger et al, 1991). For example, Martikainen and coauthors (1992) wrote, "Tiredness may take the form of sleepiness." According to Glaus (1993), on aspect of fatigue is the "dull, sleepy" factor. The Piper Fatigue Self-Report Scale include "sleepy" and "drowsy" as fatigue sensations (Piper et al, 1989). The idea that fatigue may be caused by insufficient sleep (Jamar, 1989) may spring from this confusion in terminology. So it is entirely possible that individuals with poor sleep who also have fatigue will interpret their tiredness as being caused by insufficient sleep and attempt to increase their sleep. Insomnia may even contribute to *causing* depression. In a study involving almost 8,000 community respondents, people who still had insomnia a year after an initial interview were 40 times more likely to be depressed. This last finding (Ford and Kamerow, 1989), that insomnia may trigger depression, is particularly difficult to reconcile with other findings about the connection between sleep and depression. For example, sleep deprivation is used to treat depression, but sleeping afterward causes the depression to return (Wiegand et al, 1987). Excessive sleep is found in patients with bipolar depression, in young depressed patients, and in patients with seasonal affective disorder (SAD). If insomnia truly represents insufficient sleep, then one would expect depressed people to sleep less, not more, than normal people.

Dr. Winningham: Taking this a step farther, are you suggesting that insomnia, depression, and excessive sleep may be related?

Dr. Olders: What if, contrary to what most people believe, insomnia (or at least, the most common form known as primary or psychophysiological insomnia) actually is the result of trying to sleep *more* than one needs (Chambers and Keller, 1993)?

What is known is that insomniacs get into bed early, stay in bed late, and nap (Spielman, Saskin, and Thorpy, 1987). They spend *more time in bed* than normal subjects (Middelkoop et al, 1996), they underestimate the amount they actually sleep (McCall and Edinger 1992), but they sleep as much as normal people (Pace-Schott et al, 1994). The amount of daytime sleep is directly related to sleeping problems (Bazargan, 1996). In fact, voluntarily extending sleep is known to cause insomnia (Aserinsky, 1969). Conversely, *reducing time in bed* is a very effective treatment for insomnia (Bliwise et al, 1995; Spielman, Saskin, and Thorpy, 1987) even when it is due to chronic pain (Morin, Kowatch and Wade, 1989).

Following this line of reasoning, we can see that insomnia and hypersomnia are similar in that both represent excessive sleep. The finding that depressed people are likely to have either hypersomnia or insomnia is not contradictory. It is possible that the element of

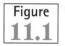

Figure 11.1   A Historical Perspective on Getting Up Early

The quotations and proverbs that follow suggest that for hundreds of years, the emphasis was on early rising. The earliest recorded reference to "early to bed" appeared in 1639.

As the olde englysshe proverbe sayth in this wyse,
who soo woll ryse erly
shall be holy helthy and zely.

(zely = happy, fortunate)
Wynkyn de Worde,
A Treatyse of Fysshynge wyth an Angle, 1496

Diluculo surgere saluberrimum est.
(to rise early is very healthy)
William Lily (ca. 1468–1522),
Latin Grammar, 1513

At grammar-scole I lerned a verse, that is this,
Sanat, sanctificat, et ditat surgere mane.
That is to say,
Erly rysyng maketh a man hole in body, holer in
soule, and rycher in goodes.
Anthony Fitzherbert (1470–1538),
The Book of Husbandry, 1523

Six hours in sleep, in law's grave study six,
Four spend in prayer, the rest on Nature fix.
Sir Edward Coke (1549–1634)

To business that we love we rise betime,
And go to 't with delight.
William Shakespeare (1564–1616),
Antony and Cleopatra

Ryse you early in the morning,
for it hath propertyes three:
Holynesse, health, and happy welth,
as my Father taught mee.
Hugh Rhodes, *Boke of Nurture*, 1577

Earley to bed and earely to rise,
makes a man healthy, wealthy, and wise.
John Clarke (1596–1658),
in *Paroemiolgoia Anglo-Latina*, 1639

One hour's sleep before midnight is worth
two hours after.
John Rays (1627–1705),
A Compleat Collection of English Proverbs, 1670

Plough deep while sluggards sleep.
Benjamin Franklin (1706–1790), maxim
prefixed to *Poor Richard's Almanac*, 1757

The early bird catches the worm.
unknown

My formula for success?
Rise early, work late, strike oil.
J. Paul Getty

insomnia that triggers depression may be excessive sleep. By extension, if fatigue is itself a form of depression, then excessive sleep may also trigger fatigue.

Dr. Winningham: Help me with something: We hear a lot today about people who are overworked and sleep deprived. Is this a modern phenomenon? In the days before electric lights, didn't people go to bed earlier and get up later? Isn't it likely that throughout the ages, most people got more sleep every night?

Dr. Olders: I don't believe that people necessarily slept a great deal more in years past than they do today. Consider the sixteenth-century maxim by Sir Edward Coke (see Figure 11-1): "Six hours in sleep, in law's grave study six, Four spend in prayer, the rest on Nature fix." Here's another from the eighteenth century: "Six hours sleep for a man, Seven for a woman, And eight for a fool." If people went to sleep at sunset, in the summertime when nights are short at high latitudes, they would get little sleep. What is more likely is that many people stayed up past sunset for much of the year, using the light from the stars, the moon, or a cooking fire for social gatherings with music making and storytelling. The more intense light provided by candles, gas, and now electricity is necessary for the evening activities of only a very few people, even today. And those activities (chiefly reading) are optional in any case.

Daytime sleepiness, other than the normal sleepiness in the early afternoon, may be a sign that the person is getting insufficient sleep. But it could also be a side effect of medication, or a symptom of narcolepsy or sleep apnea. It is certainly possible, and even likely, that many people in the United States and Canada are getting insufficient sleep in general. But these are people who are burning the candle at both ends, who are often highly productive and lead full, energetic lives. They are unlikely to listen to the message to get more sleep. The people who take this message to heart are the fatigued insomniacs who are already getting more sleep than they need!

Dr. Winningham: If you have had the right amount of sleep, shouldn't a person awaken in the morning "bright-eyed and bushy-tailed" as the saying goes? Isn't morning sleepiness a sign of insufficient sleep?

Dr. Olders: I rarely come across people who feel clear and alert when they first wake up. Usually, people feel very sleepy, and it may be that this sleepiness increases the longer you have slept! If people are sleepy when they first awaken (for me, until I'm actually drinking my first coffee), they may interpret their sleepiness as tiredness, and decide that they haven't had enough sleep. If they sleep in, they will have overslept, and they will encounter sleep difficulties that night (Helmus et al, 1996).

Dr. Winningham: Could you briefly clarify, then, what you would use as criteria for sleep disturbance?

Dr. Olders: I would ask the following questions: Do they have frequent difficulty with falling asleep, staying asleep, or waking earlier than desired? Do they experience distress due to these symptoms? Has there been a significant change in sleep patterns from when they were well, even if they are not distressed about it?

Dr. Winningham: Thank you. Back to the sleep-depression discussion. What mechanisms do you propose may be behind this?

Dr. Olders: Suppose that we accept the hypothesis that excessive sleep could trigger fatigue and even depression in predisposed individuals. Is this due to a particular aspect or characteristic of sleep? Let's look at the data on which we base our assumptions. We know that sleep, when monitored by measuring the electrical signals from the brain and from eye muscles (polysomnography), can be divided into five stages: stages 1 and 2 represent light sleep;

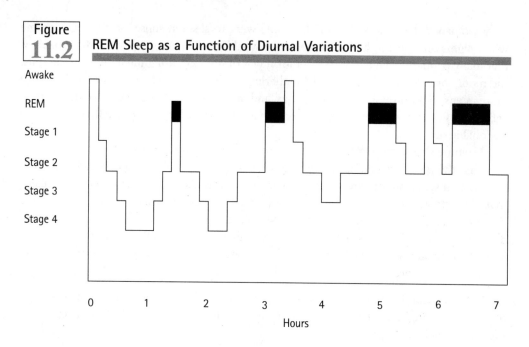

Figure 11.2   REM Sleep as a Function of Diurnal Variations

stages 3 and 4, called *slow wave sleep,* are deep restorative sleep; and rapid eye movement (REM) sleep is the last stage.

REM sleep typically starts about 90 minutes after we first fall asleep and recurs periodically throughout our sleep. REM sleep, which occupies about 20% to 25% of our total sleep time, is when we do most of our dreaming. This type of sleep appears to be essential for consolidation of long-term memory in our brains (Karni et al, 1992).

A lot of evidence suggests that REM sleep is linked to depression. For example, REM sleep is increased during depression (Lauer et al, 1995; Nofzinger et al, 1995) and in relapse of depression following successful treatment (Kupfer et al, 1991). Short REM latency and a shift of REM into the first part of the night are also markers for depression (De la Fuente et al, 1992; Lauer et al, 1995). Selective REM sleep deprivation is an effective antidepressant treatment (Klysner, Geisler, and Andersen, 1985). REM sleep is suppressed by antidepressant treatments including tricyclic medications such as nortriptyline and amitriptyline, the newer antidepressants including venlafaxine (Salin-Pascual, Galicia-Polo, and Drucker-Colin, 1997), and the selective serotonin reuptake inhibitors (SSRIs) like paroxetine (Saletu et al, 1989), and electroconvulsive therapy (Cohen and Dement, 1966). Psychostimulants that suppress REM sleep include methylphenidate (Chatoor et al, 1983) and dextroamphetamine (Saletu et al, 1989), exercise (Driver et al, 1988), and bright-light treatment used for SAD. One can predict the amount of clinical improvement that a depressed patient will eventually experience with tricyclic antidepressant treatment by measuring the amount of REM sleep suppression after the first dose (Höchli et al, 1986).

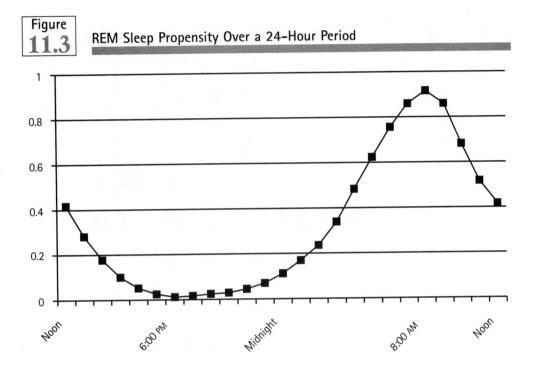

Figure 11.3 REM Sleep Propensity Over a 24-Hour Period

Conversely, the antihypertensive medication reserpine, which has depression as a side effect, is known to increase REM sleep (Faber and Havrdova, 1981). A depressed person who gets better with sleep deprivation will relapse if they have a nap, which includes REM sleep (Wiegand et al, 1987). Wiegand and colleagues (1987) proposed what they call "the depressiogenic sleep theory"; that is, *too much REM sleep may induce depression.* Given what I said earlier about the possibility that fatigue in cancer and other conditions is a mild form of depression, my proposal is to extend Wiegand's theory to include fatigue as a consequence of excessive REM sleep.

People often ask, If sleep is good for you, isn't it a good idea to get as much as you can? I ask them in turn, Is there anything that they can think of that we need, where some is good, for which excessive amounts do *not* lead to problems? Too much food causes obesity; too much sunlight causes skin cancer and cataracts; too much oxygen causes blindness in premature infants; too much water can result in seizures! And too much REM sleep may cause fatigue and depression.

Dr. Winningham: You've talked about REM sleep as a *stage* of sleep that possibly promotes depression and fatigue. How would cancer patients (or anyone else who becomes fatigued or depressed) get too much REM sleep? It sounds like sleep *patterns* are involved.

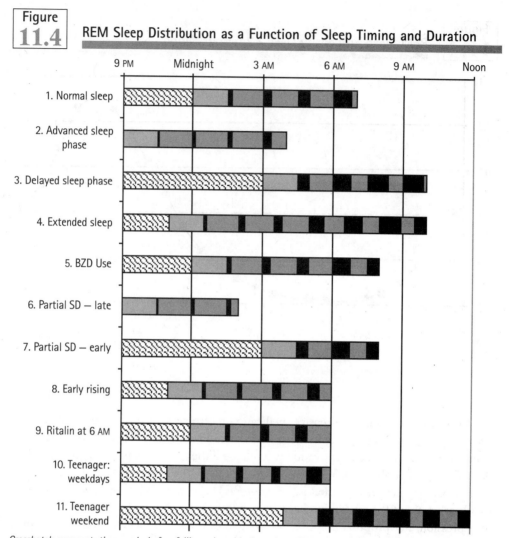

Figure 11.4 — REM Sleep Distribution as a Function of Sleep Timing and Duration

Crosshatch represents time awake before falling asleep; black portions, REM sleep; and gray portions, non-REM sleep (i.e., stages 1 through 4). BZD = benzodiazepine; SD = sleep deprivation.

Dr. Olders: To answer this question, we need to consider how REM sleep is *distributed* during sleep (see Figure 11-2). Normally, the first REM period occurs about 90 minutes after sleep onset; subsequent REM periods recur with a cycle length of about 90 minutes, but each REM interval throughout the night is longer than the previous one. It appears that REM sleep propensity has a diurnal variation (Akerstedt et al, 1993): It increases through the night (Carskadon and Dement, 1985), peaking at about 8:30 AM (Taub, Hollingsworth and Bruce, 1983), and then decreases through the day (Webb and Agnew, 1968) to reach a

Table 11.1	REM Sleep as a Function of Timing Versus Duration					
	Time of Sleep Onset	Awakening Time	Total Sleep (hr)	REM Sleep (hr)	REM (% of Total Sleep)	Change in REM (%) From Baseline
1. Normal sleep (baseline)	Midnight	7 AM	7	1.75	25%	0%
2. Advanced sleep phase	9 PM	4 AM	7	0.67	10%	-62%
3. Delayed sleep phase	3 AM	10 AM	7	2.96	42%	69%
4. Extended sleep	11 PM	10 AM	11	3.48	32%	99%
5. BZD use	Midnight	8 AM	8	2.25	28%	28%
6. Partial SD-late	9 PM	2 AM	5	0.33	7%	-81%
7. Partial SD-early	3 AM	8 AM	5	1.74	35%	-1%
8. Early rising	10:30 PM	5:30 AM	7	1.10	16%	-37%
9. Ritalin at 6 AM	Midnight	6 AM	6	0.99	17%	-43%
10. Teenager: weekdays	11 PM	6 AM	7	1.31	19%	-25%
11. Teenager: weekend	4 AM	Noon	8	3.58	45%	105%

BZD = benzodiazepine; SD = sleep deprivation.

minimum between 6:00 and 8:00 PM. A set of hypothetical values is plotted in Figure 11-3. Using these hypothetical values for REM sleep propensity, it is possible to demonstrate visually how REM sleep distribution varies as sleep timing and duration change in different situations (see Figure 11-4).

For each of the conditions shown in Figure 11-4, the total sleep time and the REM sleep time, based on the hypothetical values for REM sleep propensity, are calculated and shown in Table 11-1. In Table 11-1 and Figure 11-4, "normal sleep" is taken to consist of seven hours, from midnight to 7:00 AM. Advanced sleep phase, experienced to a greater or lesser degree by many elderly people, results in a 62% decrease in REM sleep for the conditions in our "thought experiment." Many people with advanced sleep phase offset the loss of REM sleep by returning to bed in the morning.

The delayed sleep phase syndrome (DSPS) experienced by some teenagers and young adults who find it next to impossible to get up early in the morning causes a 69% increase in REM sleep compared to normal sleep in our thought experiment, even though the total number of sleep hours is the same. DSPS, it should be noted, results in poor morning alertness, and in one study 75% of sufferers were or had been depressed (Regestein and Monk, 1995). Late sleeping, by itself, may aggravate or precipitate depression (Globus, 1969; Wehr et al, 1979), whereas delayed sleep can lead to feelings of depression, as well as decreased alertness, happiness, and energy (David et al, 1991). Could these effects be related to excessive REM sleep?

Staying in bed past the usual time of getting up results in longer sleep duration. Unfortunately, sleeping nine hours or longer is associated with poorer physical health (Belloc and Breslow, 1972) and with higher mortality (Wingard and Berkman, 1983). In nursing home residents, increasing impairment in activities of daily living correlates with longer sleep times (Meguro et al, 1990). The thought experiment demonstrates that extended sleep doubles REM sleep.

Continuing with this thought experiment, the amount of REM sleep varies more with the *timing* of sleep than with its *duration*. This may explain why late partial sleep deprivation, but not early partial sleep deprivation, can be an effective treatment against depression and premenstrual syndrome (Parry et al, 1995). The antidepressant response correlates with shorter REM duration (Sack, 1988). Even advancing the sleep phase by several hours without reducing sleep time has an antidepressant influence (Sack et al, 1985).

The sleep habits of some teenagers may also help explain their mood switches. For example, my daughter, who typically goes to bed at 11:00 PM on school nights and gets up before 6:00 AM, seems to have plenty of energy for the long commute, her classes, after-school sports and extracurricular activities, homework, and chatting with friends. On weekends, however, if she remains in bed until noon, she remains listless all afternoon, getting little accomplished, "comes alive" at 11:00 PM, and wants to party. It seems that the longer the time elapsed between the "depressiogenic" REM sleep of the morning, the better she feels.

Dr. Winningham: For years I've been concerned about the "get more rest" advice given to people with cancer. When I started my research back in 1981, that was common advice. I told cancer patients to take one or two short—20 to 30 minutes maximum—naps per day and to maintain regular sleep patterns. That advice was treated with so much incredulity that I reluctantly started saying 30 to 45 minutes maximum. I'm sorry I ever changed. One thing was certain: The people I observed who spent more time in bed went downhill quickly. I always wondered whether it was bed rest, the cancer, or treatments. The purpose of the exercise programs I developed was to counter the effects of the decreased activity. Can you elaborate on the application to cancer patients of what you just suggested?

Dr. Olders: Certainly. We can use our thought experiment to explain how cancer patients might be getting excessive REM sleep: sleeping too long, or simply sleeping late in the morning. For example, sleeping 11 hours, from 11:00 PM until 10:00 AM, doubles the amount of REM sleep, as does sleeping only 8 hours, from 4:00 AM until noon. Just adding one extra hour of sleep in the morning, which might result from using sleeping medication such as benzodiazepines, can increase REM sleep by 28%. Could this help to explain why taking sedative or hypnotic medication greatly increases the risk of becoming depressed (Patten, Williams, and Love, 1996)?

Dr. Winningham: And of course, the experience of cancer interferes with normal sleep patterns in so many ways. As I've pointed out for years, many people deal with fatigue by getting more rest, which results in more fatigue! It's nice to run into someone else who can give concrete reasons why this is counterproductive. It's quite logical and there are so many reasons. It's quite destructive. I think one of the few benefits of managed care is that patients don't spend as much time in the hospital lying in bed and watching television at all hours.

Dr. Olders: That's right. Why would cancer patients sleep longer or later in the morning? One reason is increased opportunity. Cancer patients frequently stop working, particularly when in active treatment, when fatigue is most severe (Smets et al, 1998). Hospitalized patients may have little to do other than sleep. Some patients use sleep as a way to escape boredom or the psychological distress caused by receiving their diagnosis, or to find respite from physical pain or other symptoms such as nausea or dyspnea. In addition, interferons and interleukins produced by the illness or as a result of the acute inflammatory response during cancer treatment induce sleepiness (Darko et al, 1992; Modofsky, 1993). Finally, opioids, antidepressants, many antiemetics, and antiepileptic medications used for pain control cause drowsiness.

This becomes a trap: Sleeping longer is likely to lead to insomnia (Aserinsky, 1969). Insomniacs, believing that their sleep difficulty means they're not getting enough sleep, attempt to sleep longer by spending more time in bed and napping more (Spielman, Saskin, and Thorpy, 1987). They are also more likely to take hypnotic medications. All these strategies may worsen their insomnia.

Sleeping longer, and in particular, sleeping later or returning to bed after breakfast increases the amount of REM sleep. I would like to hypothesize that this excessive REM sleep causes fatigue, or increased fatigue and other depressive symptoms. In individuals who are predisposed to clinical depression (on a genetic basis, for example), too much REM sleep may trigger a full-blown depressive episode.

What evidence is there for this hypothesis? It is known that ill people sleep more (Guilleminault and Mondini, 1986) as do cancer patients receiving treatment (Greenberg et al, 1993; Jamar, 1989). As the number of hours of daytime rest increases, so does physical fatigue (Kobashi-Schoot et al, 1985), which may be promoted by the excessive rest (Graydon et al, 1995; Winningham, 1991). Fatigue leads patients to attempt to sleep even more (Dodd, 1984); excessive sleep leads to insomnia (Spielman, Saskin, and Thorpy, 1987), which frequently coexists with fatigue in cancer patients (Degner and Sloan, 1995; Graydon, 1994; Irvine et al, 1994; Knobf, 1986; McCorkle and Quint-Benoliel, 1983; Sarna, 1993).

While there is a large body of mostly indirect evidence that excessive REM sleep can cause depression, and lots of convincing data that REM sleep suppression is an effective antidepressant treatment, there is little research on the influence of REM sleep on fatigue. Students whose sleep was prolonged to ten hours or more developed a "worn out" syndrome, described by the terms "tired, lethargic, in an irritable mood, fuzzy thinking, difficulty getting started" (Globus, 1969). The impaired mood and performance caused by sleep prolongation are hypothesized to be due to augmentation of REM sleep (Taub, 1980). Long sleepers have poorer psychological adjustment compared to short sleepers (Montplaisir, 1984). Melatonin, which increases sleep duration, also increases self-reported fatigue (Dollins et al, 1994).

Fatigue and hypersomnia are related in human immunodeficiency virus (HIV)–infected individuals (Darko et al, 1992), in chronic fatigue syndrome patients (Morris, Weardon, and Battersby, 1997), and in patients with infectious mononucleosis (Guilleminault and Mondini, 1986). In cancer patients receiving radiotherapy, fatigue correlated highly with number of hours of daytime rest (Kobashi-Schoot et al, 1985). A questionnaire study of cancer

Swiss Cheese Memory—Part One

About ten years ago, I enrolled at a major university to pursue a master's degree in political science with an emphasis on political economy. After several quarters, during which I worked in a paint factory and also taught, I had emergency surgery for cancer.

I had always been physically vigorous–never an illness–I was a really big guy and could work like a horse (with apologies to the horse). Not long after beginning chemotherapy, I began to experience physical symptoms. My little fingers and ring fingers, and the sides of my hands above those fingers and on up my forearm, began to tingle periodically, like they were asleep. Then similar symptoms began to show up in my feet and legs. As the nerves continued to deteriorate, the burning and tingling pain increased in intensity and became constant. Other physical symptoms began to manifest themselves: sleep apnea, loss of balance, and tremendous exhaustion–the word fatigue *doesn't do it justice. It took great concentration just to keep from falling flat on my face if I just stepped on a pebble, or walked on an uneven surface. It was all I could do to get to school. I was sleeping 12 to 14 hours a day. I was taking elevators instead of stairs because to climb one flight of stairs (20 steps) at school required more energy than I had.*

The worst part was the cognitive problems resulting from lack of energy. My brain just wasn't working right. I developed what my wife referred to as "Swiss cheese memory." I could read and retain the conceptual material in the philosophy of science and political science courses, but the high-level math in the graduate courses was impossible. It was so confusing.

Homework for Economics 666 went something like this: I attended the lectures and read the chapters. Sometimes I seemed to read the chapters again and again without remembering the material. Later, I would try to work the practice problems. For an hour or so I would practice the techniques involved in matrix math with total partial differential equations, "Jacobians," "transforms," whatever material was in the chapter. Satisfied that I could work the problems, I would take a nap before supper. When I woke up an hour later, I could remember having studied and successfully worked the problems an hour before, but when I went back, I had no memory of how to solve the problems. When I would go back through the chapter, the material was vaguely familiar, but I couldn't use the mathematical rules to manipulate the data.

After three or four painstaking reviews of each chapter, I would have a reasonably good grasp of what I was supposed to be able to do. I understood the relationship between the mathematical concepts and the questions they were supposed to answer. I still could not manage to keep in my memory the techniques, rules,

patients showed that the later patients got out of bed in the morning, the greater their fatigue (Olders, submitted for publication, 1999). High-fatigue patients were also more depressed, had more insomnia, used more sleeping medication, and spent more time in bed, compared to low-fatigue patients.

Dr. Winningham: You have presented a good argument for considering "sleep therapy" interventions in cancer. This is a brave new world in developing our CRFS arsenal. How-

---

and processes required to figure out the math. They just didn't stick. I had always done well in courses like this before; in fact, I tutored others. I was familiar with the background material. Yet now, I was putting in five or six times the effort and failing miserably. It was humiliating.

It was unthinkable to me: I was failing my economics class and there was nothing I could do about it. . . . Nobody understood, and no one could explain to me why all this was happening. Since no one seemed to be interested, they clearly had no suggestions about anything I might do to improve. I could not study any harder. Then I started becoming depressed. Piled on top of the physical problems, it only made the fatigue worse. For whatever reason—and I believe it was the terrible fatigue— that part or aspect of the memory I needed to permanently store those mathematical skills was simply inaccessible. After several tries at Economics 666, I dropped out of graduate school, one class and one thesis short of a degree.

For most of my adult life, I have had considerable self-confidence . . . a belief in my own abilities: I always felt like, come what may, I could overcome, persevere, tough it out, see it through. . . . I knew I was pretty smart. Now, in addition to my Swiss cheese memory, I had a Swiss cheese self-concept. I was flawed, defective, damaged goods . . . weak . . . vulnerable! It was very frightening. I felt victimized and I was too easily fatigued and mentally exhausted to do much about it.

I continued to have more surgeries. There were many complications. I had terrible reactions to the anesthetics. Grinding fatigue became so much a part of my life that it was hard to remember a time when I could do things without effort. Vague memories of vigor and effortless living taunted me.

That's been a number of years. All I can say is, if you haven't experienced it, you can't possibly understand what it's like. . . . I hear others talk about their cancer fatigue, and I can really identify with what they're saying. Then I look at the fatigue questionnaires. I must tell you folks: You just aren't getting it. Those questionnaires are make-believe. What we have experienced is actually much, much worse. And it doesn't always go away. Remember that.

Could I go back now and do the math and get the degree? I don't know. And frankly, the distasteful and depression-laced memories of having experienced several abject failures in those days were so demoralizing that I have been afraid to try. I am not sure whether my "math memory" has recovered; certainly it doesn't appear that the holes in my gradually recovering Swiss cheese self-confidence are entirely healed.

Cancer survivor

ever, I'm thinking about the bone marrow transplant patients or those on biological agents for whom an overwhelming fatigue seems to be an inherent part of the treatment. I suspect you are not talking about these patients. After all, some of them have trouble with even small amounts of exertion.

Dr. Olders: I think that the fatigue many of them experience is what I refer to as "acute fatigue," which all of us experience after physical exertion. But in their case, because of the result of anemia, dehydration, extreme deconditioning, interleukins, and interferons, it surpasses the fatigue experienced by healthy individuals and the recovery is much slower. In distinction, the fatigue that I am talking about I refer to as *chronic fatigue*, because it seems to be there even without any exertion.

Dr. Winningham: I agree with you, and this kind of deconditioning happens very rapidly–it starts within 24 hours of bed rest (note further comments on this in Chapters 2 and 18). I think a lot of what people feel when they first try ambulating is the acute effect of dehydration and cardiovascular deconditioning that contributes to orthostatic hypotension. To counter this effect in astronauts, National Aeronautics and Space Administration (NASA) researchers developed a fluid bolus drink they nicknamed "Astro-aid." Astronauts drink it shortly prior to reentry to help them adapt to gravitation effects. I think the idea of a fluid bolus–whether by intravenous line or by mouth–prior to ambulation would be worth investigating in very deconditioned patients. We would need to experiment with the timing required from bolus to ambulation, contraindications, and so forth.

Dr. Olders: That's interesting. Regarding the disease and deconditioning-related fatigue: Attempting to reverse the deconditioning to improve exercise tolerance is the key. When a person is not experiencing chronic fatigue, however, I wouldn't want to fiddle with his or her sleep. For people who both have chronic fatigue and suffer from acute fatigue due to deconditioning, anemia, etc., I would want to make sure the chronic fatigue is addressed first, so that the patient will have the motivation to exercise or work with physiotherapy. I feel that the kind of fatigue that worsens as the day wears on may be either sleepiness, acute fatigue, or both, probably superimposed on chronic fatigue.

By the way, regarding those patients who as a result of their treatment are unable to stand: When I say, "Get up," I really mean wake up and stay awake. I see palliative patients who are entirely bed bound and obviously are not going to get up out of bed. This is where Ritalin comes in handy, because it keeps people awake and more alert in the morning even when they stay lying down. Coffee can also be a great help!

Dr. Winningham: You mentioned a few criteria for sleep disturbances earlier. Could you please elaborate on how you would perform a differential diagnosis on a fatigued cancer patient?

Dr. Olders: When a cancer patient presents with complaints of fatigue, depression, or sleep disturbance, I include in my psychiatric history taking the patient's psychiatric history, family psychiatric history, usage of alcohol or illicit or street drugs, medications, allergies, medical history, history of present illness, relationships, history of psychotrauma or severe stress (other than cancer), religious or spiritual values, and mental status. (Figure 11-5 presents a pocket guide abbreviating the interview questions that can be copied for personal, clinical use.) In addition, I address more specific issues or questions:

- *Fatigue/tiredness (differentiated from drowsiness/sleepiness)*–how often, what time of day or evening, how distressing, impact on life (work, play, relationships).
- *Are you depressed?* This single question has been shown to outperform the Beck Depression Inventory in correctly identifying persons with depression (Chochinov et al, 1997). If the answer is yes, rule out a history of depression, bipolar depression, or dysthymia using DSM-IV criteria.
- *Time of going to bed, time of waking in the morning. What does the person do after waking?* Stay in bed? Get up and have breakfast? Read the newspaper? Follow up with the question, "And what do you do after that?" It no longer surprises me to find individuals frequently going back to bed after breakfast, or after getting the kids off to school.
- *Time of getting out of bed for the day.* If the person tells you they wake up early, but further questioning reveals he or she remains in bed or goes back to bed, find out when the person gets up for good.
- *Daytime naps*–what time of day, how long, how often, how long before they fall asleep.
- *Sleep habits before the illness (when working and doing well).* This is usually a baseline for sleep duration and timing. For example, a patient who went to bed at 11:00 PM and was up at 5:00 AM when working will be spending too much time in bed and getting up too late if they start getting up at 6:30 AM while continuing to go to bed at 11:00 PM.
- *Quality of sleep.* If the person seems to have a sleep disturbance, I ask how long it takes to fall asleep, whether the patient wakes during the night, the reasons for waking, the number of times, and how long it takes to fall asleep again.
- *Daytime drowsiness/sleepiness*–how often, what time of day or evening, how distressing, occurrence of accidents or near-accidents due to drowsiness. This is very important. It is critical that patients know when medications can contribute to drowsiness. Failure to identify and appropriately refer people who subsequently have accidents can engender civil and possibly criminal liability for health care providers.
- *Use of sleeping aids*–prescribed medications (including using somebody else's pills), over-the-counter (OTC) drugs, herbal and other "natural" products, alcohol, or other substances.
- *Frequency of sleep problems*–difficulty falling asleep, difficulty staying asleep, waking too early, inability to get up.

Figure 11.5 — Olders Interview Guide for Fatigue, Depression, and Sleep Disturbances

Olders Fatigue, Depression, and Sleep Disturbance Screen

Pocket guide for interviewing patients with complaints of fatigue, depression, or sleep disturbances.

General Psychiatric History Taking

History of present illness

Past psychiatrichistory (Consider possibility of clinically significant but undiagnosed conditions.)

Family psychiatric history (Also ask about family history of violence or abuse.)

Use of alcohol and/or illicit/street drug use (also ask re "natural" or herbal products that may have psychotropic implications.)

Medications (prescribed, "borrowed," and over-the-counter [OTC])

Allergies (include environmental, prescription and OTC meds, and adverse reactions to dental or surgical anesthetics)

Past medical history

Relationships

History of psychotrauma, severe stress (separate from dx of cancer)

Religious/spiritual values

Mental status

Specific Questions

Fatigue/tiredness (differentiated from drowsiness/sleepiness)

How often? Time of day or evening? How distressing?

Impact on life (work, play, relationships, spiritual undertakings)?

Ask: *"Are you depressed?"*

Yes or No. If answer is Yes, question further for typical symptoms of depression, dysthymia, or bipolar disorder, using DSM-IV criteria as a guide.

Time going to bed?

Time waking in the morning?

What does the person do after waking?

Stay in bed? Get up and have breakfast? Read the newspaper? Follow up question, "And what do you do after that?'"

Watch for reports of going back to bed afterward.

Time getting out of bed for the day?

If the person says they wake up early, but further questions reveal they remain in bed or go back to bed, find out when they get up for good.

Daytime naps

What time of day? How long? How often? How long to fall asleep?

Where do they nap (bedroom, couch, recliner)?

Sleep habits before onset of illness (when working and doing well)

Use as baseline for sleep duration and timing. Ask about "shift" work.

Quality of sleep?

Restless? Agitated? Solid? Uninterrupted?

How does the person feel on awakening?

Groggy? Clear headed and rested? Disoriented? No energy? Weak? Headache?

If sleep disturbance is reported or suspected, ask . . .

Frequent difficulty falling asleep, staying asleep, or waking earlier than desired. How often, distress due to these symptoms, significant change in sleep patterns from when well, even if not distressed.

Daytime drowsiness/sleepiness

How often? What time of day or evening? How distressing? Accidents/near accidents due to drowsiness

Failure to identify and appropriately refer cases who subsequently have accidents can engender civil and possibly criminal liability.

Use of sleeping aids

Prescribed meds (including "borrowed" from someone else), OTC meds, herbal/natural products, alcohol, or other substances

Frequency of sleep problems

How distressed by sleep problem

Use of stimulants (coffee, tea, caffeinated soft drinks)

What? How much? How often?

Attitudes toward sleep

If you feel sleepy, does that always mean you're not getting enough sleep?

If you feel fatigued, does that mean you need more sleep?

If you sleep poorly at night, do you make up for it by sleeping late or by taking a long nap?

If you've slept poorly, would you go into work late or call in sick?

Physical exam, lab tests, consultations

As indicated, based on the differential diagnosis

Thyroid stimulating hormone (TSH) and Vitamin B_{12} levels should be routinely requested for depressed patients.

For patient with excessive daytime sleepiness not ascribable to medications such as hypnotics, sedatives, opioids, antidepressants, anticonvulsants, or other sedating drugs, and where the history or information obtained from a bed partner suggests sleep apnea, a referral to a sleep disorders specialist or sleep laboratory is indicated.

Consider psychiatric consultation where appropriate.

Collect 24-hour sleep/rest log for 14 continuous days.

- *Level of distress due to the sleep problem.*
- *Use of stimulants (coffee, tea, caffeinated soft drinks).*
- *Attitudes toward sleep.* For instance, if they feel sleepy, does that always mean they're not getting enough sleep? If they feel fatigued does that mean they need more sleep? If they sleep poorly at night, do they make up for it by sleeping late or by taking a long nap? If they've slept poorly, would they go in to work late or call in sick?
- *Sleep log or diary* (Figure 11-6 is a sleep log for patients). Ask patients to record daily, for a period of two weeks, the following: sleep medications taken, time into bed, time of "lights out," how long it takes to fall asleep, how many awakenings occur, how many minutes were they awake, time of morning waking (after which they couldn't sleep), time of arising, time returning to bed (if applicable), time arising for the day, daytime naps (when, how long), sleepiness during the day (rated on a scale from 1 to 5), fatigue during the day (rated on a scale from 1 to 5), coffee (number of cups), tea, caffeinated soft drinks.
- *Physical examination, laboratory tests, consultations.* As indicated, based on the differential diagnosis, thyroid-stimulating hormone (TSH) and vitamin B_{12} levels are routinely measured in depressed patients in our clinic. For patients with excessive daytime sleepiness not ascribable to medications such as hypnotics, sedatives, opioids, antidepressants, anticonvulsants, or other sedating drugs, and where the history, obtained from a bed partner, suggests sleep apnea, a referral to a sleep disorders specialist or sleep laboratory is indicated.

Dr. Winningham: I doubt whether even a small fraction of people suffering from the CRFS are getting an evaluation like the one you just described. It doesn't even sound complicated. We could probably design a questionnaire patients could fill out at their leisure and bring into the clinic. Once again, it comes back to what we learned from the NASA bed rest studies during the past 40-plus years: If you take a healthy young athlete and put him to bed, he will deteriorate, physically, and start exhibiting signs of depression, cognitive impairment, nausea, lethargy, and a host of other symptoms. Figures 11-5 and 11-6 are provided to help readers gain experience in asking these questions. Given answers relating to the above questions or issues, how do you formulate a diagnosis?

Dr. Olders: When fatigue and other depressive symptoms are present in the context of people who spend more time in bed than they need (the presence of primary insomnia or hypersomnia is an indicator), especially when they are getting out of bed later than usual or returning to bed in the morning, it may be that excessive REM sleep is causing their symptoms.

Dr. Winningham: Excuse me . . . so those simple questions can help to discriminate between a behaviorally treatable fatigue or depression and one where the fatigue has other causes. What else?

Figure 11.6 Sleep Log for Fatigue, Depression, and Sleep Disturbances

Name _____

Sleep Journal for 12 Noon to 12 Noon Starting Date ___/___/___

12N 1p 2p 3p 4p 5p 6p 7p 8p 9p 10p 11p 12a 1a 2a 3a 4a 5a 6a 7a 8a 9a 10a 11a 12N

Codes:

B = Mark time lying in bed with solid line

C = Mark time lying on couch or recliner with solid line

N = Nap (daytime sleep)

Mark times at beginning and end with slash marks

Mark time actually napping/sleeping at beginning and end on above solid or wavy line (depending on where you were) with an "X"

B = |———X———X———✳✳✳✳✳———X—|

Ex NB = 3:00 PM through 5:00 PM, x from 4:00 through 4:50 PM

Sleepy = SL <——————>   Fatigued = F <——————> for the duration of the event

Mark any other symptom like Pain as Pain <——————>   Nausea = <——————>

SM = Sleep Medications Taken (Specify how much of what & when). Number each amount taken

ST = Stimulants (coffee, tea, caffeinated soft drinks, pills - how much and when). Number each specific intake throughout the day.
Ex. ST1 = 1 12 oz Coke, St2 = 1 cup coffee

Comments:

Dr. Olders: Benzodiazepines, particularly when taken during the day, or long-acting benzodiazepines such as clonazepam taken anytime, may contribute directly to feelings of fatigue and lacking energy. Because these medications promote sleep, they may cause patients to sleep later than usual. Daytime drowsiness due to medication may also result in napping. Extra sleep, particularly when close to the REM sleep peak at about 8:30 AM, will result in excessive REM sleep and thus lead to more fatigue.

Dr. Winningham: You've presented a convincing argument. What kinds of treatments or interventions do you recommend?

Dr. Olders: The first is early rising to reduce REM sleep. As demonstrated earlier, timing of sleep has a very powerful influence on the amount of REM sleep obtained. Getting up early is an effective technique to reduce REM sleep. REM sleep deprivation has an antidepressant effect, and to the extent that fatigue is a depressive symptom, an antifatigue effect. I counsel patients to get up at 6:00 AM, or simply to go back to the sleeping pattern they followed when well.

Dr. Winningham: That is important. Often, hospitalized patients get in the habit of watching late night television, a habit they continue when they go home. I often wish we could pull the plug on telephones and televisions at 10:00 PM. What else do you recommend?

Dr. Olders: Hypnotic medications are a critical issue. Getting up early may be extremely difficult for people taking benzodiazepines. It is important to convince patients of the necessity to taper and eventually discontinue these medications, not only because they perpetuate the fatigue, but also because they can be dangerous of their own accord. This is especially true of elderly patients. The risk of falls, automobile accidents, cognitive impairment, disinhibition, depression, and dependence are all increased. Unfortunately, most people, including physicians, are unaware that benzodiazepines quadruple the risk of becoming depressed for hospitalized patients (Patten, Williams, and Love, 1996). For individuals taking benzodiazepines for insomnia, therapeutic alternatives include sleep hygiene, sleep restriction (described below), and trazodone. Trazodone, being an antidepressant, will not increase the risk of depression as benzodiazepines do, and in doses of 25 or 50 mg at bedtime it will promote sleep. If benzodiazepines are being used for anxiety, one can propose antidepressants, exercise, or relaxation training instead. Again, trazodone in low doses may help control agitation.

Dr. Winningham: What sleep recommendations do you present?

Dr. Olders: If insomnia is a problem, the following can be helpful:

- Arise at the same time each day, whether you have slept well or not, or even if you have not slept at all.

- Limit daily in-bed time to a "normal" amount. This depends on age, and on what worked for the individual when well. I usually recommend seven hours for middle-aged adults, six hours for people in their 60s or early 70s, and five to six hours for elderly clients.
- Limit or discontinue use of drugs that act on the central nervous system (e.g., caffeine, nicotine, alcohol, and stimulants).
- Cut out daytime naps, if they exceed 15 or 20 minutes.
- Establish physical fitness with a routine of exercise early in the day, followed by other activity.
- Avoid evening stimulation; substitute either listening to the radio or leisure reading for watching television.
- Try a warm 20-minute body bath or soak near bedtime.
- Eat on a regular schedule; avoid large meals near bedtime.
- Practice an evening relaxation routine.
- Maintain comfortable sleeping conditions.
- Spend no longer than 20 minutes awake in the bed.
- Adjust your sleep hours and routine to optimize your daily schedule and living situation.
- Use the bedroom only for sleeping or making love, so as to train yourself not to be in bed while awake.

By far the most effective and long-lasting treatment for insomnia is sleep restriction (Morin et al, 1999), also called *sleep compression*. The way you do it is you take patients' estimates of how many hours of actual sleep they get in 24 hours. They should then spend only that many hours in bed each night. Once they have been sleeping well for a week at a given stage, increase the time in bed by a half hour.

Dr. Winningham: Naps are often a source of confusion. You just said to eliminate naps longer than 20 minutes in duration. People take extended daily naps of several hours. I have had people tell me they need daytime naps of several hours, but I see no miraculous improvement. I am convinced it makes things worse and impairs nighttime sleep. I have told people to use an inexpensive watch with an alarm or a kitchen timer to keep naps short. Could you elaborate?

Dr. Olders: Timing is critical. Short naps are refreshing, relieve drowsiness (Harrison and Horne, 1996), and increase alertness and feelings of well-being. Longer naps induce sluggishness and torpor, referred to as *sleep inertia*, and may also impair nighttime sleep. This is how I handle it: When patients feel drowsy or sleepy, they should take a *brief nap;* that is, lie down for not more than 15 or 20 minutes. A kitchen timer may indeed be useful for waking up. If they have not fallen asleep after 15 minutes, they do not need a nap. Period. If they fall asleep after 5 or 10 minutes and sleep for only a few minutes, they will be able to get going again easily.

Dr. Winningham: Dr. Olders, some professionals are now using psychostimulants to enhance cognitive awareness. You mentioned the use of psychostimulants to treat fatigue and depression in patients with cancer.

Dr. Olders: Psychostimulants, particularly methylphenidate (Ritalin), are widely used to treat attention deficit disorder, but they may also be helpful in treating fatigue and depression in patients with cancer or other illnesses. It has been used for years to treat apathy and withdrawal in poststroke and dementia patients (Galynker et al, 1997; Watanabe et al, 1995).

A retrospective study of elderly depressed stroke patients showed that 53% of patients treated with methylphenidate had complete remission of symptoms, with an average peak response time of 2.4 days. In comparison, 43% of nortriptyline-treated patients required an average of 27 days to remission (Lazarus et al, 1994). Of depressed, hospitalized oncology patients at the Massachusetts General Hospital, 73% showed marked or moderate depressive symptom improvement with dextroamphetamine or methylphenidate, usually within 2 days (Olin and Masand, 1996). In patients with malignant glioma, methylphenidate, 10 mg given twice daily, led to improved gait, increased stamina, and motivation to perform activities (Meyers et al, 1998).

Dr. Winningham: How does methylphenidate work to reduce depression and fatigue? I have heard it interferes with onset of sleep. Doesn't that create a problem?

Dr. Olders: Besides its direct REM-suppressant effects, methylphenidate also helps keep people awake (Bishop et al, 1997), which further reduces REM sleep, particularly if it is administered early in the morning so it doesn't interfere with sleep onset in the evening. I have obtained excellent results in treating fatigue in both inpatients and outpatients by administering 5 to 20 mg at 6:00 AM.

Dr. Winningham: Another drug being used for cancer patients is pemoline (Cylert). In the United States, pemoline is a schedule IV drug while methylphenidate is a schedule II drug. Pemoline requires monitoring of hepatic enzymes. There are few data on the use of these drugs in cancer patients. Recent work supported by the National Institute on Drug Abuse at the National Institutes of Health indicates that the abuse risk for methylphenidate in patients for whom it is appropriate is very low despite its similarity to other stimulants like cocaine and amphetamines. The oral form of methylphenidate does not reach peak concentrations in the brain until 60 minutes after ingestion, compared to 9 minutes for the intravenous form and 5 minutes for cocaine (Volkow et al, 1998).

To be honest, when I first heard about using methylphenidate and pemoline in this way, I was not enthusiastic. I could not find clinical trials on the use of these medications in the cancer patients who were demanding them. I am particularly concerned about the potential for interactions with other drugs they may be taking. In addition, psychostimulants are appetite suppressants and may contribute to weight loss if misused. Treatment for breast cancer is associated with weight gain. When I first heard of breast cancer patients on the West Coast demanding methylphenidate, I wondered if they were also considering weight control. This could potentially be associated with psychostimulant abuse even after treatment. However, after I thought about it, I asked myself, "How is fatigue different from pain?" We do not hesitate to treat pain or nausea with appropriate pharmacological interventions. If fatigue is indeed viewed as a syndrome, there is room for many interventions. Considering the seriousness and universality of the CRFS, I now think the appropriate use of psychostimulants warrants investigation. What other interventions do you think may help?

Dr. Olders: There is no doubt that light is the most important cue for adjusting our circadian biological clocks. Individuals who are insufficiently exposed to light, especially morning light, may develop DSPS. This can occur if people keep their bedrooms dark, if windows are small, or views are obstructed with trees, fences, walls, etc. Encourage patients to keep their drapes or blinds open at night while they're asleep. Natural light wakes them up in the morning. As a matter of good hygiene, when buying or renting housing, look for bedrooms that receive plenty of natural light.

Dr. Winningham: How about foods or OTC interventions? What should we be looking for?

Dr. Olders: Caffeine is important because it may induce its own metabolism. In fact, individuals who use small amounts, or who use it irregularly, may have more severe and longer-lasting insomnia or anxiety than those who consume larger quantities on a daily basis. Caffeine acts as a mood elevator. In the ongoing Nurses' Health Study involving about 86,000 nurses in the United States, those who drank no coffee committed suicide at 2.9 times the rate of those who drank two or more cups daily (Kawachi et al, 1996). I encourage *consistent* caffeine consumption (e.g., two cups of coffee daily).

I also encourage people to engage in cardiovascular (i.e., aerobic) exercise. Exercise has been associated as a useful treatment for depression and fatigue. Exercise has also been associated with improved sleep if patients do not exercise too near to bedtime. The exercise I recommend is at an intensity that raises your heart rate and causes you to breathe harder–but not enough to become out of breath. For someone who is ambulatory but deconditioned, walking with one's arms swinging is vigorous enough, thank you! I also work with elderly people, many of whom are in exercise programs where they sit and lift their arms or legs. Even for people with joint or muscle injuries, aqua fitness programs can provide sufficiently vigorous exercise.

Dr. Winningham: There is little doubt that there are multiple positive emotional as well as physiological consequences of safe aerobic activity. Pinto and Maruyama (1998) wrote a concise review article about exercise in breast cancer survivors. What do you consider the most important, practical intervention?

Dr. Olders: Of all the above interventions, the one that is most crucial for the successful treatment of cancer fatigue, in my clinical experience, is having the patient get up early. Many can-

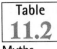

Table 11.2 Sleep: Popular Myths and the Facts	
Myths	**Facts**
I won't have enough energy to function if I haven't had a good night's sleep.	Partial sleep does not impair exercise performance (Meney et al, 1998).
If I've slept poorly, I should make up for it by sleeping late.	Sleeping late may aggravate or precipitate depression (Globus, 1969; Wehr et al, 1979).
If some sleep is good for you, more sleep is better.	Longer sleep is associated with poorer physical health and increased mortality (Belloc and Breslow, 1972; Wingard and Berkman, 1983), and causes insomnia (Aserinsky, 1969).
After a poor sleep, the fatigue I experience is from lack of sleep.	Insomniacs have less daytime sleepiness (Middelkoop et al, 1996) and better reaction times at night (Bonnet and Rosa, 1987), indicating sufficient sleep.
I haven't slept a wink all night! No wonder I'm tired!	People with insomnia underestimate the amount they sleep (Frankel et al, 1976), in some cases to extremes (McCall and Edinger, 1992).
I'm too depressed to get out of bed.	Total sleep deprivation takes away depression (Gill et al, 1993) as does late partial sleep deprivation (Sack et al, 1988).
You can't convince me that my getting up late has anything to do with feeling tired.	A study in cancer outpatients showed that the later people got up, the more fatigue they experienced (Olders, personal conversation 1999).

cer patients are quite willing to try any approach that will relieve their lack of energy and motivation. They may be skeptical, initially, about any possible benefits from getting up early, but they frequently become enthusiastic supporters of the principle when they experience a rapid improvement (often the same day) when they get out of bed at 6:00 AM. Unfortunately, there are significant numbers of cancer patients who hold dear to a number of false beliefs and attitudes. Table 11-2 lists several popular myths and the facts. When an empathetic presentation of the facts still fails to convince, it may be necessary to involve family members who will undertake to get the patient up and keep them up each morning.

Dr. Winningham: It all sounds rather like "tough love," and it's so different from conventional attitudes. It reminds me of the resistance I first encountered in proposing exercise programs for cancer patients! I found encouragement from the patients' physicians to be a strong influencing factor in converting patients and families. I just reviewed a series of fatigue inventories and in no place did I find questions that asked about specific sleep patterns, or whether patients tried a sleep hygiene plan.

Dr. Olders: Figure 11-1 contains a collection of time-honored sayings on how people have viewed sleep throughout the ages. It is clear that sleep has been a controversial topic for a long time.

As for patients who insist they cannot get up early, or when a trial of early waking fails, an alternative is methylphenidate. I get more consistent results when the medication is taken at 6:00 AM, instead of the more usual 8:00 or 9:00 AM. A second dose at noon, recommended by some, seems to make little difference in my experience. Starting at 5 mg, the single daily dose can be increased to 10 mg after two or three days, with further increases depending on clinical response.

It's rare to find inpatient settings that are sufficiently staffed to provide the one-on-one intervention often required to wake a hospitalized patient at 6:00 AM and keep them awake during the morning. Accordingly, for hospitalized or bed-bound patients, I start with methylphenidate as a first intervention.

When depressive symptoms are prominent, or when methylphenidate even at larger doses fails to improve patients' fatigue, I will start with or add to the methylphenidate an antidepressant, such as paroxetine, which I also give at 6:00 AM. Consider a tricyclic antidepressant such as desipramine for patients with anorexia or nausea, which may be worsened with SSRIs.

Check TSH levels; even mildly abnormal levels should be treated when fatigue or depression is present. We also use intramuscular vitamin B_{12} when blood levels are even marginally low. Vitamin B_{12} supplementation may play a role in treating DSPS (Ohta et al, 1991; Okawa et al, 1990).

While my clinical experience certainly suggests that the hypothesized link between excessive REM sleep and cancer fatigue is well founded, further research is essential to confirm that a link exists. Only randomized controlled trials can adequately determine whether getting up early or early-morning psychostimulant treatment, or both, is a useful intervention. Clearly, if excessive REM sleep can be shown to cause cancer fatigue, it strongly suggests that the fatigue (as distinct from sleepiness) that plagues sufferers from many other illnesses has a similar origin, and should respond to the same treatments and preventive approaches. This is an important public health issue, given the lost productivity due to illness-related fatigue as well as costs for its medical treatment.

Dr. Winningham: From a syndrome perspective, it is reasonable that sleep interventions be considered in all fatigued cancer patients. There is no doubt that some patients are affected by profound chemical changes in their bodies. As you share this, I find myself reflecting on all the patients I remember talking with–and I ask, Could they have handled the restrictions you are suggesting they place on their sleep? On the other hand, people were equally incredulous when I suggested exercise to improve functioning and well-being in cancer patients in the early 1980s. What you are saying is going to take a real adjustment in attitude.

Since syndromes are, by definition, multifactorial, it would be logical that there are also several possibilities for interventions. It is unlikely that there is one cure for some fatigued cancer patients. Our best approach should be to find several strategies, each of which help somewhat. I think this could become one of the most powerful tools in our arsenal. Like exercise, it may not be magical for everyone, but it may be useful for many patients in controlling some of the most devastating side effects, and, like exercise, it has a powerful physiological as well as emotional effect. Can you explain how light exposure and times influence the mechanisms you outlined above?

Dr. Olders: Well, a condition in which fatigue and lack of energy figure prominently is seasonal affective disorder (SAD). That morning treatment with bright light if effective implies a connection between SAD and circadian rhythms. It is often assumed that the farther north one lives, the higher the risk of SAD because the amount of daylight in winter decreases as one goes north. However, Iceland has little SAD even though it is quite far north, at 64 degrees latitude. Iceland has two peculiarities that might explain its low incidence of SAD. First, Icelanders stay on Standard Time all year-round. Second, even though this island by its longitude should be in a time zone two hours earlier than Greenwich Mean Time (GMT), the residents actually adhere to GMT. In early November, the sun rises for Icelanders after 9:00 AM, almost three hours later than for Montrealers at the same time of year.

What is the possibility that the switch from Daylight Savings Time to Standard Time may be the trigger for SAD in North America? Consider the facts: The time switch takes place on the last weekend of October each year, and results in everyone getting up an hour later with respect to the time of sunrise, thereby acutely increasing their REM sleep. Would we all feel better, more energetic, if we stay on Daylight Savings Time all year-round? What about going to double Daylight Savings Time, so we all get up an hour earlier in relation to sunrise?

Dr. Winningham: What about the use of antidepressants?

Dr. Olders: Tricyclic antidepressants should be avoided in the elderly. The anticholinergic effects impair memory, increase risk of orthostatic hypotension, and can have untoward effects on the heart. SSRIs may be sedating in some individuals. They are the preferred treatment for panic disorders and phobic disorders. If these disorders interfere with sleep, they may help insomnia.

Dr. Winningham: Recommendations about drugs and dosages change with regularity. The National Cancer Institute's PDQ (Physician's Data Query) Web site provides a continual update on topics specific to mental health and related pharmacological interventions. Rather than making recommendations or listing values here, clinicians and researchers are encouraged to refer to this site on a regular basis: <http://cancernet.nci.nih.gov/clinpdq/supportive.html>. Since depression is reported to be the most common DSM-IV diagnosis in cancer patients, DSM-IV diagnostic criteria are presented in Table 11-3 with specific implications for cancer patients.

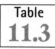

Table
11.3

Diagnostic Criteria for Depression: Implications for Fatigue and Cancer

Criterion A

5 or more of the following symptoms during same 2-week period and a change from prior functioning: At least (1) depressed mood or (2) loss of pleasure or interest in life must be present.

Characteristics

1. Daily depressed or irritable mood, most of the day, by subjective report
2. Notably diminished interest in most activities (can be objective or subjective report)
3. Significant nondieting weight gain or loss (5% change in body weight in a month); can also be reflected in marked increase or decrease in daily appetite
4. Daily insomnia or hypersomnia
5. Daily psychomotor slowing or agitation (objective, not just subjective feelings)
6. Daily fatigue or loss of energy
7. Feelings of worthlessness or inappropriate guilt (not just over illness)
8. Daily decreased ability to focus or concentrate, indecisiveness (subjective or objective report)
9. Recurrent thoughts of death, suicidal ideation with or without a specific plan; not just fear of death

Implications for Fatigue and Cancer

1. Fatigue can appear as a depressive feeling as well as irritability. Keeping a sleep diary as well as noting the time of day the patient feels best may help in making the diagnosis as well as developing priorities.
2. Diminished activities may become evident to family members before the patient becomes aware of them.
3. It is important to note the source of the weight loss. Gastrointestinal problems (nausea, vomiting, and diarrhea), increased bed rest, glycogen depletion, and fatigue (decreased fluid intake) can result in several pounds of water loss secondary to dehydration. In addition, many medications can dull the sense of thirst. Medications can also contribute to weight gain. Source of weight gain or loss should be investigated and corrected.
4. Precancer sleep patterns should be maintained. Naps should be limited to 1 or 2 for a limited period of 15–20 minutes each per day to minimize disturbance to nighttime sleep cycles. Change in sleep patterns may become obvious to family members before the patient notices them.
5. Ask a trusted family member or friend to observe and help with activity. If the person responds to a strenuous day, such as a treatment day, or a surgical procedure by sleeping late or sleeping longer, 2 or even 3 days of aggravated exhaustion may ensue. These cyclic changes are physiologically based and will be delayed (i.e., after the stressful event is over). It is essential to return to regular sleep hours as soon as possible.
6. Watch for changes in activity based on nadirs, anemia, and stressors.
7. It is common for patients, especially women, to express guilt about not fulfilling their social roles as a parent or spouse. In addition, relatives may lay guilt trips on the patient, accusing them of malingering or using their cancer for secondary gain.
8. The impaired ability to concentrate or focus is one of the common characteristics of cancer-related fatigue. This may particularly show itself in the inability to keep track of money (e.g., balancing a checkbook, paying bills, keeping track of bank accounts, paying taxes), appointments, and time. Studies show that this cognitive impairment may be long lasting and may be associated with specific cancer treatments.
9. Be aware of the patient's prior experience with cancer, knowledge of pain control, fear of the course of the disease, fear of loss of independence, and other issues that may be related to fear of death but appear as suicidal/death ideation. Also be aware of possible retraumatization experiences related to prior intense life experiences that may contribute to feelings of hopelessness.

Criterion B

Not part of a mixed episode.

Characteristics

1. Both manic and major depressive episode for 1 week or more
2. Severe enough to impair functioning, characteristics of harm, or psychotic features
3. Symptoms not due to the physiological effect of a substance or general medical condition (e.g., hyperthyroidism)

Implications for Fatigue and Cancer

Family as well as personal history should be carefully screened for a history of DSM-IV diagnoses. Note that patients and their families may not admit to mental illness in the family because of the stigma; indeed, they may accept such behaviors as "normal." Ask about violence, substance use and abuse, and estranged family relationships as a round-about way to get at this issue. Where there is special concern, based on clinical symptoms, a genogram may be a subtle and less threatening way of identifying family histories with suicides, depression, and substance abuse. History is critical because use of corticosteroids or antidepressants in an individual with a history of or potential for mania can contribute to a full-blown psychotic manic episode. In addition, a rapid decrease in such medications may precipitate a profound and unexpected depression.

Criterion C

Symptoms cause significant impairment in functioning.

Implications for Fatigue and Cancer

Regardless of whether the impairment is caused by fatigue or whether it is caused by depression, any symptoms that contribute to functional impairment can often lead to increased fatigability and depression and should be treated aggressively.

Criterion D

Symptoms are not due to direct physiological effects of substance or medical condition (e.g., hypothyroidism).

Implications for Fatigue and Cancer

1. After corticosteroid treatment, patients often talk about "crashing," a profound exhaustion, possibly accompanied by depression.
2. In cancer, it is common for other, less life-threatening conditions to be minimized as "just part of the cancer." These conditions, however, may have a significant effect on mood and functioning. Hypothyroidism can present with many minor subjective, and apparently unrelated symptoms including fatigue, paresthesias, difficulty focusing, clinical presentation of asthma, repeated infections, and sensory changes. This may lead to patients' complaints not being taken seriously or being categorized as depressed, anxious, or malingering.

Criterion E

Symptoms cannot be accounted for by a more obvious or significant cause (e.g., grief), last 2 months or more, or result in functional impairment, suicidal thoughts, psychosis, or decreased psychomotor activity.

Implications for Fatigue and Cancer

When the symptoms are unresolved or become severe, the patient should be referred to a psychiatrist for treatment and should be given the opportunity for psychotherapy as appropriate. Unresolved past experiences can be a source of retraumatization and hopelessness that should be identified and promptly treated. Do not wait for such conditions to spontaneously improve.

Note: The DSM-IV specifies that these criteria do not include symptoms that are clearly due to a general medical condition or mood incongruent delusions or hallucinations.

Source: Adapted by Maryl L. Winningham (1999) from *Diagnostic and Statistical Manual of Mental Disorders: DSM-IV.* 4th ed., American Psychiatric Association (Copyright, 1994), Washington, DC. Used with permission.

I'd like to change the topic, if I may. Research as well as clinical observation has validated the high incidence of nightmares in individuals who have been traumatized. However, over the past few years, I've run into an interesting phenomenon you may be able to help explain: people who have gone through a period of enormous trauma–prolonged stress in their lives–who say they never dream. They describe their sleep, usually five to six hours per night, as "one unbroken darkness." Given their background, it would be expected they would have nightmares, but they don't. They say if they do dream, it is in the form of brief, realistic little "dreamlets" on the fringes of awakening. I have no doubt psychoanalysts would be quite frustrated by this. (The poet Elias Canetti wrote, "All the things one has forgotten scream for help in dreams.") But these people claim to have no nightmares. In fact, some have told me they do not think they even turn or move at night (a feature of REM sleep), because they wake up with numbness on the side of the body on which they slept. What is interesting is that, as a whole, they seem to be busy, creative, and dynamic. There seems to be no cloud over them. However, I have noticed when they get cancer or some chronic illness that is emotionally and physically very draining, they can decompensate quite quickly. I am concerned about these people, particularly in view of the reported higher suicide rate among Holocaust and other major trauma survivors. The literature talks about a higher risk of depression, especially in women, in homes where there was violence and sexual abuse. We have refugees and former victims of human rights violations among us. Although these people can look pretty normal in everyday life, they have been tortured and scarred. They spend a good deal of their energy trying to adapt to a new setting, to a new country, while ignoring or overcoming their past. It's almost as if they are trying to outrun the past while desperately holding on to the here and now. But then the past comes nipping at their heels. As I talked with others about this, I realized this is a population we seem to have overlooked.

There is a great deal about cancer and its treatment milieu that can retraumatize someone who has hidden wounds. In countries where there is repression and persecution, physicians and nurses are often the assistants in the white coats who assist in torture. The health care system is full of authority figures–but then, so was their former life. Procedures we put patients through are humiliating (but so are abuse and torture), painful, freedom limiting (NPO means "no water, no food"), and include invasions of privacy and dignity. They may have been raped, both men and women. But how is that different, to a tired, elderly, or confused mind, from vaginal, prostate, or rectal examinations? Cancer is a life-threatening experience, but they've been there before, often asking, "Why me?" with no clear answer.

As a group, they are unlikely to talk about their former experiences. As someone once suggested, "Paranoia is a normal response to a paranoid society." They may lack insight into their reaction to past experience, although they may be otherwise intelligent and alert. They may do well for as long as 30 or 40 years, then crash. During the process of diagnosis and treatment for cancer, they may become incredibly depressed, or be confronted by post-traumatic stress disorder (PTSD)–like responses.

How do you reach out to them? I have been able to find little in the literature about this phenomenon. Could it be that the worst, the unimaginable, the most inhumane things had already happened? Had the stuff of nightmares come true already? When they were willing to talk with me about it, in every case, they suddenly appeared to be dissociative, with flat affect. Is it possible that by staying so busy, they have erected a mental barrier to the horrors of their past that not even the weakness of sleep can breach? Could there really be people who do not dream? What about the lack of nightmares? How do they survive and carry on normally for so long? Even as thought experiments are used to explore scientific issues, I use poetry to explore issues of deep human significance. I used the poem "Repression" to gain insight into this problem (see page xii). What are your thoughts?

Dr. Olders: I was touched by the poem. I think it has more to do with not remembering dreams than with not dreaming at all. I don't profess to have any sort of expertise when it comes to dreams, but my take on this goes as follows: For most people, most dreams, including nightmares, occur during REM sleep. REM sleep tends to occur more during the later part of the night, peaking (see Figures 11-3 and 11-4 and Table 11-1) around 8:30 AM. If you get up early, you will have less REM sleep, hence less dreaming. With the deconditioning and physical exhaustion of illness, they may spend more time in bed, sleep more, and have more time for REM sleep than previously.

Dr. Winningham: That sounds reasonable. Also, people who are very active usually don't sit around after they wake up trying to remember dreams. They usually get right into the activities of their day.

Dr. Olders: To remember a dream consciously seems to require waking up during the dream or perhaps shortly afterwards. If you are sleeping seven or eight hours, chances are excellent that you will wake up briefly several times during the night, particularly toward the end of your sleep, when there is less deep sleep. The busy, creative people you have known who don't seem to dream are sleeping only five or six hours, if I remember correctly. If they are a little sleep deprived, they will be sleeping deeply (i.e., more slow wave sleep for a larger proportion of their sleep), less likely to wake up, and therefore less likely to remember their dreams. They are probably also getting up early.

Dr. Winningham: Perhaps in response to debilitating illness, they start sleeping more, or change their sleep patterns, thus opening themselves up for breakthrough nightmares and memories. I have a friend whose mother lived through some unspeakable experiences during World War II. Several years ago, she suffered anoxic damage to her brain. Since then, she seems to be trapped in an in-again, out-again twilight of reliving the horrors. I wonder if the strange behavior of elderly, confused patients finds a basis in earlier, traumatic experiences. One of my former students, now a hospice nurse, suggested this might be the basis for the "sundown syndrome."

Lawrence Langer, the Holocaust scholar, has written about this existential confusion and isolation in his book *Admitting the Holocaust: Collected Essays* (1995). Cancer also has a

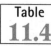

Table 11.4	Posttraumatic Stress Disorder (PTSD): Issues Relevant to Cancer and Fatigue

Criterion A

Exposure to a traumatic event with 2 characteristics.

Characteristics

1. Person experienced or was involved in event(s) characterized by actual or threatened serious harm or death to physical integrity of self or others.
2. Response included intense fear, helplessness, or horror. This may be manifested by agitated or disorganized behavior.

Issues Relevant to Cancer and Fatigue

1. Threat of disfigurement, loss of life, independence, and social roles can profoundly influence cancer survivors. Much depends on their past experiences and vulnerability. Keep in mind that vulnerability is not always obvious. Individuals who appear to be carefree, independent, or insensitive may be at greatest risk. Most significantly, the threat is relative, not absolute, depending on background and the perceived current type and degree of threat.
2. Response may not be obvious, nor may it be immediate. The need to focus on immediate lower survival needs (on Maslow's hierarchy) may force the person to postpone or suppress dealing with feelings and emotional response. Since disorganized or agitated behavior is also characteristic of cognitive fatigue in cancer, this may be misinterpreted or misunderstood by both patients and professionals. Such behavior should be carefully examined as to cause.

Criterion B

This traumatic event is reexperienced as 1 or more of the characteristics.

Characteristics

1. Recurrent, intrusive, and threatening recollections of the event(s).
2. Recurrent nightmares.[b]
3. Feeling as if the traumatic experiences were recurring (may include sense of reliving the experience, hallucinations, or dissociative "flashback" episodes).
4. Intense emotional distress upon reexposure to internal or external cues that recall some aspect of the traumatic place or event.
5. Physiological reactivity on exposure to those cues.

Issues Relevant to Cancer and Fatigue

1. The need for recurrent follow-up examinations and diagnostic tests, and the fear of associated recurrence, extend the risk of the traumatic events.
2. See note.[b]
3. Patients describe a literal "flashback" experience while on the way to the clinic, entering the building, smelling certain clinic-associated odors, undergoing CT scans, preparing for bone marrow biopsies, or thinking of follow-up treatments. Be aware of patients describing their experience of cancer and cancer treatment with such terms as *rape*.
4. These flashback or associated reliving experiences may occur without warning; they may be self-reinforcing, producing a feedback loop of avoidance behavior (see criterion C below).
5. The link between the stimulus and the response may not be evident. Patients who are identified as suffering from this problem should be referred for professional therapy and possible treatment with appropriate psychotropic medications.

Criterion C

Persistent avoidance of anything associated with the trauma and numbing of responsiveness (not present prior to the trauma) with 3 or more of the characteristics.

Characteristics

1. Avoidance of thoughts, feelings, or conversations about anything associated with the trauma.
2. Avoidance of places, events, or people that may arouse memories.
3. Selective inability to recall a significant aspect of the trauma.

4. Diminished interest or participation in related activities or events.
5. Feeling of detachment or estrangement from others.
6. Limited affect (may be perceived by other than patients).
7. Sense of doom or shortened life span.

Issues Relevant to Cancer and Fatigue

1. & 4. Patients may also avoid support groups, association with former clinical employees, or any literature or information sources, or show disinterest in follow-up monitoring.

2. & 3. Indicators of this problem may include avoidance of follow-up appointments, repeated "forgotten" clinic visits, or inability to remember significant aspects of treatment, allergies, or prior medical conditions. (Patients who are potential candidates for this problem may actually be identified by themselves, family or clinical personnel as "tough," "coping well," "a real survivor," "responsible," or "nothing gets me/her/him down.")

5. & 7. The feeling of detachment, estrangement, or sense of doom may be interpreted by the person as "destiny" or "karma." It is critical to be sensitive to cultural background in evaluating potential risk among patients.

5., 6., & 7. These characteristics have been described in Holocaust survivors and those who have survived incredibly traumatizing experiences. Be alert for body marks, comments, cultural affiliation, or any other identifiers that may hint of someone at high risk. Referral for specialized therapy is critical since there may be a higher risk of suicide.

Criterion D

Persistent evidence of posttraumatic arousal (2 or more characteristics)

Characteristics

1. Insomnia.
2. Irritability or unpredictable explosive anger.
3. Trouble focusing or concentrating.
4. Hypervigilance.
5. Exaggerated startle reaction.

Issues Relevant to Cancer and Fatigue

Notice the presence of irritability and trouble concentrating on this list as well as the criteria for depression. These appear to be frequent long-term characteristics of fatigue.

Criterion E

Duration of the disturbance (B, C, and D) 1 month or more.

Issues Relevant to Cancer and Fatigue

The disturbance may manifest for the first time even several years after cancer treatment. Some patients may interpret this as a sign of cancer recurrence or of impending doom.

Criterion F

.   Disturbance results in significant clinical distress or impairment related to some significant aspect of life.

Issues Relevant to Cancer and Fatigue

The effects of PTSD can be summarized as functional impairment, impaired ability to pursue self-care activities, increased time spent sleeping, and continued emotional distress. This should be recognized as a reason for referral for treatment as soon as the condition is suspected.

---

[a] less than 3 months (acute) or more than 3 months (chronic). "With delayed onset" means onset of symptoms is at least 6 months after the stressor.

[b] Some patients with extremely traumatic backgrounds have been reported to have suppressed dream recall. See discussion in this chapter.

Source: Adapted from the DSM-IV criteria for posttraumatic stress disorder (American Psychiatric Association, 1994).

"why me" stage where many people try to find meaning in their experience. Flint (1995) found that women who participated in support groups attended to their grieving process more, and were willing to look for meaning as part of their adjustment process. But what about those who were more closed (i.e., those who did not participate)? She observed that it seemed to reflect their mother's values of closedness. They were less likely to attend to grieving and did not look for meaning. What if they were afraid to look? What if their past experiences had already told them there was no meaning, that they could expect only lone-liness, isolation, and bewilderment?

Countless studies indicated that people who develop PTSD were more likely to have suffered abuse and trauma when they were young. Although this phenomenon has been studied most commonly in Vietnam veterans and Holocaust survivors, it also applies to sur-vivors of childhood violence and physical, verbal, and sexual abuse. Table 11-4 presents the DSM-IV characteristics of PTSD with special implications for people with cancer.

Several years ago, Oppenheim (1996), a practicing physician, published an article enti-tled, "7 Ways Doctors Torture Their Patients." He was serious about the title. He had taken an honest look at the health care system and realized there are many ways we torment our patients. We don't mean to; we just don't think about it. We don't realize how the everyday part of our work looks to "outsiders," especially those who are our "victims." Patients do not come into the clinic with labels tattooed on their foreheads (although some still have tat-tooed numbers on their arms). It is important to pay special attention to individuals with backgrounds of childhood violence and abuse, imprisonment, psychiatric hospitalization (in some countries that was how political dissidents were dealt with), refugee status, and expe-riences as political prisoners. Be cautious whenever people show signs of aggression, or passivity, watching for signs of dissociation. Watch for small scars on the body that may present evidence of cigarette burns and other forms of torture. It is also important to remember that a practiced torturer does not have to leave physical scars in order to break someone. Torture scars are either the result of a sloppy interrogation or to make the per-son a living lesson to others. Sleep deprivation over a few days, especially when the victim is deprived of normal light-dark, day-night signals, is sufficient to break anyone.

For health care personnel who may wish to learn more about this, the American Asso-ciation for the Advancement of Science has prepared material on how best to provide health care to meet these patients' special needs. I would like to recommend *Serving Sur-vivors of Torture* by Randall and Lutz (1991). Medications may be prescribed to keep per-sons from violent decompensation. Antidepressants, medications for bipolar disorder, anxiolytics, and others may help persons during cancer treatment. They often need psy-chotherapy to help them through this period. Of people who have experienced great trauma in the past, I have heard it said, "Men become violent, women become depressed." Unfortunately, our society is more threatened by the violence and ignores the depression. There is also tremendous stigma in our culture, as well as others, associated with being the victim of dehumanizing trauma as well as obtaining psychiatric help. For many immigrants, English is not their native language, making communication even more difficult.

There is another barrier to helping people with these experiences: Most Americans cannot begin to conceptualize the inhumane experiences others may have survived. Years ago, when I lived in Europe, I met people who had lived under both the Nazi and Communist regimes. The mass rape and pillage they experienced by both armies was beyond comprehension. Can you imagine how the experiences of cancer can retraumatize someone like that? Veterans of war also frequently have had overwhelming, unimaginable experiences. Often, these are the patients who don't seem to care, who appear hostile, the patients who don't communicate or cooperate, the people with walls. They may even be afraid to report symptoms, especially pain. As the population ages, we can expect to encounter more patients with this kind of background. They are already vulnerable, and the fatigability associated with cancer may be life-threatening to them.

There is another area I would like to address. It is mentioned in several other chapters of this book (especially Chapters 17 and 23). The problem of acute as well as chronic *cognitive impairment* is being increasingly recognized as a short-term phenomenon as well as among long-term survivors. In some cases, it may be part of the "fuzzy thinking" associated with depression and hypersomnia. However, it is clear there are other influences, often related to treatments, that leave people impaired for years afterwards, sometimes for life. There are several reasons for this:

1. People are having to work throughout their treatments. High-functioning individuals seem to be especially sensitive to cognitive losses. They may have increasing difficulty with planning, functioning independently, following through on projects, forgetting meetings and appointments, and short-term memory. Sometimes people even lose their jobs because of this. The cognitive effects of fatigue in cancer, especially as a long-term issue, have not been addressed adequately. Superficially, they do not seem to qualify for Americans with Disabilities Act protection, nor are they able to access the disability system.

2. Psychometric tests are becoming increasingly sensitive. This is critical since these deficits may not correlate with any objective imaging or chemistry diagnostic techniques. Even now, the tests still don't pick up on difficulties with everyday living that may develop, including handling money and paying bills. Organizational abilities like money management and keeping track of dates are central to independent, adult living. While compiling this book, I heard many times, "I didn't realize I hadn't paid the bills until the gas/electricity were shut off. People think I'm being irresponsible, but I'm trying harder than ever before in my life."

3. Patients may be aware something is wrong, but they may not even be aware they are suffering through a comparative deficit, particularly if people do not explain the characteristics and how their lives may be affected.

4. There has been scant research on developing means of helping cancer patients adapt to these deficits so they can remain productive following the termination of their treatment. The use of psychostimulants, used with other disorders, may help support developments in behavioral training.

5. More cancer patients are surviving longer; however, the therapies exact their toll on the body. In all the other major chronic illnesses, medications work with the body. In cancer, the treatments usually work *against the body,* exerting a toxic effect on normal as well as malignant cells. The therapies can have a long-term effect on the nervous system that impairs general physical functioning as well as cognitive functioning. Hence, the ability to prolong life must be supported by the rehabilitative therapies (Meyers et al, 1998).

There are several established sources from which we can draw as we develop interventions to help people cope effectively. As pointed out in Chapters 17 and 23, select techniques used for people who have suffered mild traumatic brain injury (MTBI) may be helpful. Certainly there are common characteristics in some of the limitations. In a recent study using methylphenidate (Ritalin) therapy, brain tumor patients showed improved moods, cognition, and function (Meyers et al, 1998). In another study of patients with primary malignant brain tumors, postacute traumatic brain injury rehabilitation seemed to offer a cost-effective means of optimizing functioning (Sherer, Meyers, and Bergloff, 1997).

Dr. Olders: I'd like to interject something here. The fact that cognitive impairment seems to respond to methylphenidate suggests that it may also have something to do with depression, just as fatigue does. We know that in elderly patients, depression can produce a pseudo-dementia, which at times is indistinguishable from a true dementia like Alzheimer's disease. Total sleep deprivation has been used as a diagnostic test for this kind of cognitive impairment, in cases where there had been no response to other antidepressants (Williams, Yeomans, and Coughlan, 1994). It sounds possible to me that in some cancer patients, getting too much REM sleep might produce cognitive dysfunction more so than fatigue or frank depression. Getting up early might be a useful intervention for these people also.

Children with attention deficit and hyperactivity disorder (ADHD) may sleep more than normal children (Tirosh et al, 1993). This may help to explain the therapeutic effectiveness of methylphenidate in ADHD. To the extent that cancer patients sleep excessively, they might experience some of the same symptoms as ADHD patients, and respond to the same sort of interventions. It would also be worthwhile, I think, to see what effect getting up early has on people with ADHD.

Dr. Winningham: Thank you! Ideally, every oncology clinic should have a consulting board-certified neuropsychologist with experience in working with cancer patients and their families. However, this is not an ideal world. In areas where such consultation and rehabilitation are not available, primary health care providers can encourage patients to work on organizational skills and MTBI-type rehabilitation tasks. Two books that are excellent resources are *The Rehabilitation of Brain Functions: Principles, Procedures, and Techniques of Neurotraining* by Craine and Gudeman (1981) and *The Thinking Skills Workbook: A Cognitive Skills Remediation Manual for Adults* by Carter, Caruso, and Languirand (1984). Patients who have undergone procedures like bone marrow transplantation or who have received some kind of high-dose chemotherapy find themselves physically and mentally impaired afterward (Ganz, 1998; Schagen et al, 1999; van Dam et al, 1998). Family members might even be taught to work with patients to redevelop or sharpen cognitive skills.

Other rehabilitation techniques are those used in people who have ADHD. Although it seems quite remote to suggest that someone with long-term cognitive fatigue has anything in common with ADHD, there are some important similarities. For example, trouble initiating and following through on tasks, irritability, trouble with memory, and trouble prioritizing are common to MTBI and ADHD. Organizational techniques used with them may be especially helpful for cancer survivors who still suffer from the cognitive "blahs."

Sleep hygiene, a structured lifestyle, good nutritional intake, and regular moderate exercise can help minimize deficits while promoting functioning and feelings of well-being in all three groups of patients. Organizational and management training may also facilitate more successful on-the-job performance. Use of medications to help with cognitive clarity may also help. In short, the fatigue experience of cancer represents a significant challenge for employees (Mock, 1998).

During the time I was working on this book, I was considering what could be done to help cognitively impaired patients organize. Missed appointments, confused times and dates, and difficulty keeping track of seemingly simple things make cancer survivors with cognitive impairment look careless or immature. Although identifying and carrying out priorities were identified as big problems, the use of commercial planners and personal information managers usually did not work in the long run; neither did making lists of priorities. Not only did *others* around them not understand, but also *they* did not understand themselves. There is a special planner/organizer for adults and children with ADHD that incorporates a conceptually different approach than anything I have seen before. The psychologist Janice Goldstein, who is the codeveloper of this product, is a breast cancer survivor! She said she found some of the techniques she taught her patients to be useful when she was going through cancer treatment. The SpectraPlanner is organized in a way that uses appealing color coding and a unique spatial orientation that facilitates an overview of activities. For research or clinical application, information about how and where to order the SpectraPlanner is located at the end of this chapter. This is what Goldstein had to say about how the planner was developed:

> The SpectraPlanner was conceived by myself and a colleague, Kate Goldfield, in our work with individuals who have attentional and organizational problems. I am a psychologist who has spent a great deal of my career trying to understand the relationship between

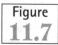

Figure 11.7 — Proposed ICD-10 Criteria for Cancer-Related Fatigue (1998 Draft)

A. Six (or more) of the following symptoms have been present every day or nearly every day during the same 2-week period in the past month, and at least one of the symptoms is (1) significant fatigue.

1. Significant fatigue, diminished energy, or increased need to rest, disproportionate to any recent change in activity level;
2. Complaints of generalized weakness or limb heaviness;
3. Diminished concentration or attention;
4. Decreased motivation or interest to engage in usual activities;
5. Insomnia or hypersomnia;
6. Experience of sleep as unrefreshing or nonrestorative;
7. Perceived need to struggle to overcome inactivity;
8. Marked emotional reactivity (e.g., sadness, frustration, or irritability) to feeling fatigued;
9. Difficulty completing daily tasks attributed to feeling fatigued;
10. Perceived problems with short-term memory;
11. Post-exertional malaise lasting several hours;

B. The symptoms cause clinically significant distress or impairment in social, occupational, or other important areas of functioning.

C. There is evidence from the history, physical examination, or laboratory findings that the symptoms are a consequence of cancer or cancer therapy.

D. The symptoms are not primarily a consequence of co-morbid psychiatric disorders such as major depression, somatization disorder, somatoform disorder, or delirium.

Source: From Cella, D., Peterman, A., Passik, S., Jacobson, P., and Breitbart, W. (1988). Progress toward guidelines for the management of fatigue. *Oncology, 12* (11A), 373. Used with permission.

how people learn and how they organize their time. I noticed the substantial impact that attention and concentration had on an individual's success in careers and in relationships with others. My understanding of the impact of attention and concentration became even clearer during my own treatment for breast cancer. During that time I realized even further how much more difficult it is to maintain a sense of organization when one is struggling with the lethargy and exhaustion created by chemotherapy and radiation. With both these professional and personal experiences in hand, my colleague and I tried to come up with a hands-on tool.

Thus evolved the SpectraPlanner. Spectra uses a unique color-coded format and logical top-to-bottom design to facilitate personal organization for teens as well as adults. It has stickers that help individuals to actively plan their time and think ahead about what may be coming up. The "week to do" stays in view all week long and the "month to do" stays in view for the month. This helps with the "out of sight, out of mind" problem of short-term memory impairment.

This is an example of what we need to prevent impairments from becoming disabilities, and disabilities from becoming handicaps. This is more than just a quality of life issue,

| Figure 11.8 | Diagnostic Interview Guide for Cancer-Related Fatigue (1998 Draft) |

Note: Capitalized text represents instructions to the interviewer. Text in quotations represents statements to be read verbatim to the respondent.

1. "Over the past month, has there been at least a 2-week period when you had significant fatigue a lack of energy, or an increased need to rest every day or nearly every day?"   CIRCLE ONE: YES   NO
IF NO STOP HERE, IF YES, CONTINUE.

"For each of the following questions, focus on the worst 2 weeks in the past month (or else the past 2 weeks if you felt equally fatigued for the entire month)."

2. "Did you feel weak all over or heavy all over? (every day or nearly every day?)"   CIRCLE ONE: YES   NO

3. "Did you have trouble concentrating or paying attention? (every day or nearly every day?"   CIRCLE ONE: YES   NO

4. "What about losing your interest or desire to do the things you usually do? (every day or nearly every day?)"   CIRCLE ONE: YES   NO

5. "How are you sleeping? Did you have trouble falling asleep, staying asleep, or waking too early? Or did you find yourself sleeping too much compared to what you usually sleep? (every night or nearly every night?)"   CIRCLE ONE: YES   NO

6. "Have you found that you usually don't feel rested or refreshed after you have slept (every day or nearly every day?)"   CIRCLE ONE: YES   NO

7. "Did you have to struggle or push yourself to do anything? (every day or nearly every day?)"   CIRCLE ONE: YES   NO

8. "Did you find yourself feeling sad, frustrated, or irritable because you felt fatigued? (every day or nearly every day?)"   CIRCLE ONE: YES   NO

9. "Did you have difficulty finishing something you had started to do because of feeling fatigued? (every day or nearly every day?)"   CIRCLE ONE: YES   NO

10. "Did you have trouble remembering things? For example, did you have trouble remembering where your keys were or what someone had told you a little while ago? (every day or nearly every day?)"   CIRCLE ONE: YES   NO

11. "Did you find yourself feeling sick or unwell for several hours after you had done something that took some effort? (every day or nearly every day?)"   CIRCLE ONE: YES   NO
IF LESS THAN SIX ITEMS INCLUDING #1 ARE MARKED YES, STOP HERE.

12. "Has fatigue made it hard for you to do your work, take care of things at home, or get along with other people?"   CIRCLE ONE: YES   NO
IF #12 IS NO, STOP HERE.

13. IS THERE EVIDENCE FROM THE HISTORY, PHYSICAL EXAMINATION, OR LABORATORY FINDINGS THAT THE SYMPTOMS ARE A CONSEQUENCE OF CANCER OR CANCER THERAPY?   CIRCLE ONE: YES   NO
IF #13 IS NO, STOP HERE.

14. ARE THE SYMPTOMS PRIMARILY A CONSEQUENCE OF COMORBID PSYCHIATRIC DISORDERS SUCH AS MAJOR DEPRESSION, SOMATIZATION DISORDER, SOMATOFORM DISORDER, OR DELIRUM?   CIRCLE ONE: YES   NO
IF #14 IS YES, PATIENT <u>DOES NOT MEET CRITERIA</u> FOR CANCER–RELATED FATIGUE.
IF #14 IS NO, PATIENT <u>MEETS CRITERIA</u> FOR CANCER–RELATED FATIGUE.

Source: From Cella, D., Peterman, A., Passik, S., Jacobson, P., and Breitbart, W. (1988). Progress toward guidelines for the management of fatigue. *Oncology, 12* (11A), 375. Used with permission.

it is an economic exigency in our current health care environment, and interventions like this may prove to be quite cost-effective.

Diagnostic Interview Guide for Cancer Fatigue (1998 Draft)

One development that may be especially helpful is the use of established, recognized diagnostic criteria and a diagnostic interview guide for cancer fatigue. Recently Cella and colleagues (1998) proposed draft criteria for an International Diagnostic Classification (ICD-10) diagnosis of cancer fatigue (see Figure 11-7). The medicolegal ramifications of this development are significant because it would allow cancer fatigue to be recognized by the medical and disability system (see Chapter 14 for further discussion about this). In the same publication, this team published a one-page diagnostic interview guide for fatigue that could be used both in clinical practice and for screening in research (see Figure 11-8). They emphasized this guide is a draft. It could be a critical unifying factor in research and clinical practice.

Where Do We Go From Here

This chapter has examined a number of unusual topics with reference to the CRFS. Yet, all of them can be part of the weary effects of the CRFS. Sleep disturbances, fatigue, depression, PTSD, retraumatization, and cognitive impairments suggest still other dimensions related to the CRFS and hold the possibility of innovative interventions. The implications of this discussion should challenge researchers and clinicians in new directions; this in turn should place new instruments in the hands of clinicians to address the CRFS in an inexpensive and practical manner. In patients who appear to be suffering from any of these problems, screening instruments included in this chapter as well as a good psychiatric history are of vital importance.

Cognitive fatigue, also discussed in other chapters in this book, is being increasingly recognized as a long-term source of distress. Without reinventing the wheel, techniques developed for treating other patient populations may be applicable to cancer survivors. A few recent studies point to the urgent need for additional research on risks and interventions related to this problem.

Endnote

1. The historical precedence for using "thought experiments" as a technique for presenting logical links in science originated with Galileo Galilei (ca. 1600) and is presented in Chapter 2. Rogers, E. M. (1960) *Physics for the Inquiring Mind: The Methods, Nature, and Philosophy of Physical Science.* Princeton, NJ: Princeton University Press, 8–9.

References

Abbey, S. E., and Garfinkel, P. E. (1991). Neurasthenia and chronic fatigue syndrome: The role of culture in the making of a diagnosis [see comments]. *American Journal of Psychiatry, 148,* 1638–1646.

Akerstedt, T., Hume, K., Minors, D., and Waterhouse, J. (1993). Regulation of sleep and naps on an irregular schedule. *Sleep, 16,* 736–743.

American Psychiatric Association (1994). *Diagnostic and statistical manual of mental disorders: DSM-IV.* 4th ed. Washington, DC: American Psychiatric Association.

Aserinsky, E. (1969). The maximal capacity for sleep: Rapid eye movement density as an index of sleep satiety. *Biological Psychiatry, 1,* 147–159.

Bazargan, M. (1996). Self-reported sleep disturbance among African-American elderly: The effects of depression, health status, exercise, and social support. *International Journal of Aging and Human Development, 42*(2), 143–160.

Belloc, N. B., and Breslow, L. (1972). Relationship of physical health status and health practices. *Preventive Medicine, 1,* 409–421.

Bishop, C., Roehrs, T., Rosenthal, L., and Roth, T. (1997). Alerting effects of methylphenidate under basal and sleep-deprived conditions. *Experimental and Clinical Psychopharmacology, 5,* 344–352.

Bliwise, D. L., Friedman, L., Nekich, J. C., and Yesavage, J. A. (1995). Prediction of outcome in behaviorally based insomnia treatments. *Journal of Behavior Therapy and Experimental Psychiatry, 26,* 17–23.

Bonnet, M. H., and Rosa, R. R. (1987). Sleep and performance in young adults and older normals and insomniacs during acute sleep loss and recovery. *Biological Psychology, 25*(2), 153–172.

Breitbart, W., and Holland, J. C. (Eds.) (1993). *Psychiatric aspects of symptom management in cancer patients.* Washington, DC: American Psychiatric Press.

Brunier, G. M., and Graydon, J. (1993). The influence of physical activity on fatigue in patients with ESRD on hemodialysis. *ANNA Journal, 20,* 457–461.

Buchwald, D., Pascualy, R., Bombardier, C., and Kith, P. (1994). Sleep disorders in patients with chronic fatigue. *Clinical Infectious Diseases, 18*(suppl 1), S68–S72.

Buchwald, D., Sullivan, J. L., and Komaroff, A. L. (1987). Frequency of chronic active Epstein-Barr virus infection in a general medical practice. *Journal of the American Medical Association, 257,* 2303–2307.

Carskadon, M. A., Brown, E. D., and Dement, W. C. (1982). Sleep fragmentation in the elderly: Relationship to daytime sleep tendency. *Neurobiology of Aging, 3,* 321–327.

Carskadon, M. A., and Dement, W. C. (1985). Sleep loss in elderly volunteers. *Sleep, 8,* 207–221.

Carter, L. T., Caruso, J. L., and Languirand, M. A. (1984). *The thinking skills workbook: A cognitive skills remediation manual for adults.* Springfield, IL: Charles C Thomas.

Cauch-Dudek, K., Abbey, S., Stewart, D. E., and Heathcote, E. J. (1998). Fatigue in primary biliary cirrhosis. *Gut, 43,* 705–710.

Cella, D., Peterman, A., Passik, S., Jacobsen, P., and Breitbart, W. (1998). Progress toward guidelines for the management of fatigue. *Oncology, 12,* 369–377.

Chambers, M. J., and Keller, B. (1993). Alert insomniacs: Are they really sleep deprived? *Clinical Psychology Review, 13,* 649–666.

Chatoor, I., Wells, K. C., Conners, C. K., et al. (1983). The effects of nocturnally administered stimulant medication on EEG sleep and behavior in hyperactive children. *Journal of the American Academy of Child Psychiatry, 22,* 337–342.

Chochinov, H. M., Wilson, K. G., Enns, M., and Lander, S. (1997). "Are you depressed?" Screening for depression in the terminally ill [see comments]. *American Journal of Psychiatry, 154,* 674–676.

Cohen, H. B., and Dement, W. C. (1966). Sleep: Suppression of rapid eye movement phase in the cat after electroconvulsive shock. *Science, 154*(747), 396–398.

Craine, J. F., and Gudeman, H. E. (1981). *The rehabilitation of brain functions: Principles, procedures, and techniques of neurotraining.* Springfield, IL: Charles C Thomas.

Darko, D. F., McCutchan, J. A., Kripke, D. F., et al. (1992). Fatigue, sleep disturbance, disability, and indices of progression of HIV infection. *American Journal of Psychiatry, 149,* 514–520.

David, M. M., MacLean, A. W., Knowles, J. B., and Coulter, M. E. (1991). Rapid eye movement latency and mood following a delay of bedtime in healthy subjects: Do the effects mimic changes in depressive illness? *Acta Psychiatrica Scandinavica, 84,* 33–39.

Degner, L. F., and Sloan, J. A. (1995). Symptom distress in newly diagnosed ambulatory cancer patients and as a predictor of survival in lung cancer. *Journal of Pain and Symptom Management, 10,* 423–431.

De la Fuente, J. M., Staner, L., Kerkhofs, M., et al. (1992). Polysomnographic characteristics in recurrent brief depression: A comparative study with major depression and controls. *Acta Psychiatrica Belgica, 92,* 179.

Dodd, M. J. (1984). Patterns of self care in cancer patients receiving radiation therapy. *Oncology Nursing Forum, 11*(3), 23–27.

Dollins, A. B., Zhdanova, I. V., Wurtman, R. J., et al. (1994). Effect of inducing nocturnal serum melatonin concentrations in daytime on sleep, mood, body temperature, and performance. *Proceedings of the National Academy of Sciences USA, 91,* 1824–1828.

Driver, H. S., Meintjes, A. F., Rogers, G. G., and Shapiro, C. M. (1988). Submaximal exercise effects on sleep patterns in young women before and after an aerobic training programme. *Acta Physiologica Scandinavica Supplement, 574,* 8–13.

Faber, J., and Havrdova, Z. (1981). Differential effect of REM stimulating and REM inhibiting drugs (reserpine and amitriptyline) on memory. *Activitas Nervosa Superior, 23,* 169–171.

Flint, T. (1995). "Breast cancer support groups: Differences between attenders and nonattenders." Doctoral dissertation, University of Utah, Salt Lake City, Utah.

Ford, D. E., and Kamerow, D. B. (1989). Epidemiologic study of sleep disturbances and psychiatric disorders. An opportunity for prevention? [see comments]. *Journal of the American Medical Association, 262,* 1479–1484.

Frankel, B. L., Coursey, R. D., Buchbinder, R., and Snyder, F. (1976). Recorded and reported sleep in chronic primary insomnia. *Archives of General Psychiatry, 33*(5), 615–623.

Galynker, I., Ieronimo, C., Miner, C., et al. (1997). Methylphenidate treatment of negative symptoms in patients with dementia. *Journal of Neuropsychiatry and Clinical Neurosciences, 9,* 231–239.

Ganz, P. A. (1998). Cognitive dysfunction following adjuvant therapy of breast cancer: A new dose-limiting toxic effect. *Journal of National Cancer Institute, 90,* 182–183.

Gill, D. S., Ketter, T. A., and Post, R. M. (1993). Antidepressant response to sleep deprivation as a function of time into depressive episode in rapidly cycling bipolar patients. *Acta Psychiatrica Scandinavica, 87*(2), 102–109.

Glaus, A. (1993). Assessment of fatigue in cancer and non-cancer patients and in healthy individuals [see comments]. *Supportive Care in Cancer, 1,* 305–315.

Globus, G. G. (1969). A syndrome associated with sleeping late. *Psychosomatic Medicine, 31,* 528–535.

Graydon, J. E. (1994). Women with breast cancer: Their quality of life following a course of radiation therapy. *Journal of Advanced Nursing, 19,* 617–622.

Graydon, J. E., Bubela, N., Irvine, D., and Vincent, L. (1995). Fatigue-reducing strategies used by patients receiving treatment for cancer. *Cancer Nursing, 18,* 23–28.

Greenberg, D. B, Gray, J. L., Mannix, C. M., et al. (1993). Treatment-related fatigue and serum interleukin-1 levels in patients during external beam irradiation for prostate cancer. *Journal of Pain and Symptom Management, 8,* 196–200.

Guilleminault, C., and Mondini, S. (1986). Mononucleosis and chronic daytime sleepiness. A long-term follow-up study. *Archives of Internal Medicine, 146,* 1333–1335.

Harrison, Y., and Horne, J. A. (1996). Long-term extension to sleep–are we really chronically sleep deprived? *Psychophysiology, 33,* 22–30.

Helmus, T., Rosenthal, L., Bishop, C., Roehrs, T., Krsevska, S. and Roth, T. (1996). Nocturnal sleep latencies among alert, alert-deprived and sleepy subjects. *Electroencephalography and Clinical Neurophysiology, 99,* 10–15.

Höchli, D., Riemann, D., Zulley, J., and Berger, M. (1986). Initial REM sleep suppression by clomipramine: A prognostic tool for treatment response in patients with a major depressive disorder. *Biological Psychiatry, 21*(12), 1217–1220.

Irvine, D., Vincent, L., Graydon, J. E., et al. (1994). The prevalence and correlates of fatigue in patients receiving treatment with chemotherapy and radiotherapy. A comparison with the fatigue experienced by healthy individuals. *Cancer Nursing, 17*(5), 367–378.

Jamar, S. C. (1989). Fatigue in women receiving chemotherapy for ovarian cancer. In S. G. Funk, E. Tornquist, M. Champagne, L. Archer Copp, and R. Wiese, (Eds.), *Key aspects of comfort: Management of pain, fatigue, and nausea* (pp. 224–228). New York: Springer.

Karni, A., Tanne, D., Rubinstein, B. S., et al. (1992). No dreams, no memory: The effect of REM sleep deprivation on learning a new perceptual skill. *Society for Neuroscience Abstracts, 18,* 387.

Kawachi, I., Willett, W. C., Colditz, G. A., et al. (1996). A prospective study of coffee drinking and suicide in women [see comments]. *Archives of Internal Medicine, 156*(5), 521–525.

Knobf, M. T. (1986). Physical and psychologic distress associated with adjuvant chemotherapy in women with breast cancer. *Journal of Clinical Oncology, 4*(5), 678–684.

Kobashi-Schoot, J. A., Hanewald, G. J., van Dam, F. S., and Bruning, P. F. (1985). Assessment of malaise in cancer patients treated with radiotherapy. *Cancer Nursing, 8*(6), 306–313.

Kupfer, D. J., Ehlers, C. L., Frank, E., et al. (1991). EEG sleep profiles and recurrent depression. *Biological Psychiatry, 30*(7), 641–655.

Langer, L. L. (1995). *Admitting the Holocaust: Collected Essays.* New York: Oxford University Press.

Lauer, C. J., Schreiber, W., Holsboer, F., and Krieg, J. C. (1995). In quest of identifying vulnerability markers for psychiatric disorders by all-night polysomnography. *Archives of General Psychiatry, 52*(2), 145–153.

Lazarus, L. W., Moberg, P. J., Langsley, P. R., and Lingam, V. R. (1994). Methylphenidate and nortriptyline in the treatment of poststroke depression: A retrospective comparison. *Archives of Physical Medicine and Rehabilitation, 75*(4), 403–406.

Leibenluft, E., and Wehr, T. A. (1992). Is sleep deprivation useful in the treatment of depression? *American Journal of Psychiatry, 149*(2), 159–168.

Mahowald, M. W., Mahowald, M. L., Bundlie, S. R., and Ytterberg, S. R. (1989). Sleep fragmentation in rheumatoid arthritis. *Arthritis and Rheumatism, 32*(8), 974–983.

Martikainen, K., Hasan, J., Urponen, H., et al. (1992). Daytime sleepiness: A risk factor in community life. *Acta Neurologica Scandinavica, 86*(4), 337–341.

McCall, W. V., and Edinger, J. D. (1992). Subjective total insomnia: An example of sleep state misperception. *Sleep, 15*(1), 71–73.

McCorkle, R., and Quint-Benoliel, J. (1983). Symptom distress, current concerns and mood disturbance after diagnosis of life-threatening disease. *Social Science and Medicine, 17*(7), 431–438.

Meguro, K., Ueda, M., Yamaguchi, T., et al. (1990). Disturbance in daily sleep/wake patterns in patients with cognitive impairment and decreased daily activity. *Journal of the American Geriatric Society, 38*(11), 270–276.

Meney, I., Waterhouse, J., Atkinson, G., Reilly, T., and Davenne, D. (1998). The effect of one night's sleep deprivation on temperature, mood, and physical performance in subjects with different amounts of habitual physical activity. *Chronobiolical Int, 15*(4), 349–363.

Meyers, C. A., Weitzner, M. A., Valentine, A. D., and Levin, V. A. (1998). Methylphenidate therapy improves cognition, mood, and function of brain tumor patients. *Journal of Clinical Oncology, 16*(7), 2522–2527.

Middlekoop, H. A., Smilde-van den Doel, D. A., Neven, A. K., et al. (1996). Subjective sleep characteristics of 1,485 males and females aged 50–93: Effects of sex and age, and factors related to self-evaluated quality of sleep. *Journal of Gerontology. Series A, Biological Sciences and Medical Sciences, 51*(3), M108–M115.

Mock, V. (1998). Breast cancer and fatigue: Issues for the workplace. *American Association of Occupational Health Nurses Journal, 46*(9), 425–431.

Moldofsky, H. (1992). Evaluation of daytime sleepiness. *Clinics in Chest Medicine, 13*(3), 417–425.

Moldofsky, H. (1993). Fibromyalgia, sleep disorder and chronic fatigue syndrome. *Ciba Foundation Symposium, 173,* 262–271.

Montplaisir, J. Y. (1984). Insomnia: A therapeutic dilemma. *Annals of the Royal College of Physicians and Surgeons of Canada, 17*(5), 405–409.

Morin, C. M., Colecchi, C., Stone, J., et al. (1997). Behavioral and pharmacological therapies for late-life insomnia: A randomized controlled trial [see comments]. *Journal of the American Medical Association, 281*(11), 991–999.

Morin, C. M., Kowatch, R. A., and Wade, J. B. (1989). Behavioral management of sleep disturbances secondary to chronic pain. *Journal of Behavioral Therapy and Experimental Psychiatry, 20*(4), 295–302.

Morris, R. K., Wearden, A. J., and Battersby, L. (1997). The relation of sleep difficulties to fatigue, mood and disability in chronic fatigue syndrome. *Journal of Psychosomatic Research, 42*(6), 597–605.

Nail, L. M., Jones, L. S., Greene, D., et al. (1991). Use and perceived efficacy of self-care activities in patients receiving chemotherapy. *Oncology Nursing Forum, 18*(5), 883–887.

Nofzinger, E. A., Reynolds, C. F., III, Thase, M. E., et al. (1995). REM sleep enhancement by bupropion in depressed men. *American Journal of Psychiatry, 152*(2), 274–276.

Nofzinger, E. A., Thase, M. E., Reynolds, C. F. D., et al. (1991). Hypersomnia in bipolar depression: A comparison with narcolepsy using the multiple sleep latency test. *American Journal of Psychiatry, 148*(9), 1177–1181.

Ohta, T., Ando, K., Iwata, T., et al. (1991). Treatment of persistent sleep-wake schedule disorders in adolescents with methylcobalamin (vitamin B_{12}). *Sleep, 14*(5), 414–418.

Okawa, M., Mishima, K., Nanami, T., et al (1990). Vitamin B_{12} treatment for sleep-wake rhythm disorders. *Sleep, 13*(1), 15–23.

Olin, J., and Masand, P. (1996). Psychostimulants for depression in hospitalized cancer patients. *Psychosomatics, 37*(1), 57–62.

Oppenheim, M. D. (1996). 7 ways doctors torture their patients. *Hippocrates,* 10, 61–65.

Pace-Schott, E. F., Kaji, J., Stickgold, R., and Hobson, J. A. (1994). Nightcap measurement of sleep quality in self-described good and poor sleepers. *Sleep, 17*(8), 688–692.

Parry, B. L., Cover, H., Mostofi, N., et al. (1995). Early versus late partial sleep deprivation in patients with premenstrual dysphoric disorder and normal comparison subjects. *American Journal of Psychiatry, 152*(3), 404–412.

Patten, S. B., Williams, J. V., and Love, E. J. (1996). Self-reported depressive symptoms following treatment with corticosteroids and sedative-hypnotics. *International Journal of Psychiatry in Medicine, 26*(1), 15–24.

Pinto, B. M., and Maruyama, N. C. (1999). Exercise in the rehabilitation of breast cancer survivors. *Psycho-Oncology, 8*(3), 191–206. [MEDLINE record in process]

Piper, B. F., Lindsey, A. M., Dodd, M. J., et al. (1989). The development of an instrument to measure the subjective dimension of fatigue. In S. G. Funk, E. Tornquist, M. Champagne, L. Archer Copp, and R. Wiese (Eds.), *Key aspects of comfort: Management of pain, fatigue, and nausea* (pp. 199–208). New York: Springer.

Regestein Q. R., and Monk, T. H. (1995). Delayed sleep phase syndrome: A review of its clinical aspects. *American Journal of Psychiatry, 152*(4), 602–608.

Sack, D. A., Duncan, W., Rosenthal, N. E., et al. (1988). The timing and duration of sleep in partial sleep deprivation therapy of depression. *Acta Psychiatrica Scandinavica, 77*(2), 219–224.

Sack, D. A., Nurnberger, J., Rosenthal, N. E., et al. (1985). Potentiation of antidepressant medications by phase advance of the sleep-wake cycle. *American Journal of Psychiatry, 142*(5), 606–608.

Saletu, B., Frey, R., Krupka, M., et al. (1989). Differential effects of a new central adrenergic agonist–modafinil–and D-amphetamine on sleep and early morning behaviour in young healthy volunteers. *International Journal of Clinical Pharmacology Research, 9*(3), 183–195.

Salin-Pascual, R. J., Galicia-Polo, L., and Drucker-Colin, R. (1997). Sleep changes after 4 consecutive days of venlafaxine administration in normal volunteers. *Journal of Clinical Psychiatry, 58*(8), 348–350.

Sarna, L. (1993). Correlates of symptom distress in women with lung cancer. *Cancer Practice, 1*(1), 21–28.

Schagen, S. B., van Dam, F. S., Muller, M. J., Boogerd, W., Lindeboom, J., and Brunning, P. F. (1999). Cognitive deficits after postoperative adjuvant chemotherapy for breast carcinoma. *Cancer, 85*(3), 640–650.

Schramm, E., Hohagen, F., Kappler, C., et al. (1995). Mental comorbidity of chronic insomnia in general practice attenders using DSM-III-R. *Acta Psychiatrica Scandinavica, 91*(1), 10–17.

Sharpley, A., Clements, A., Hawton, K., and Sharpe, M. (1997). Do patients with "pure" chronic fatigue syndrome (neurasthenia) have abnormal sleep? *Psychosomatic Medicine, 59*(6), 592–596.

Sherer, M., Meyers, and Bergloff. (1997). Efficacy of postacute brain injury rehabilitation for patients with primary malignant brain tumors. *Cancer, 80*(2), 250–257.

Smets, E. M., Visser, M. R., Willems-Groot, A. F., et al. (1998). Fatigue and radiotherapy: (A) Experience in patients undergoing treatment. *British Journal of Cancer, 78*(7), 899–906.

Spielman, A. J., Saskin, P., and Thorpy, M. J. (1987). Treatment of chronic insomnia by restriction of time in bed. *Sleep, 10*(1), 45–56.

Taub, J. M. (1980). Effects of ad lib extended-delayed sleep on sensorimotor performance, memory and sleepiness in the young adult. *Physiology and Behavior, 25*(1), 77–87.

Taub, J. M., Hollingsworth, H. H., and Bruce, N. S. (1983). Effects on the polysomnogram and waking electrocorticogram of ad-libitum extended-delayed sleep. *International Journal of Neuroscience, 19*(1–4), 173–178.

Tirosh, E., Sadeh, A., Munvez, R., and Lavie, P. (1993). Effects of methylphenidate on sleep in children with attention-deficient hyperactivity disorder. An activity monitor study. *American Journal of Diseases in Children, 147*(12), 1313–1315.

van Dam, F. S., Schagen, S. B., Muller, M. J., Boogerd, W., v d Wall, E., Droogleever Fortuyn, M. E., and Rodenhuis, S. (1998). Impairment of cognitive function in women receiving adjuvant treatment for high-risk breast cancer: High-dose versus standard-dose chemotherapy. *Journal of the National Cancer Institute 90*(3), 210–218.

Volkow, N. D., Wang, G. J., Fowler, J. S., Gatley, S. J., Logan, J., Ding, Y. S., Hitzemann, R., and Pappas, N. (1998) Dopamine transporter occupancies in the human brain induced by therapeutic doses of oral methylphenidate. *American Journal of Psychiatry, 155*(10), 1325–1333. Web site accessed August 4, 1999 <http://www.pslgroup.com/dg/ble8a.htm>.

Watanabe, M. D., Martin, E. M., DeLeon, O. A., et al. (1995). Successful methylphenidate treatment of apathy after subcortical infarcts. *Journal of Neuropsychiatry and Clinical Neurosciences, 7*, 502–504.

Webb, W. B., and Agnew, H. W. (1968). Measurement and characteristics of nocturnal sleep. In L. E. Ab, and B. F. Riess (Eds.), *Progress in clinical psychology* (pp. 2–27). New York: Grune & Stratton.

Wehr, T. A., Wirz-Justice, A., Goodwin, F. K., et al. (1979). Phase advance of the circadian sleep-wake cycle as an antidepressant. *Science, 206*(4419), 710–713.

Wiegand, M., Berger, M., Zulley, J., et al. (1987). The influence of daytime naps on the therapeutic effect of sleep deprivation. *Biological Psychiatry, 22*(3), 389–392.

Williams, C. J., Yeomans, J. D., and Coughlan, A. K. (1994). Sleep deprivation as a diagnostic instrument. *British Journal of Psychiatry, 164*(4), 554–556.

Wingard, D. L., and Berkman, L. F. (1983). Mortality risk associated with sleeping patterns among adults. *Sleep, 6*(2), 102–107.

Winningham, M. L. (1991). Walking program for people with cancer: Getting started. *Cancer Nursing, 14*(5), 270–276.

World Health Organization (1992). *International diagnostic classification (ICD-10)*. Geneva: World Health Organization. Web site access: <www.who.int/msa/mnh/ems/icd10/cliexamp.htm>.

Resources

Breitbart, W. (1995). Identifying patients at risk for, and treatment of, major psychiatric complications of cancer. *Supportive Care in Cancer 3*(1), 45–60.

Breitbart, W., and Holland, J. C. (1988). Psychiatric complications of cancer. *Current Therapy in Hematology-Oncology, 3,* 268–274.

Breitbart, W., and Passik, S. D. (1993). Psychiatric aspects of palliative care. In D. Doyle, G. W. Hanks, and N. MacDonald (Eds.), *Oxford textbook of palliative medicine* (pp. 609–626). New York: Oxford University Press.

Freemon, F. R. (1972). *Sleep research: A critical review.* Springfield, IL: Charles C Thomas.

Goldberg, L., and Elliot, D. (1994). *Exercise for prevention and treatment of illness* (pp. 310–315).

Holland, J. C., and Rowland, J. H., (Eds.) (1989). *Handbook of Psycho-oncology: Psychological care of the patient with cancer* (pp. 470–491). New York: Oxford University Press.

Kazak, A. E., Stuber, M. L., Barakat, L. P., et al (1996). Assessing posttraumatic stress related to medical illness and treatment: The Impact of Traumatic Stressors Interview Scale (ITSIS). *Families, Systems, and Health, 14,* 365–378.

Kryger, M. H., Roth, T., and Dement, W. C. (1989). *Principles and practice of sleep medicine.* Philadelphia: W. B. Saunders.

Randall, G. R., and Lutz, Ellen L. (1991). *Serving survivors of torture.* Washington, D.C.: American Association for the Advancement of Science (AAAS). [For a copy of this book, send a check for $22.00 (includes $4.00 shipping and handling) to American Association for the Advancement of Science Books, P.O. Box 753, Waldorf, MD 20604. For further contact with the AAAS and to request a list of related books, call 202-326-6790.

Razavi, D., and Stiefel, F. (1994). Common psychiatric disorders in cancer patients: I. Adjustment disorders and depressive disorders. *Supportive Care in Cancer, 2*(4), 223–232.

SpectraPlanner. Goldstein, J. and Goldfield, K. North Andover, MA 01845. Tel. 978-682-1579. Web address: <http://www.andovercounseling.com>.

Winningham, M. L. (1994). Exercise and cancer. In L. Goldberg and D. Elliot (Eds.), Exercise for prevention and treatment of illness (pp. 301–315). Philadelphia: F. A. Davis.

Karen Rabus, 55-year-old
Carmel, Indiana breast cancer survivor

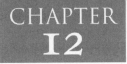

Clinical Issues in Allergy and Immunology

Renata J. M. Engler
Maryl L. Winningham

Why don't health care professionals understand about cancer fatigue? Members of a support group responded:
"You don't ask the right questions."
"They ask questions in front of your relatives so you don't feel free to talk."
"They put words in your mouth."
"It's kinda embarrassing to talk about, especially in front of other people."
"You wouldn't understand."
"I don't know any words that describe this."
"You've never gone through it yourself or you would understand. Then we wouldn't need words."
"Somehow, I never feel it when I'm in the clinic. I don't remember about it until I get home. Then I crash."
"Because there aren't any lab tests for it. All you seem to understand are lab tests."

Dr. Winningham: Several years ago, you helped me with an ovarian cancer survivor who was experiencing debilitating recurring infections. She was always "dragging," as she put it. She could barely make it to the end of the day. She had completed her therapy with a good prognosis, but was having trouble in her job as a teacher because of the exhaustion the infections wrought. She was referred to me because other clinicians thought an exercise program might help her. This poor woman could barely make it across the parking lot! I would like to start this chapter by presenting her case. I'm going to include some of her comments and observations because they reflect the stressors she encountered in trying to get an appropriate diagnosis and treatment.

A 46-year-old, white, single female teacher, was three months premature at birth and weighed 3 pounds. She stated that after struggling for the first few months her general health had been excellent most of her life. She had had all the usual childhood illnesses and rarely missed more than one or two days of school per year except for an allergic reaction (localized urticaria and edema) to a bee sting at four years old and a tonsillectomy at nine years old. She denied having drug, food, or environmental allergies, as well as any known combination of sensitivities. She denied having any systemic problems. Later in the interview, she remembered having had repeated sinus infections in college that were finally treated with surgery. She stated she entered puberty about the age of 13 or 14 years and has always had a male body fat pattern. Her menstrual cycle was regular and unremarkable (every 21 days).

Five years prior to the onset of cancer, when she was 37 years old, she was diagnosed with endometriosis. A laparoscopy showed a lot of adhesions; the pathology report findings were negative. At 41 years old, she started getting an intense, knife-like pain in her right side without attributable cause. At first, the pain came and went without predictability. With time, the pain became increasingly frequent, becoming so severe she had trouble walking. She said she remembers going down the hall at school, leaning against the wall. She kept a journal, looking for a pattern. Whenever she went back to her family physician, he would write her a prescription for ibuprofen, two 800-mg tablets as needed, and send her on her way. She said she would rock on her hands and knees with pain. Once more she saw the family physician. This time when he palpated her lower abdomen, something burst. The patient finally called a gynecologist and read the report to him over the phone on a Friday night. She had just been released from the hospital. He told her to come in at 6 AM the next day—he seemed to know what it was. The oncologist was with him.

Surgery revealed a large, right ovarian malignancy pressing against a nerve. She received postsurgical chemotherapy consisting of vincristine, actinomycin D, and cyclophosphamide, six rounds at one-month intervals. (She observed, "You go in, sit in a chair, and hear all the side effects—they go on for about an hour. When you leave, you don't

About the Contributor

Renata J. M. Engler, a colonel in the U.S. Army, is a person of remarkable compassion and insight into the everyday struggles of her patients. Her background includes a bachelor of arts in biology from Stanford University (1971) followed by a medical degree from Georgetown School of Medicine (1975). She is board certified in internal medicine as well as allergy and immunology, with special certification in clinical and laboratory immunology. She is the founder and director of the adult and pediatric immunodeficiency clinic at Walter Reed Army Medical Center (1984 to the present) and has been both a provider and an advocate for the special needs of patients with chronic fatigue syndrome.

As a clinician, educator (currently running a fellowship training program in allergy-immunology), and lecturer, she is highly regarded among her colleagues, both locally and nationally. She has served on the Board of Allergy and Immunology and has been an active member of the Clinical and Laboratory Immunology Committee of the American Academy of Allergy, Asthma, and Immunology. She participated in the formulation of the published "Practice Parameters for the Diagnosis and Management of Immunodeficiency" (1996).

Her personal, frequently agonizing experience taking care of her parents for over 20 years has given her rare insight into the perspective of both the patient/consumer and the caregiver/health care provider.

remember a thing because you're so exhausted.") Six months after the completion of chemotherapy, she started having severe abdominal and back pain. She first went to see her family practice physician, who told her she had the flu. She received no treatment. Finally, one night, the pain was so severe she went to the emergency department. She was admitted for treatment of dehydration and for intravenous antibiotics for a significant kidney and bladder infection. These infections persisted on and off for about a year. She also had a flare-up of her sinus infections, three separate episodes, treated with intravenous antibiotics. She also had a lot of pulmonary infections after her cancer, with a persistent and chronic cough. Because of her exposure to children at the school where she taught, she easily acquired multiple infections.

She started becoming resistant to each of the antibiotics she was given. She stated she was becoming very run down and discouraged from the recurrent infections. Her family physician reminded her of how lucky she was to have survived cancer. (She said she wanted to hit him, but she was too fatigued.)

Because the chemotherapy had altered her sense of taste, her diet was poor. For instance, she stated water tasted "furry," so she avoided it. Mint flavors burned her mouth (toothpaste was a problem). Many fruits and vegetables, particularly those with a strong citrus taste, were offensive to her. She became extremely exhausted and discouraged. That's when I first saw her. Rather than sit in the office, I interviewed her as we slowly walked in a park. This enabled me to observe her cardiorespiratory response to exertion. She had an extremely poor tolerance to activity as evidenced by shortness of breath and a high pulse even after brief, low-intensity exertion. I felt that getting the chronic infections cleared up constituted a higher priority than starting an exercise program. That's when I turned to you.

These responsibilities have taught her the most about everyday life from the patient's perspective, and have contributed to her unique empathy and ability to advocate for the complex, chronically ill patient.

Over the years, she has seen many chronic fatigue syndrome patients including those with a history of cancer and other chronic illnesses. When I first talked with Renata, she stated: "I get many of my patients referred by psychiatrists." When asked for an explanation, she responded, "Other physicians refer them to psychiatrists because their symptoms appear to reflect a psychiatric disorder. The psychiatric evaluation suggests appropriate reactive depression related to the physical symptom complex, not endogenous depression. Medication may help some of the associated sleep problems; however, it does not relieve the clinical symptoms or functional deficits associated with the fatigue syndrome. The psychiatrists send them to our service saying, 'This guy doesn't have just a psychiatric problem, there must be something organic.' "

Renata is also interested in research relating to alternative medicines that may boost patients' feelings of energy and well-being. This interview focuses on select issues in allergy and immunology as they relate to cancer patients' fatigue.

When you and I first discussed this case, we identified several different issues that may have implications for clinical immunology, allergy, and the cancer-related fatigue syndrome (CRFS). I would like to review a number of these issues and then conclude by reviewing this patient's case and discussing the specific issues that influenced her health.

Dr. Engler, this book will be read by individuals from very diverse backgrounds. Some readers will be health care professionals with a highly sophisticated understanding of the immune system. Sometimes they may have difficulty understanding how their discipline relates to cancer patients' everyday living, or communicating their knowledge in a way that nonprofessionals can understand. Others may not know much about the immune system or how it is generally related to the CRFS. Can you use everyday English to explain the fundamentals of how the immune system works?

Dr. Engler: As you know, I am a U.S. Army physician, so I'd like to explain this in military terms: The immune system is actually a network of cells, like soldiers in an army. The army has individuals trained in a lot of different roles. The soldiers include the infantry of neutrophils and the "special forces" of lymphocytes. Lymphocytes consist of B cells, T cells, and natural killer cells (NKCs). This army is designed to police every nook and cranny of your body for possible threats or foreign invasion. These cells localize in specialized tissues like the thymus gland (the higher-education center for T cells) and lymph nodes (like police stations or holding cells where the "bad guys" are processed). If the threat is big enough, a larger attack is mounted. Sometimes, however, the body is not able to sufficiently defend itself from an attack.

The defenses of the body against infection or injury (including a healthy skin barrier and healthy mucosa in the mouth, nose, lungs, and gut) go beyond the immune system. They consist of the sum of all the components working together in harmony or balance to result in good health. Immunology is ultimately the first and, in my view, the premier holistic medical science. The immunologist must be aware of all the factors that can interrupt the balance and how this imbalance contributes to a clinical problem. It is the clinical manifestation of this imbalance that is viewed as some kind of illness.

An external insult, such as a long-term, ongoing infection, can chronically activate or anger the immune system. The body is adversely affected by the overactive immune response. Interestingly, immunology is viewed as high-tech medicine, but the earliest medical history bears witness to the awareness of fundamental truths about the body's defenses as the key elements for wellness.

Dr. Winningham: What can we do to keep our immune system as healthy as possible?

Dr. Engler: In our day of sophisticated medicine, we need to remember unsophisticated but common-sense living. A healthy life includes eating right, getting the right amount of sleep, thinking good thoughts, and getting a reasonable amount of exercise. Each of these things, when missing from our lives, adversely affects the immune defenses. The golden middle way (sometimes called the *golden mean*) is essential to optimizing wellness; it means nothing to excess, a balanced lifestyle, and positive mental outlook.

Dr. Winningham: That sounds a lot like what Henry Olders said in the chapter preceding this one. We spend so much on health care "fixes" and expensive "cures" but the simple things are often neglected, aren't they?

Dr. Engler: Isn't that remarkable? Many intelligent folks have forgotten these truths or distained them with scornful sophistication. Exposure to tobacco smoke chronically damages the mucosal defenses; it fills the blood with carbon monoxide, thereby chronically depriving tissues of optimum oxygenation. It destroys the vacuum cleaner system of the airways and suppresses the fight of some of the immune cells. Is it any surprise that its use leads to an increased risk of infections and cancer or that its chronic use may lead to fatigue? Many of my patients are initially angry when I suggest that tobacco use and excess alcohol can cause fatigue and decreased quality of life! Some who have been most upset with my suggestions have steamed off, cooled down, and then followed through with the advice. Later, they come back to thank me for challenging them to confront the truth.

Dr. Winningham: We hear a lot today about food supplements or natural treatments versus traditional medicines. It always amazes me when people decry traditional medicine as "stuffing a lot of chemicals in your body." They don't seem to realize that water is a chemical, vitamin C is a chemical, herbal remedies are chemicals, and even a tomato is made up of many chemicals. In earlier conversations, you told me you were open to researching and incorporating select alternative treatments into the practice of traditional medicine. I know you have been interested in research on alternative treatments that may promote immune functioning. Can you share some thoughts on this matter?

Dr. Engler: First, let me explain my biggest worry: I am *very* concerned about safety issues. You know the old maxim in medicine, "First do the patient no harm." Traditional medicines are subjected to close scrutiny for safety, proper use, and efficacy, at the cost of millions of dollars. On the other hand, our supermarkets, health food stores, and over-the-counter pharmacy shelves are full of food supplements or alternative or complementary medicines. Did you know that those products have had no testing at all? Some are mislabeled, some have unlabeled and even dangerous impurities, and many have no proven efficacy. In spite of this, the public is rushing to buy them and self-experiment, totally unaware that this entails risk (in some cases), as well as some potential benefit. Some of them also interfere with treatment for cancer such as chemotherapy.

I think people would be surprised to learn that many of these agents have a *negative* effect on the immune system. Some are even toxic! It worries me. Why are folks willing to blindly try some untested "snake oil," but are unwilling to get a flu shot that has been demonstrated to boost the immune system and prevent illness or even death? We need to be open to nontraditional methods, but they must be tested to ensure public safety. I would like to see more clinical trials in the United States that investigate alternative medications, some of which have a good track record in Asia and Europe.

Now, if you'll let me digress a little, I'm *really* going to get on my bandwagon: Are we all careful enough about what may be impairing our health? Are we proactive enough about using the tools and aids that can safely enhance our health? In the quest for the Madison Avenue image of adolescent feminine beauty, women diet to the point of neglecting their nutrition. As a result, the richest country in the world has a lot of self-imposed *malnutrition!* It's self-imposed starvation in the name of beauty. Sadly, it is not just a problem in developing countries, as we may think. What is the most common cause of immunodeficiency in the world? Malnutrition! But there are other types of malnutrition in our society: Love, harmony, friendship, positive family relationships, beauty, soothing music, laughter, and so many other attributes of spiritual wholeness feed the soul as well as the body. These also nurture the immune system, but we rarely think of these as immunological nutrients.

Dr. Winningham: It's funny, but if you weren't so well regarded in the field of immunology, readers might think they were listening to a crackpot! Love, harmony, friendship, etc, are usually not mentioned as part of the health care system. I think it is this very lack of regard for the important things in life that has driven people to look for answers in alternative treatments.

You've made a very important point. We get up in the morning to an alarm clock, groggy because we've had too little sleep. We take a handful of expensive supplements with a cup of coffee for breakfast (we're trying to lose weight). We have a knock-down, drag-out fight with our spouse or yell at the children. After that, we get in a car and sit in traffic, inhaling carbon monoxide and high levels of particulate matter. We become angry at other drivers. By the time we reach work, we're ready to kill another driver who beats us into a parking place we've spotted. . . . And that's just the beginning of the day!

I'd like to remind you of an article you showed me several years ago. It was entitled "Occasional Notes: Healing by Design" (Horsburgh, 1995) and talked about the emotional and physiological stressors imposed by the confused design and conditions in many of our hospitals and clinics. There are several great quotes that go a long way toward linking the stress and the exhaustion that result from having to deal with health care environments and buildings. The author spoke of "the thoughtless juxtaposition of new and old buildings" as being "notoriously Labyrinthine." He then continued by describing "the riot of signs and profusion of colored lines on the walls and floors of many hospitals" that "give testimony to the difficulty patients have in finding their way." He discussed such architectural concepts as *orientation, connection, scale,* and *symbolic meaning.* He quoted Frank Lloyd Wright, the visionary architect, as saying, "Hospital patients should never be imbued with the idea that they are sick. . . . Health should be constantly before their eyes" (Cunningham, 1948). He said that in 1948, over 50 years ago!

Dr. Engler: Wasn't that article remarkable? We could learn so much by looking to the past.

Dr. Winningham: I think it's important to examine the effect of cancer as the *experience* versus cancer as the *disease*. Let's go back to the effects of all this added to the disease and its treatment as people experience cancer. How would you apply this to the CRFS?

Dr. Engler: With cancer, as with any chronic illness, there are many ways in which the immune system is compromised. First, a lot of medication is required and it may cause impaired nutrient absorption or functioning. The illness and treatment(s) often interfere with proper eating as well as appetite. For instance, in a hospital, we may have people taking nothing by mouth for certain procedures. We see it as standard operating procedure and routine. The body sees it as starvation and reacts accordingly. Disease and treatment also interfere with normal activity, thus robbing us of many of the experiences that make us happy or give us a sense of self-worth. Being a patient is a humiliating experience that deprives us of dignity and autonomy. There is the fear, the anxiety, the uncertainty.

Cancer directly assaults every front of our immune wellness. First, the cancer itself may severely hamper the immune system's key functions and that is why so many patients with cancer suffer severe, potentially life-threatening infections. The cancer itself, in conjunction with the immune response, may produce hormone-like chemicals called *cytokines* that suppress appetite or cause profound feelings of malaise or fatigue.

> *Hospital patients should never be imbued with the idea that they are sick. . . . Health should be constantly before their eyes.*
>
> Frank Lloyd Wright, 1948

The battle for adequate nutrition is monumental for the person with cancer. Having been the principal caregiver in my late father's battle with multiple myeloma, I lived with an intimate awareness of the daily struggle to eat enough and drink sufficient fluids. I think there were more than a few moments when my father hated my nagging him about eating and drinking, but I was a relentless coach. Toward his last days, however, I understood and respected his decision, "enough is enough." For those of us who love the patient, we experience a daily struggle with doing the right thing versus the compassionate perspective of "enough is enough."

Malnutrition is common, both during the peak cancer treatment and afterward because of some of the problems described earlier in the case study. Hydration is also a constant struggle. I cannot emphasize enough that people, like flowers, need water to bloom. People have the misconception that coffee or caffeinated soft drinks count as liquids when in fact, they dehydrate through their diuretic actions. Chicken, whole-grain rice, vegetable broths, herbal teas, and juice are some of the tools to get the hydration job done, but don't forget the elixir of life—water. Water, juice, broth—preferably liquids containing electrolytes such as sodium and magnesium—are essential in the diet since their absence can cause feelings of fatigue, profound weakness, or muscle cramps. If all this sounds like a full time job, it is. Being a patient is hard work. Being a caregiver is the hardest work I have ever had to do . . . and my physician training years were considered quite hard (100-120 hours of work per week). In her wonderful book, *Helping Yourself Help Others,* Rosalyn Carter (1994) pointed out the desperate need to build loving networks of support to facilitate one another's wellness.

Dr. Winningham: Thank you. . . . I would like to change the subject again, if I could. People commonly confuse definitions of fatigue. For instance, chronic fatigue syndrome is quite different from cancer fatigue. In Chapter 1 of this book, I proposed that we call the cancer type of long-term fatigue the cancer-related fatigue syndrome, to clearly differentiate it and to demonstrate that it is really a mixture of phenomena. This has also been proposed by others (William Breitbart, MD, personal conversation, 1999). Wendy Harpham (1995), who wrote the introduction to this book, coined the term *postcancer fatigue* (PCF). Depending on the reference and disciplinary perspective, various definitions are posited and then categorized in terms of physiological versus psychosocial, and normal physiological versus pathological, and according to specific causes. I would like to clarify some of these definitions for our readers.[1]

Fatigue is commonly classified in terms of duration. Sometimes I've seen acute fatigue described in terms of months ($<$ 3 months or 6 months). Chronic fatigue is described as lasting longer. Now that's a little silly. Does that mean that you don't have chronic fatigue if your fatigue is cyclic or periodic for years but lasts several weeks each time? It seems more practical to express acute and chronic fatigue in terms of recovery. That's how the early medical physiologists like Walter Cannon approached it. You recover from acute fatigue through normal mechanisms like sleep and replenishment of food and fluids, through restoring the environmental milieu. With chronic fatigue, the individual never feels replenished or rested. Chapters 2, 6, 10, 16, and 18 in this book discuss some of the various mechanisms of normal physiological fatigue such as activity/inactivity, the sources of energy, appropriate amount and timing of sleep, and neuromusculochemical deficit. Smeeding (see Chapter 6) reviews the history of fatigue research, which alternated between biological and psychological mechanisms depending on the social demands that supported the science (i.e., war, industrial demands, space programs).

The term *chronic fatigue syndrome* (CFS) is defined by the U.S. Centers for Disease Control and Prevention (CDC) according to criteria established by a committee of experts in 1988, and revised in 1993 (Fukuda et al, 1994; Komaroff, 1997). Other names formerly used or confused with CFS have included chronic Epstein-Barr virus disease, chronic fatigue immune dysfunction syndrome, epidemic neuromyasthenia, and myalgic encephalomyelitis.

In contrast to conditions that are defined by a specific pathological problem or organism, CFS is defined by what it is *not*. Results of screening tests for common exclusionary conditions (like some of those just mentioned) are negative. The testing process usually begins when the patient visits the health care provider with a complaint of severe and debilitating fatigue. A complete history and physical examination including assessment of vital signs (pulse and respiratory rate, temperature, and blood pressure), complete blood cell count (erythrocytes, macrophages, neutrophils, basophils, eosinophils, B lymphocytes, T lymphocytes), and erythrocyte sedimentation rate should be performed. Other blood tests include measurement of alanine aminotransferase, plasma total protein, albumin, globulin, alkaline phosphatase (ALK), calcium, phosphorus, glucose, blood urea nitrogen (BUN), electrolytes, creatinine, and thyroid-stimulating hormone (TSH); assessment for malabsorption conditions and malnutrition; and urinalysis. Indeed, the CDC report that set the most recent standards stated that more than 90% of patients presenting with severe fatigue will have normal values for these laboratory tests. Tests for Epstein-Barr virus, enterovirus infections (poliomyelitis, aseptic meningitis, encephalitis), retroviruses, and *Candida albicans* have not been helpful. Studies on NKCs and various cytokines (interleukin-1, -6) have not shown a consistent difference between CFS and control groups. Finally, no cell marker assay (T cells) has been identified to serve as a diagnostic tool for CFS. That doesn't mean there is no physiological marker; it merely means we haven't discovered it yet.

If initial test results suggest an alternative explanation for the fatigue, additional laboratory testing may be required to confirm the diagnosis. Based on the CDC criteria, it is obvious that if cancer exists, the diagnosis of CFS becomes a moot point. Normally, if no cancer or any other specific cause for chronic fatigue is identified here, the additional criteria that must be met include the following:

1. Unexplained fatigue is not associated with ongoing exertion, is not relieved by rest, and results in a substantial reduction in previous activity. There is no indication that "sedentary" individuals are more prone to get CFS.
2. A mental status exam shows no psychiatric abnormalities.
3. Four or more of the following symptoms must be concurrently present for six months or longer:

   - impaired memory or concentration
   - sore throat
   - tender cervical or axillary lymph nodes
   - muscle pain
   - multijoint pain
   - new headaches
   - unrefreshing sleep
   - postexertional malaise

The fatigue cancer patient's experience is not, *by definition, chronic fatigue syndrome, although the lived experiences may be very similar.*

If a patient's fatigue is not severe enough, or if the symptom criteria for CFS are not met, he or she is classified as having idiopathic chronic fatigue.

There are all kinds of remedies being hawked to desperate individuals as a cure for CFS. It is important to be aware that CFS is a distinct diagnosis and seems to bear no pathological similarity to the CRFS. Although there is not complete agreement among

CFS experts, the CFS Web site by the CDC (see Resources list at end of chapter) with the consensus report has a great deal of information that could serve as a model for us as we begin to seriously categorize and study the CRFS.

As mentioned earlier, Wendy Harpham (1995), internist and cancer survivor, wrote about PCF in her book *After Cancer*. She also proposed, similarly to CFS, that the diagnosis of PCF be made only after all other causes are ruled out. She is quite concerned about the late effects of cancer that could contribute to persistent, postcancer fatigability. In their chapter in Norris's *Concept Clarification in Nursing*, Hart and Freel[1] (1982) did a nice job of pulling together a historical overview, abbreviating the various definitional approaches, and identifying clinical implications.

You and I talked about blood transfusions and anaphylaxis or other autoimmune responses. I remember when I first worked in hospitals, I was shocked by how cavalier blood transfusions were treated. I was studying physiology in graduate school and working nights as a nursing assistant. I couldn't figure out why patients had to always have prophy-

Swiss Cheese Memory—Part Two

After 8 months of surgery, complications, and more surgery, I thought I should be getting back on my feet. The cancer-related activities such as dressing changes, treatments, and struggles just to function as a normal human being seemed to be over. But they weren't. I was trying to be normal, but I noticed that things were sliding. Little tasks and little chores that would normally have been taken care of in about 15 minutes at some point during the day were not getting the 15 minutes they needed: They were getting pushed back because the big things were taking more time and energy.

Being a believer in action and organization, I decided I needed to "get organized." I just must not be paying attention—I must have gotten lazy over the past months. So I started each morning by writing a list for myself of the things I needed to do that day. Ah, the glorious list, my saviour. If I would only make a list, everything could get done! Make a list. So I made lists . . . very good lists.

For a while, I believed the new, "organized" approach would let me get back on top of things. But it didn't work. I couldn't figure out why. As fatigue increased, I began routinely to come to the ends of days with things still on the list. I was puzzled. For a while I clung to the belief that this was just a short-term thing. Of course, I would adjust. Hadn't I always been able to conquer things by willpower? But something was wrong: As weeks passed, the number of things left on the list at the end of the day kept growing. I pushed myself. . . . And then I really pushed myself. And I still couldn't get it all done.

The lists started to evolve. They began to get shorter. I was prioritizing. I was eliminating the "nonessentials." I had bills to pay, so work got first commitment of my energy. Social contacts and time for friends were among the first things to get dropped. Somehow they didn't seem so important, so motivating. Not only was I too busy, but also I was too exhausted. Social activities took a lot of energy. Finally, time with my family started being eliminated as I worked into the evenings struggling to complete what I

lactic diphenhydramine (Benedryl) to prevent allergic reactions–especially in view of the chance of life-threatening anaphylaxis–and acetaminophen (Tylenol) to treat febrile reactions, before receiving transfusions if they were so safe. Studies have demonstrated how immunologically threatening transfusions are to the human body. Unnecessary transfusions contribute to the risk of increased hospitalization, increased costs, impaired immunological response, and even cancer recurrence (Blumberg, 1997; Heiss et al, 1994; Suzuki, 1998). Nutritional and growth factors should be considered as alternatives whenever possible. Blood transfusions and related treatments such as packed red blood cells should only be used as a last resort. When is it ever safe to place tissue from one body into another? Only during the miracle of pregnancy is one body in another not a threat to health. This is another example of the need for a commonsense approach to medicine. After all, cancer patients are often immunocompromised as it is.

There are an increasing number of biological agents being developed and marketed to treat cancer. These agents can extend life in patients who even five years ago had no hope.

---

couldn't finish in the daytime. Should I have quit my job and spent my energy on the things that "really mattered?" That is an option only available to the rich.

The fatigue got worse. I was going to bed at 9:30 PM so tired I could hardly crawl. When I got up at 7:30 AM, I hardly had enough energy to shower, dress, and feed myself. By a year later, I was taking 2-hour naps in the early afternoon. Fifteen months later, I was taking two 2- to 3-hour naps a day. I was angry with myself. I became angry with everybody else. The lists kept getting shorter and I still couldn't get it all done. I was depressed. I felt like I was letting down the people who depended on me, who trusted me. I felt I was failing my friends, I was failing my family, I was failing myself.

One night about 8:30 PM, I was sitting at the desk in my study. I was looking at the list of 14 tasks, major and minor, and it still had 8 things on it. Three of those were left over from the day before, one from the day before that. There was nothing I could do about the things on that list. I was having trouble reading the list. I was so exhausted that my hand shook from the effort of holding up the paper.

There were tears running down my face and I couldn't stop them. The anger and depression turned to grief and despair. All the drives and desires I had always possessed were still there, but the capacity to fulfill them was gone. Things were not going to get better; they were going to get worse. The routine of two years before, school and work in the daytime and fun and games with my friends and family at night, was gone forever. I have never been able to find words to express the depth of loss that I felt that night. Technically speaking I was still alive, but I was dying in parts and pieces and the loss of those pieces was breaking my heart.

Cancer survivor

In some cases, they even seem to result in cure. However, the side effects of these treatments are difficult for patients to endure. To describe a flu-like syndrome is putting it mildly. I am especially seeing an increasing number of long-term, negative treatment effects on physical functioning and cognition in cancer patients. Even treatments that have been used for years are being found to have enduring, impairing effects. I think that makes an even greater case for the wisdom you talked about, especially during recovery, so patients can be returned to as full a life as possible.

You were on the committee that prepared the paper titled, "Practice Parameters for the Diagnosis and Management of Immunodeficiency" published in the *Annals of Allergy, Asthma, and Immunology* (AAAI) (Shearer et al, 1996). We would like to encourage clinicians who deal with cancer patients to get a copy of this resource. Ideally, according to the AAAI practice parameters, patients who exhibit immunological deficits should be referred to an immunologist for testing. But in this day of managed care, that may not happen. Regardless of the environment, there are certain triggers that should signal referral. What would you like to share with oncologists, nurses, and primary care practitioners?

Dr. Engler: It's important to understand that independent of the treatment, the general effects of the chronic illness and the accompanying nutritional compromise contribute to immunosuppression. Add onto this the malignancy and exposure to the customary multiple immunosuppressive therapies such as radiation or chemotherapy, and it is not surprising that cancer patients may develop a clinically significant secondary or acquired immunodeficiency. This may manifest as increased frequency of infections such as sinusitis and bronchitis or fungal infections.

Some patients, particularly those with malignancies involving the lymphoid cell lines, actually develop an inability to make antibodies to certain infections such as pneumococcal pneumonia. Like the patients with a congenital inability to make specific antibody to certain antigens (whether vaccine antigens or live infectious organisms), patients with secondary hypogammaglobulinemia (low antibody levels) may benefit from immunoglobulin replacement therapy or antibiotic prophylaxis or both. Obviously, it is important that the antibiotic prophylaxis be known to be effective against the specific troublesome organism(s).

In some cases, the problem may reverse with time and recovery, but some patients have a permanent defect that waxes and wanes in severity. Measuring blood antibody levels alone may not detect the defect; rather, *a more specific evaluation is required to determine antigen-specific functional deficiency.* A significant cellular immunodeficiency, such as is seen in patients with the acquired immunodeficiency syndrome (AIDS), may also be associated with cancer and its therapies. A panel of delayed-type hypersensitivity skin tests (like the tuberculin PPD skin test) using common recall antigens such as tetanus, mumps, and *Candida* can define T-cell or cellular immunity. Be certain the patient has not been receiving high-dose corticosteroids at the time of this testing. Finally, acute illnesses and immunosuppressive drugs can make this test temporarily abnormal.

Dr. Winningham: We need to be responsible about health care costs, but we need to balance that with quality health care. Unnecessary referrals to specialists (and the requisite diagnostic procedures required by specialists) are stressful on both the economic system and the patient. What would you say should be an indication for appropriate referral to a specialist?

Dr. Engler: According to recommended guidelines in the AAAI 1996 article, the following situations should trigger referral:

1. All patients with recurrent infections should be considered for referral to an allergist or immunologist for evaluation of immunodeficiency.
2. Because immune defects are a form of chronic disease, communication on a continuing basis between the referring physician and the allergist or immunologist is essential.
3. In certain circumstances, the allergist or immunologist and the primary care or oncology practitioner will need to consult specialists in infectious diseases, ear-nose-throat, metabolism, hematology/oncology, pulmonology, gastroenterology, surgery, and other fields.

When patients present with chronic or repeated infections, measuring blood antibody levels alone may not detect the defect; rather, a more specific evaluation is required to determine antigen-specific functional deficiency.

Dr. Winningham: How would you treat antigen-specific functional deficiency?

Dr. Engler: If making the diagnosis is difficult, treatment is even more so! Of course, optimal nutrition is important. Even treatments such as gamma globulin can be prohibitively expensive! There may be some gentle immune adjuvants available among the herbal therapies such as *Eleutherococcus senticosus maxim* (Siberian ginseng) that can ameliorate the problem, but it remains a complex challenge for the oncologist and immunologist. Unfortunately, over-the-counter sources of some of these herbal products carry no guarantee of safety or purity. Further research needs to be done to evaluate the potential benefits of some of the agents that make claims to improve the problem but may, in fact, only deplete the wallet! As I mentioned before, one of the biggest problems is finding pure sources of these drugs because the vitamin-supplement industry does not have to comply with standards that traditional medications require. This is an area where a lot of research is needed.

All of these compromises to the immune system are associated with fatigue symptoms. Recurrent infection or flu-like illnesses frequently impact most on quality of life because of the drain in energy that results. Also, it is frequently forgotten from the old surgical literature that tissue injury and healing require a great deal of energy and high protein intake and are associated with an increased need for appropriate restful healing time. A cancer being killed by therapy and the body's need to repair after the treatment is completed are every bit as big an insult as major surgery! The demand for patience and self-tolerance during the healing period is really the hardest part of enduring the course of any illness. We expect instant cures and are disappointed when medicine doesn't work that way. It's amazing that we've forgotten much of the research done and wisdom learned already years ago!

Dr. Winningham: That's interesting. People have come to me and said, "Gee, I finished with treatment, the cancer seems to be gone, but I feel rotten. I don't have any energy." Even before asking about their nutritional, sleep, and exercise patterns, I ask, "How long has it been since you finished your treatment?" Not infrequently I get answers like, "two weeks ago," "two months ago," and the like. I tell people, the first six months is just for your body to get over the initial shock. Give yourself as long as two years for long-term recovery and healing. In the meanwhile, let's examine the nutrition, sleep, and activity patterns. The biggest sin besides doing nothing, physically, is overdoing it. I think it sets people up for recurrences, especially when they engage in chronic, high-intensity exercise. High-tech medicine doesn't substitute for wisdom and patience in healing, does it?

Dr. Engler: No . . . Yet, the positive way in which the patient approaches this challenge also has an impact on the progress and the healing forces from the immune system. How often do we see patients with the same severity of disease, the same quality of laboratory abnormalities, yet very different functionality and healing dynamics? Although the medical establishment makes patients feel passive in their health care, the wise healer knows that empowering the patient as a full partner in the journey toward healing is a powerful therapeutic strategy in itself!

Dr. Winningham: You once told me about a common problem you encounter in people who are referred to you with chronic fatigue problems. Can you repeat what that is?

Dr. Engler: One of the biggest obstacles to solving a long-term fatigue problem is the lack of organized medical records. People who come to me have usually seen a number of other specialists. Their records are scattered all over the place. They can't even tell me what test they had, where, when, and what the results were.

For cancer survivors, in particular, start assembling your medical records. You need the following:

- a standard medical and health history that is up-to-date
- the name of the hospital/physician/clinic where you had various procedures done
- address, telephone, and fax numbers for that place
- list of procedures done, when, where, and the results
- information on treatments received (like antibiotics, for example) and the response
- a complete list of all medications taken in the past including herbal and over-the-counter remedies, and the response to each
- information on allergies and exposures to pollution or wastes
- list of other health problems besides infections

Keep this information in chronological order. Update it every time something relevant happens. Putting it on a computer is nice because you can go back later and fill in things you forgot.

Dr. Winningham: And now about the outcome with the patient described at the beginning:

> Immunological testing confirmed a gamma globulin deficiency, as you suggested. It was obviously clear from her food aversions that she also had nutritional deficiencies. Vitamin B_{12} is so critical to the immune system; in addition, some chemotherapeutic agents rob the body of B_{12} as a tumor-arresting mechanism. B_{12} is found in red meat, but she had an aversion to the taste of red meat, of protein. Her avoidance of certain fruits and vegetables guaranteed a vitamin C deficiency. I'm sorry she had not received a nutritional consult much sooner. She received gamma globulin for several months.
>
> It has been several years now, and only in the past year has she stated that she has been feeling better. She says she only gets "the crud" (as the teachers call it) when there is something special going around with the children. She told me that just last week she was able to drink her first full glass of water since her chemotherapy. There also has been some neurological improvement in her taste buds. In terms of her cancer, she is doing well with no sign of recurrence.

Endnote

1. Scholars, researchers, and students of clinical fatigue are urged to read the fatigue chapters in C. M. Norris's (1982) book, *Concept Clarification in Nursing*, for good literature reviews and related concept discussion.

References

Blumberg, N. (1997). Allogeneic transfusion and infection: Economic and clinical implications. *Seminars in Hematology, 34*(3 Suppl 2), 34–40.

Carter, R., and Golant, S. K. (1994). *Helping yourself help others: A guide for caregivers.* New York: Random House.

Cunningham, R. M. (1948). Frank Lloyd Wright on hospital design: A *Modern Hospital* interview with the world famous architect. *Modern Hospital, 71,* 4.

Fukuda, K., Straus, S. E., Hickie, I., Sharpe, M. C., Dobbins, J. G., Kamaroff, A. L., and the International Chronic Fatigue Syndrome Study Group (1994). The chronic fatigue syndrome: A comprehensive approach to its definition and study. *Annals of Internal Medicine, 121,* 953–959.

Harpham, W. S. (1995). *After cancer: A guide to your new life* (paperback edition). New York: Harper-Collins.

Hart, L. K., and Freel, M. I. (1982). Fatigue. In C. M. Norris, *Concept clarification in nursing* (pp. 251–261). Rockville, MD: Aspen.

Heiss, M. M., Mempel, W., Delanoff, C., Jauch, K. W., Gabka, C., Mempel, M, Dieterich, H. J., Eissner, H. J., and Schildberg, F. W. (1994). Blood transfusion-modulated tumor recurrence: First results of a randomized study of autologous versus allogenic blood transfusion in colorectal cancer surgery. *Journal of Clinical Oncology, 12,* 1859–1876.

Horsburgh, C. R. (1995). Occasional notes: Healing by design. *New England Journal of Medicine, 333* 735–740.

Komaroff, A. (1997). A 56-year old woman with chronic fatigue syndrome. *Journal of the American Medical Association, 278,* 1179–1185.

Shearer, W. T., Buckley, R. H., Engler, R. J. M., Finn, A. F., Fleisher, T. A., Freeman, T. M., Herrod, H. G., III, Levinson, A. I., Lopez, M., Rich, R. R., Rosenfeld, S. I., and Rosenwasser, L. J. (1996). Practice parameters for the diagnosis and management of immunodeficiency. *Annals of Allergy, Asthma, and Immunology, 76,* 282–294.

Suzuki, I. N. (1998). Blood transfusion and postoperative serum interleukin-6 levels in colorectal cancer patients. *Hepatogasteroenterology, 22,* 1011–1013.

Resources

Norris, C. M. (1982). *Concept clarification in nursing.* Rockville, MD: Aspen.

Self-help and coping techniques used for people suffering from immunological deficits and chronic fatigue syndrome may also help people with cancer who suffer from immune deficiencies and the CRFS. Although all these techniques have not been tested, we can learn from other clinical populations and share ways cancer survivors can experiment with solutions that may work for them. Based on much of what we know about a balanced diet and nutrition, coping with long-term debilitating fatigue, and adopting a healthy lifestyle, well-developed interventions are available from other clinical areas. Here are several resources on chronic fatigue syndrome that may have some effective coping techniques:

The CDC maintains a 24-hour voice information system that provides up-to-date information on CFS: 1-404-332-4455. Web site: <http://www.cdc.gov/ncidod/diseases/cfs/facts.htm>

The American Association for Chronic Fatigue Syndrome, c/o Harborview Medical Center, 325 Ninth Avenue, Box 359780, Seattle, WA 98104. Voice: 206-521-1932. Fax: 206-521-1930. email: debrap@u.washington.edu

Other resources on everyday living with fatigue include Web sites representing members with multiple sclerosis, postpolio syndrome, lupus, arthritis, and similar chronic illnesses.

PART
III

A Global Approach to Rehabilitation

" I just ran out
of _starch_ " — nothing
to hold me up.
Feeling blah and drained
AND guilty because I
expected to be able to
keep up with working
full time.

DROOPY

Diana Dean, 67 years old, breast cancer overcomer, Indianapolis, Indiana

Fatigue and Oncology Rehabilitation: An Historical Perspective

Maryl L. Winningham
Eileen S. Donovan

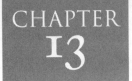

I think people associate pain with dying. . . . But I think fatigue is associated with hopelessness.

Betty R. Ferrell, 1996

Background

To understand the status of rehabilitation and its place in cancer research, it is necessary to follow several seemingly unrelated historical threads through to the end of the twentieth century. A review of the brief history of bureaucratic developments and periodic initiatives in the United States since the late 1920s contributes to an understanding of why rehabilitation with its psychosocial issues, symptom management, and palliation have not been given priority status in cancer research at the national level.

The War Against Cancer

In 1927, a West Virginia Senator offered a $5 million reward to anyone who found a cure for cancer. The implication was obvious: There was an expectation of a magic cure. Although some cancer research was included in the establishment of the National Institutes of Health (NIH) in 1930, the National Cancer Institute (NCI) Act of 1937 made it an established and recognized entity of the Public Health Service (PHS).

Carl Voegtlin was appointed first director of the NCI. He brought with him the NIH Division of Pharmacology staff to help in the organization. The next year, in 1939, a large contingent from the Harvard Office of Cancer Investigations joined them. The focus was to be on basic research–primarily pharmacological research. In fact, indicative of the priority, in 1940, when Washington governmental office buildings became too hot for people to work in, mouse research buildings were the only facilities with air conditioning! Throughout the 1940s and 1950s, Presidents Roosevelt and Truman continued to steadily support the NCI <http://rex.nih.gov>.

In 1970, at the urging of the influential Mary Lasker and her powerful associates, Texas Senator Ralph W. Yarborough, chair of the Senate Labor and Public Welfare Committee, called for an accounting of cancer research in the United States. There was political pressure for an independent budget for a separate, cancer research part of the NIH. In the contested debate, many in medical research believed that if the NCI had an independent budget, it would hinder research exchange between other branches of the NIH. As the battle heated up, the Citizen's Committee for the Conquest of Cancer, guided by Lasker and associates, took out full-page newspaper advertisements and lobbied Congress and President Nixon for an autonomous national cancer program. A supportive plea from columnist Ann Landers resulted in a flood of 300,000 letters to Congress. In the end, the negotiated terms of the act kept the NCI within the NIH, but established a bypass budget that went straight to the President and could not be controlled by political interests in the NIH or Congress.

In the same year, at an annual cancer conference sponsored by University of Texas M.D. Anderson Cancer Hospital and Tumor Institute, Mary E. Switzer, head of the government Social and Rehabilitative Services, was given an award for promoting the inclusion of cancer in rehabilitation, along with cardiac disease and stroke. According to proceedings from this meeting, Switzer quoted Will Mayo's statement in 1925, "Rehabilitation will be the masterword of medicine in the future." She then added, "I think we have a long way to go." At the same meeting, Dr. John Healey (1972, p. 268) declared: "Why is cancer ignored? Because laity, paramedical groups, and physicians alike still regard this disease, cancer, with a defeatist and fatalistic attitude. . . . Even the patient with the Biblical disease, leprosy, (is) given more rehabilitation consideration." He went on to say, "One of our immediate needs is education. All these groups (laity, paramedical groups, and physicians) must be educated . . . with the goal of making them realize that the cancer patient must be regarded in the same manner as any patient with a chronic disease–for cancer is a group of chronic diseases."

As part of his 1971 State of the Union address, President Richard M. Nixon declared the "war against cancer" and requested $100 million for cancer research. In October of that year, a portion of Fort Dietrick, Maryland, was converted into the Frederick Cancer

About the Contributor

Eileen Donovan, physical therapist, has had a long-standing commitment to working with patients with cancer. After graduating with a degree in physical therapy from the University of Texas Medical Branch at Galveston in 1967, Eileen started working at M. D. Anderson Cancer Center. She left for a brief period to work in a nursing home but soon returned "with a whole new attitude." She knew where she belonged. Her mentor was Dr. John E. Healey, one of the first leaders in oncology rehabilitation. She earned her master's degree in 1976 in allied health administration and education. She is no stranger to

Research and Development Center. When Nixon signed the National Cancer Act into law on December 23, 1971, he declared, "I hope in the years ahead we will look back on this action today as the most significant in my administration." <http://rex.nih.gov> At that time, the stated expectations and hopes were for a cure within five years. Thus, from the 1920s through the early 1970s, there was an expectation that the cure for cancer was imminent, with the focus on pharmacological solutions. This reflected twentieth-century expectations that there was a scientific magic pill for everything. This mind-set has continually dominated cancer, supported by spectacular media headlines and announcements. However, since a cure was considered imminent, there was no rationale for making significant investments in rehabilitation research and training.

As we approach the end of the century, several critical historical events and their philosophical implications have dampened this expectation:

1. No quick cure for cancer has been found. Recognition of the complexity of the many kinds of cancer, the complexity of the genetic mechanisms, and the confounding mechanisms of carcinogenesis has been the major contributor to these brakes on the hope for an imminent solution. On the positive side, what has been learned from cancer research has also been applied to the treatment of many other diseases (e.g., arthritis, human immunodeficiency virus [HIV] infection, cardiac disease, genetic mechanisms).

2. Antibiotics, the darlings of twentieth-century health care, are failing in the face of increasingly virulent, adaptive, and resistant microbes. Once again, the expectation of one-for-all solutions seem to be eluding our grasp.

3. The acquired immunodeficiency syndrome (AIDS) continues to devastate the lives of hundreds of thousands around the world. Treatments are expensive and only available to the richer Western countries, while populations in countries with lower mean per capita income are laid to waste. This has been a sobering experience in the health care community.

4. Although remarkable progress has been made with many kinds of cancer that were deadly even a few years ago, it is obvious that hundreds of thousands of individuals will continue to battle cancer, many will continue losing the battle,

cancer: Her father died of a brain tumor when she was 8 years old. She said she wondered whether she started at M. D. Anderson to "fix" him. She herself has had cancer and still has some fatigue that appears to be related to chemotherapy and menopause. Her family history of many different kinds of cancer has taught her much, and has changed the way she relates to her patients. Even on the tough days, she says she keeps coming back to her job with the thought, "Today will be the day I learn something else new and fantastic."

many will live with long-term sequelae to disease and treatment, and many thousands of health care professionals will battle with them through all these processes. This continues to result in untold suffering in four ways:

a. on the part of the patients who have to endure the physical, emotional, and financial costs of disease and treatment;
b. by patients who suffer long-term work discrimination and impairments that affect their work and social lives;
c. by their families who are distressed by their lack of control in helping their loved one; and
d. by health care providers who "burn out" as they confront an inadequate arsenal of interventions, the dehumanizing effect of diminished financial resources, and suffering on the part of those they have committed themselves to help.

5. Treatments for cancer that have resulted in remission and cure have also featured significant side effects and long-term impairment on the part of many survivors. A ground swell in the survivorship movement has demanded more than remission or cure: Survivors are no longer content to hear they should be grateful they are not dying of cancer. There is an increasing demand for attention to symptom management, subsequent functioning, and postcancer quality of life issues regardless of disease outcome. After years of focus on the management of the more obvious and acute phenomena of nausea and pain, physical impairments, the cancer-related fatigue syndrome (CRFS), and postcancer fatigue (PCF) are being identified as related problems that will not go away.

The Development of Therapies

Although the roots of health care professions like nursing, physical therapy, and dietetics go back to ancient times, most of the modern allied therapeutic professions experienced their birth or greatest development in times of war. As technological sophistication and knowledge increased, need for more sophisticated training and education led to the development of the various specialties. Nursing led the way: In the Crimean War (1854–1855), Florence Nightingale demonstrated that hygiene, shelter, and nutrition were essential adjuncts to battlefield surgery in cutting the overwhelming losses of life to postoperative complications. Her measures reduced the battlefield hospital death rate from 45% to 2%. Nightingale was also a leader in the development of public health and mathematical foundations of epidemiology, having taught herself by studying parliamentary health reports. During subsequent European wars, the International Red Cross (founded in 1863) taught fundamental nursing and relief care to leaders from all involved nations, regardless of their nationalistic allegiance.

Modern physical therapy was established in the late 1800s in Great Britain. In the United States, physicians trained female graduates of physical education programs to practice in their offices and hospitals. The great poliomyelitis epidemic that swept the eastern coast of the United States in 1916 and the entry of the United States into World War I led to the establishment of the first physical therapy school at Walter Reed Army Hospital in Washington, D.C. Therapists, called *reconstruction aides*, were needed for follow-up care, particularly prosthesis use, gait, and exercise training for amputees. Between the wars, the polio epidemics of the 1920s and 1930s gave physical therapists new challenges in developing adaptive techniques and solutions. Each subsequent war led to a greater need for the expertise of physical therapy as improvements in triage, medicine, surgery, and rapid evacuation from the front meant more soldiers, as well as civilian victims, survived with more severe impairments. Technological developments in materials resulted in concomitant improvements in assistive devices.

Occupational therapy began as a profession during World War I in response to a need for vocational rehabilitation, independent living, and work training. Vocational education focused on integrating impaired individuals into society as employed citizens. Psychotherapists and psychologists worked on overcoming war-related mental impairments. Psychopharmacological developments focused on stabilizing chemical imbalances to help individuals become more productive. Advancements in these therapies were accompanied by developments in speech, nutrition therapy, and social workers specializing in rehabilitation. With the Vietnam War, a new kind of therapist—the respiratory therapist—emerged. U.S. medics trained as respiratory therapists were soon in demand in multiple settings, as well as in other countries, teaching their art. All of these disciplines and their related technological developments had components that transferred and contributed to some aspect of cancer rehabilitation, but there was no singular focus on cancer.

With the war on cancer, there began to be hope for change. Many of today's developments related to cancer rehabilitation, including symptom management, found their roots in the early 1970s. War on Cancer funds became available for graduate, specialist, oncology-related education of nurses, therapists, physiatrists, and other paramedical professionals. Nursing, especially with the growth and development of the Oncology Nursing Society, made significant contributions to symptom management. The formation of special interest groups in several additional nursing organizations, physical therapy, and other paramedical professions also dates from this time. As each profession has matured, it has been supported by the development of standards for licensing, education, and certification to protect the public welfare.

Strangely, something went wrong. The "jump start" that oncology rehabilitation had in the 1970s stalled. Today, despite the fine work of a few "points of light" in large medical centers around the country, there are few specialized oncology rehabilitation programs in the United States. Most patients who could definitely benefit from some form of rehabilitation do not even know these resources exist and their lives could be made easier. But we are getting ahead of the story.

In the early and mid 1950s, two significant movements that developed could have and should have had a profound impact on rehabilitation oncology; however, for some reason, they did not. These movements were (1) the widespread funding of physiological research in preparation for the U.S. space program and the subsequent discoveries, and (2) the development of sports medicine and cardiovascular (and later pulmonary) rehabilitation programs.

Implications of Aeronautical and Space Research

In preparation for the physiological changes of microgravity, National Aeronautics and Space Administration (NASA) scientists as well as scientists in the Soviet Union used bed rest as a model. Over several decades of research, it became eminently clear that extended bed rest had a malignant influence on all aspects of human life: Every single organ system of the body showed rapid deterioration as a result of bed rest. In addition, potent perceptual and emotional alterations affected the well-being of the young, healthy, athletic individuals who were part of the studies. The experience of bed rest, as well as microgravity, had an overwhelming, multisystem, and long-term effect on functioning, including loss of endurance (fatigability) and strength. A significant focus of this early research, indeed, standard operating procedure in the space program, was in developing exercise programs to counteract some of the physiological entropy that rapidly and inevitably takes place. Studies of astronauts in space have validated the use of bed rest as an earth-bound model for microgravity. NASA-supported research in materials, telemedicine, electronics, and physiology turned out to be one of the greatest "bang-for-the-buck" investments U.S. taxpayers ever had. Little of this has been applied to oncology rehabilitation.

Implications of Cardiac Rehabilitation

The second major movement was the development of cardiovascular rehabilitation. As always, the mixture of politics and people was significant and makes an interesting story. Through the early 1950s, cardiac patients in the United States were often kept in bed; were stuffed with potatoes, meat, and gravy; and suffered fatal heart attacks–from blood clots that formed while the patient spent weeks in bed! In the fourth and fifth decades of the twentieth century, sports medicine was coming into its own, mostly aimed at athletes and the exceptional models of human performance. One of the leading figures in this movement was Ernst Jokl, a physician, athlete, philosopher, historian, and educator who came to the United States in the early 1950s. Jokl was significant in promoting an interest in sports medicine in the United States. He was also a "bridge" between the medical and nonmedical communities. Jokl was astute in his recognition of historical trends and credited Howard

Rusk of New York and Henry Kessler of New Jersey as being critical to the development of rehabilitation medicine (Jokl, 1964).

A pivotal event determined the expansion of rehabilitation medicine from hospital-based, physician-run programs to community-oriented, out-of-hospital programs: The American Heart Association and the American College of Cardiology voted to deny membership to nonphysician exercise leaders and physiologists. From earlier roots in another organization, the interdisciplinary American College of Sports Medicine was founded in 1954 (Berryman, 1995). Later, the American Association of Cardiovascular and Pulmonary Rehabilitation was founded, focusing more specifically on those specific areas of study and practice. Both these organizations focused on practice/clinical as well as research aspects of cardiopulmonary rehabilitation. These were the first formal, non-physician, nontherapist training programs from which many of the present-day exercise physiology programs and degrees developed. Unfortunately, exercise physiology has not developed a separate identity with specific educational standards and licensing; hence, many individuals with minimal training call themselves exercise physiologists. Over the past 45 years, cardiopulmonary rehabilitation has benefited from controlled human research, animal research, and well-developed instruments to measure outcomes. Certification and training programs for leaders–both for prevention and for rehabilitation–have become de rigeur. Remarkably, beyond the work of a few researchers, few of these developments have infiltrated oncology care.

In May 1956, under the sponsorship of the Institute of Physical Medicine and Rehabilitation, New York University–Bellevue Medical Center, leading cardiologists of the day attended a cardiovascular rehabilitation conference. The list of attendees included such renowned figures as Paul Dudley White, Howard A. Rusk, William Morris, Byran Williams, Philip R. Lee, Robert Levy, Howard Sprague, and Herman Hellerstein. A significant part of this meeting was devoted to teaching cardiac rehabilitation; however, the content was physician oriented (White et al, 1957). Two other events gave cardiac rehabilitation a boost about this time: Dwight D. Eisenhower, president of the United States, bounced back from a myocardial infarction and returned to golfing, as witnessed by an aghast press. The statistics began showing cardiac disease as a potentially preventable cause of death, and shortly thereafter, the Young Men's Christian Association (YMCA) undertook a major initiative in having exercise classes as well as rehabilitation sessions in its community centers. Out of this grew a need for trained exercise specialists, exercise physiologists.

It is important to note that the rationale for applying a cardiopulmonary rehabilitation program model to cancer patients is quite logical. At first glance, one could argue that exercise may be good for the heart, but less relevant to people with cancer. However, the greatest benefit of exercise in cardiopulmonary patients is not in the immediate effect on the heart or on the lungs; it is peripheral, promoting efficiency in the working muscle cells, the sites where oxygen is combined with fuel to produce energy. In cardiopulmonary patients, like any other human, exercise helps reduce the overall stress of exertion by improving musculoskeletal efficiency and muscular endurance. These effects, likewise, have important implications for cancer patients.

The greatest benefit of exercise in cardiopulmonary patients is not in the immediate effect on the heart or on the lungs, it is peripheral, promoting efficiency of the working muscle cells, the sites where oxygen is combined with fuel to produce energy. In cardiopulmonary patients, like any other human, exercise helps reduce the overall stress of exertion by improving musculoskeletal efficiency and muscular endurance. These effects, likewise, have important implications for rehabilitation in cancer patients.

Why should a half century of research in the space program and cardiopulmonary rehabilitation not be utilized in oncology rehabilitation? Before we "reinvent the wheel," we need to examine what has already been done that can serve as a model, practically, in terms of research and with respect to the reimbursement system. In cancer fatigue rehabilitation, as in cardiopulmonary rehabilitation, the key concept is energetics. Undertaking a detailed study of the wealth of research in the field of cardiopulmonary rehabilitation should provide a trove of protocols and research designs, as well as potential outcome measures that heretofore have eluded oncology researchers.

The War Against Cancer: The Inclusion of Rehabilitation

In the fall of 1972, at the beginning of the war against cancer, the Department of Health Education and Welfare, NIH, and NCI assembled a group of individuals who were actively working with oncology patients at that time. The purpose of the meeting was to address seven objectives of the National Cancer Program. While rehabilitation for cancer patients was not widely practiced, it was passionately advocated by John E. Healey, Guy Robbins, Herbert Dietz, and others who had been responsible for getting rehabilitation included in the National Cancer Act.

The panel's objectives included the following:

1. restoration and palliation
2. restoration: head and neck
3. physical restoration: breast, extremities, gastrointentinal, and genitourinary involvement
4. psychosocial aspects of the rehabilitation of cancer patients
5. vocational
6. educational
7. prevention, cure, and control

Healey, Robbins, and Dietz particularly lobbied to get rehabilitation included as part of objective 7. The participants' task was to brainstorm together, to develop and prioritize projects related to the panel's focus. The goals for the rehabilitation of persons with cancer were generally identified as a return to optimal physical and social functioning, an objective consistent with the definition of rehabilitation by the World Health Organization. The following are a sample of the identified high-priority projects:

- nutritional rehabilitation of persons with cancer
- multidisciplinary pain clinics
- an oncology nursing program
- improved methods of reconstruction of resected mandibles
- development of laryngeal communication prostheses
- minimization of disturbance of salivary gland function resulting from radiation therapy of head and neck cancer
- development of instructional materials for patients with breast cancer
- immediate postamputation fitting in lower-extremity cancer amputees
- prospective randomized study to define more accurately the etiological factors of lymphedema and to evaluate the methods of lymphedema management
- national and regional clearinghouses for cancer rehabilitation information
- an educational program for professional nurses working in cancer rehabilitation
- cost-effectiveness of vocational rehabilitation for cancer patients compared with people with other disabilities
- training of professional teams in cancer rehabilitation

Many of these goals have never been fully realized; indeed, the need is greater than ever. Many of the professionals who were educated in these programs and who shared in this vision are no longer actively involved in cancer rehabilitation, are nearing retirement age, or are retired. Many of the physicians who were in leadership roles are deceased. There is an urgent need for a long-term policy—not just another initiative—providing for professional training in rehabilitation and rehabilitation team building.

In the few medical centers where rehabilitation is more than a token, the physical medicine and rehabilitation departments have been the mainstay of traditional cancer treatment, with physical therapy, occupational therapy, and speech therapy. Oncology neuropsychologists are rare. Few clinical specialists in nursing currently are experienced in cancer rehabilitation.

Shortsighted and narrow-minded downsizing at many medical centers has particularly contributed to a loss of nursing clinical specialists, social workers, and dietitians at a time when they are most needed. Even worse, their clinical expertise is being lost, affecting the training of future leaders. One of the biggest problems is that oncologists, whether medical, radiation, or surgical, are not aware of the potential for rehabilitation, although it is sometimes reimbursable. In the end, it is individuals, families, and society at large that suffer from this communication gap. We will surely pay for this lack of commitment and foresight.

Another Kind of Rehabilitation: Cancer-Related Fatigue as the Focus

Despite nearly a half century of overwhelming documentation that bed rest is counterproductive to maintenance of health and functioning in humans, activity generally has been discouraged in cancer patients. When patients complained of fatigue, they were usually told to get more rest, a measure guaranteed to promote more fatigue.

The deterioration of cancer patients during their treatment was observed in early research using antineoplastic chemotherapy. In 1949, Karnofsky and Burchenal wrote an important paper describing their use of nitrogen mustard to treat a man who had a tumor. The tumor regressed. It was a pioneering step forward in the chemotherapeutic treatment of cancer. There was only one problem: The man's cancer was improved, but his performance status had declined. Hence, Karnofsky and Burchenal (1949) proposed that one of four treatment-related outcome variables include quantification of performance status. On their performance status scale, a percentage of 100 indicated normal, no restrictions whatsoever; a percentage of 0 meant dead. Later performance scales, (e.g., Zubrod, Eastern Cooperative Oncology Group, South West Oncology Group, World Health Organization) were adaptations of this original proposal. Beyond the continued application of traditional rehabilitation techniques, there is little evidence that thought was given to increasing or maintaining energetic functioning in patients.

> *Every person who is diagnosed with cancer should be considered a candidate for rehabilitation: Cancer-related fatigue and other function-limiting symptoms should be core issues in that rehabilitation. Indeed, in view of aggressive treatments and the aging population, we have no choice if we are to minimize catastrophic costs to individuals, families, and society in general. Our goal must be to keep people functioning independently while maintaining quality of life through effective symptom management.*

What Happened to Cancer Rehabilitation?

Einstein once suggested that asking the right question was as important as finding the right answer. In this case, we are led to four critical questions.

1. *Why is it that cancer-related fatigue and its relationship to decrements in perception of quality of life by patients have only recently been perceived to be a problem?* There was one big, fundamental flaw in assumptions Karnofsky and Burchenal (1949) used in using their proposed scale to evaluate functioning: In evaluating functioning, clinicians—usually physicians—assumed their observation of the patient's behavior, in the hospital or clinical setting, represented a whole and true picture of the patient's functioning. Unfortunately, they were usually deceived by their cursory observations. In fact, their very presence and the artificial clinical environment induced artifact into the "data." This is not unlike the philosophical implication of Heisenberg's uncertainty principle. Functional level was usually overestimated because the

patient was stimulated into an artifical mode of performance by the environment, anxiety, and expectations. Hence, patients were assumed to be doing better than they actually were. The error of this type of assessment of performance and functioning has only been challenged in recent years (see related discussions on arousal, epinephrine, and the reason for false perception of performance ability in Chapter 2).

The phenomenon of "rising to the occasion" involves interesting physiological changes that influence behavior. A few of the following examples can help us understand this to be part of a universal behavioral phenomenon:

- We joke about the story of the old lady carrying her piano out of the burning house.
- Anyone who has an aging Labrador or golden retriever marvels at how quickly a stiff, tired old dog can respond to the sound of the refrigerator door opening or the dog "cookie jar" opening.
- We hear about the "white coat phenomenon" where patients' blood pressures go up when the physician walks in the room.

In each case, there is a near-instantaneous alteration in behavior, a stimulation to alertness and action, that is quite different from what is observed under normal, quiet, and nonstimulating conditions.

In 1859, Florence Nightingale warned us that we should never evaluate how well patients are doing when they are excited or engaged in an animated conversation with us. Rather, she said, we should come back and see how they are doing afterward and see how they spent the night. She said that was the truest measure of functioning. It is after the patients are pronounced "doing well" that they often go home and "crash," requiring as much as two or three days for recovery. What is most remarkable is, because these events and their consequences are delayed, even patients usually do not relate the "performance" with the subsequent fatigue. It is clear we must approach functioning and fatigue from quite a different perspective.

2. *What happened to the initiative in cancer rehabilitation and why didn't it keep pace with developments in cardiopulmonary rehabilitation and sports medicine?* The answer is summed up in two words: defeatism and money. In clarifying the first, Healey's remarks earlier in the chapter were prescient: Our lack of attention to rehabilitation and the phenomena it addresses is one of ignorance and attitude. In clarifying the second, it is essential to compare the development of cancer treatment with parallel economic events. As treatments became more sophisticated and more individuals with cancer survived, or survived longer, we started experiencing catastrophic budget cutting in health care. In the absence of leadership and new ideas in the health care industry, legislators, chief executive officers, and health care insurance administrators began meeting bottom-line mandates by cutting budgets. Their approach usually started by cutting what they thought to be "nonessential"

staff (often adjunctive therapists) and reducing services. Although cardiac rehabilitation has struggled with reimbursement issues, its development and expansion had a head start during a time when more funds were available for research and program development, and there was a smaller population of patients, most of whom were economically secure, middle-class men.

Beyond the jump start cancer rehabilitation experienced in the 1970s, there was not the same impetus to sustain this development. Unfortunately, in view of an aging population and more cancer survivors, we need creativity to address our problems with health care costs. It is urgent that we keep cancer survivors, regardless of the phase of their disease and treatment, independent and functional. Cut-rate budgets and quality of service has proved shortsighted, uncreative, and socially irresponsible.

3. *Why has the relationship between cancer-related fatigue and cancer rehabilitation not been obvious?* Once again, the answer probably is twofold. First, from the medical perspective, fatigue was viewed as an unimportant or bothersome symptom, not to be taken seriously unless, like vomiting, it contributed to a serious physiological problem. The lack of clinical evidence associated with fatigue, such as electrolyte imbalance, in most cases led to its not being taken seriously. Further, until recently, fatigue was not something that appeared to be fixable with medications. The pharmaceutical industry is big business and contributes significant amounts of money to medical centers for research. On the other hand, rehabilitation is not "big money," nor is it considered an exotic and impressive discipline in medicine. Physiatry and the adjunctive therapies have played a traditional role in the rehabilitative treatment of select cancer patients (e.g., amputees, patients with problems in lymphedema control). Chapters 15 and 16 present the conceptual perspective of physical medicine and fatigue-related interventions used in the rehabilitative therapies. It is significant that we are currently engaged in a crusade for interventions for fatigue in cancer while disregarding those techniques and approaches that have proved successful for years. Unfortunately, most patients do not have access to these interventions.

4. *What is it going to take to make health care and government leaders see the crisis in this area and take effective action?* In the early 1970s, a mass movement led by a few outstanding public figures, influenced Congress to fund cancer research. The same declaration of war is needed today on behalf of cancer rehabilitation. The cancer survivor movement has already had a powerful impact on political will. It behooves us to demonstrate what could be done to improve the everyday life of cancer survivors if rehabilitation were a significant and standard part of traditional services.

The transition step to a physiologically based, therapeutic intervention for fatigue in cancer took the form of a question:

How do you put energy into cells? How do you keep it there when people are going through treatment for cancer? This question was the object of research at Ohio State University in the 1980s. Familiar with the fatigue and loss of functioning resulting from diminished activity in patients with chronic illnesses, one of us (M.L.W.), during doctoral work in exercise science, became interested in exercise and cancer (Winningham, 1983). While studying the biochemical basis for the exercise-training stimulus, Winningham met Mary G. MacVicar, a visionary medical sociologist with rigorous doctoral training in disability and rehabilitation. MacVicar urged Winningham to focus on the rehabilitation needs of breast cancer patients, since that area had been neglected. MacVicar urged that the cardiac rehabilitation model be applied. This approach focused on a broad variety of physiological and psychological outcomes as a result of maintaining and promoting the body's own energetic capacity without inducing metabolic fatigue, stiffness, or injury. This work from more than a decade ago laid a comprehensive foundation for fatigue-related oncology exercise rehabilitation. It demonstrated that a specific kind of exercise (1) based on knowledge of the biochemical mechanisms of muscular work and recovery, (2) with appropriate clinical screening and precautions, (3) with monitoring of appropriate clinical parameters for risk, (4) by application of a prescriptive stimulus-response model, and (5) with monitoring of functional status and safety parameters as they relate to cancer patients, could increase energetic capacity and well-being. More recently, Canadian and European researchers began doing solid, empirical clinical trials on the physiological and psychosocial effects of prescriptive exercise on cancer patients. Current work by Kerry Cournyea of Alberta, Canada, Bernadine Pinto of Rhode Island, and Fernando Dimeo of Germany emphasizes rigorous research designs as a foundation laid for the future.

With the appropriate guidelines and precautions, prescriptive, dose-response exercise can contribute to more positive outcomes than any other intervention. These benefits have included improved body composition, ancillary symptom management, perceived somatic improvement, improved feelings of control, positive emotional response, improved sleep, and increase in functional capacity.

Powerful interventions carry commensurate risks if they are not conducted with appropriate clinical guidelines to ensure patient safety. In contrast to studies on pharmacological agents, there is no database on complications and interactions between cancer and exercise in patients undergoing specific antineoplastic therapies. Rehabilitative exercise functions as an endogenous drug. There is a need for studies comparing modes of exercise, testing the safety of drug-exercise interactions, developing databases of complications and contraindications, establishing definitive guidelines as to when exercise is not appropriate (contraindications), and testing models and economics of rehabilitation programs. These studies will parallel the model set forth for evaluating the effects of cardiac rehabilitation. See Chapter 18 for more on therapeutic exercise for cancer fatigue rehabilitation.

In the mid to late 1990s, the idea that exercise could be used to counter fatigue in people with the CRFS finally attracted popular attention. That is perhaps unfortunate, since the measured outcome in some studies focused on the more narrow psychosocial measures of quality of life or perceived fatigue. We must think beyond symptom management.

Researchers assessing clinical and quality control outcomes must not forget that the *process* (i.e., rehabilitation) is the means to the outcome (i.e., restoration and decreased fatigue). By focusing on the full spectrum of fatigue management measures as a standard component of rehabilitation, it is more likely that the health care system will eventually contribute to reimbursement.

To date, prescriptive, rehabilitative exercise for oncology patients is the most powerful intervention against fatigue, but it can do far more than just counter fatigue. Having the energy and endurance to participate in all the dimensions of living has significant quality of life implications.

Where Do We Go From Here?

As we go into the next millennium, it is shocking to discover that the NCI has budgeted next to nothing for research and training of rehabilitation professionals. Many of the "old time" rehabilitation therapists trained in the 1970s have retired or are approaching retirement age. Who will train the teachers and practitioners of the future? The future is here. We must act now. We have been waiting for the "magic bullet," the cure for cancer for well over 50 years. In the meanwhile, we have neglected what *can* be done to make life worth living *now*. We can wait no longer. We must move aggressively to press for new priorities in funding that would help the greatest number of individuals, with the greatest economic benefit, in the shortest period of time.

References

Berryman, J. W. (1995). *Out of many, one: A history of the American College of Sports Medicine.* Champaign, IL: Human Kinetics.

Healey, John M. (Ed.) (1972). *Rehabilitation of the cancer patient: Proceedings of the annual clinical conferences on cancer.* Sponsored by University of Texas M.D. Anderson Cancer Hospital and Tumor Institute.

Jokl, E. (1964) *The scope of exercise in rehabilitation* (p. 128). Springfield, IL: Charles C. Thomas.

Karnofsky, D. A., and Burchenal, J. H. (1949). The clinical evaluation of therapeutic agents used in cancer. In C.M. MacLeod, (Ed.), *Evaluation of chemotherapeutic agents* (p. 196). New York: Columbia University Press.

Nightingale, F. (1859). *Notes on nursing.* London: Harrison and Sons. (Reprinted in offset in 1946 by Edward Stern & Co., Philadelphia, PA.)

White, P. D., Rusk, H. A., Williams, B., and Lee, P. R. (1957). *Cardiovascular rehabilitation* (p. 155). New York: McGraw-Hill.

Winningham, M. L. (1983). *Effects of a bicycle ergometry program on functional capacity and feelings of control in women with breast cancer.* [Dissertation]. Ohio State University, Columbus, OH.

Winningham, M. L., and MacVicar, M. G. (1983). Exercise as a tension reduction mechanism in cancer patients [Abstract]. *Ohio Journal of Science, 83*(2), 75.

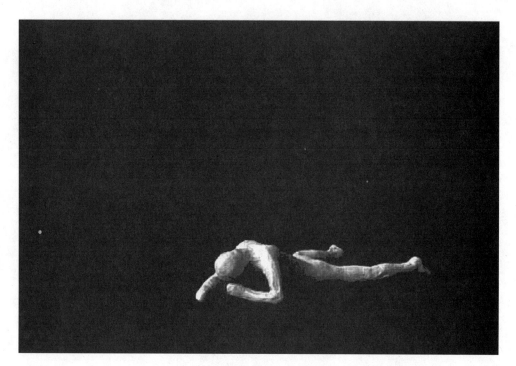

Fatigue

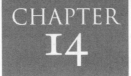
Assessing Manifestations: Quality of Life From a Quality Improvement Perspective

Maryl L. Winningham

Marilyn Bookbinder

Just going to the clinic exhausts me. There is so much activity, . . . so many questions (I know I answer the same questions five times—don't they ever talk to one another?), . . . having to undress, . . . having someone poke around to take blood while I have to act like it doesn't hurt, . . . getting dressed again. I smile and react to everyone, telling them I'm fine (do they really believe I'd be getting chemotherapy if I was fine?). Does anyone ever listen? Do any of them understand what this is like? Of course, I want them to think I'm a good patient. There is so much commotion. Later when I get home, I'm exhausted. . . . I feel like a ton of bricks hit me. All the questions I wanted to ask haunt me all night long. It takes me days just to recover from a clinic visit.

Anonymous cancer patient

Background

The present health care system will not pay for interventions relating to the cancer-related fatigue syndrome (CRFS) unless they are linked to functioning performance and traditional rehabilitation models already in existence. In other words, in the current restrictive and benighted third-party payer and disability system, it is next to impossible to obtain reimbursement, rehabilitation, or disability services for fatigue. The trend today is toward using discrete outcomes as a means of demonstrating progress, but how do we measure something that is a loss, something that is *not*? As long as we insist on looking at fatigue as a *symptom* and not as a *syndrome* with manifest functional issues, the medicolegal system will not acknowledge patients' needs. Rather, we can assess individuals in terms of *functional losses* that are also part of their suffering. As long as we make statements like, "Little is known about cancer fatigue" and "Fatigue is what the patient says it is," we are party to a lost cause. Conversely, this book shows that we know a great deal more about fatigue in general than has been thought. Further, fatigue is far more than what the patient says, particularly when the patient has trouble communicating about the experience of the CRFS using the word *fatigue!* Other chronic conditions that are acknowledged by the medicolegal system are similar to different aspects of the CRFS. Possible interventions that have been demonstrated to be beneficial with other patient populations (see Table 14-1) are the first place we should start, since they reduce the burden of proof and minimize the necessity for "fishing expeditions."

Assessing and Measuring Fatigue

As we improve in the ability to assess cancer patients with the CRFS, we can identify which of the preexisting measures and techniques for addressing outcome measures transfer from other clinical conditions to oncology patients. Only then can we present a framework for identifying, measuring, treating, and evaluating outcomes for cancer fatigue from a comprehensive perspective. By going beyond the CRFS as a mere symptom, we will be able to start measuring the very loss or gain in functioning we need to relate to the disability system. We will also be able to establish specific indicators.

When fatigue is discussed, quite often the terms *assessment* and *measurement* are used interchangeably or synonymously. The two are distinctly different, conceptually and methodologically. Clinicians *assess* cancer patients in the hospital, in the clinic, or (more rarely) at home for the impact this symptom has on a patient's life and health. *Measurement* is a term used by scientists and researchers to quantify variables associated with the CRFS. Scientific, theoretically based interventions used in research are applied to the subject in an attempt to measure and manipulate the variable.

We are still in the phase of observation and assessment when it comes to the CRFS, and those are still notoriously weak. Only recently have screening interview and diagnostic criteria been suggested. The most promising examples are Figures 11-7 and 11-8, respectively, in Chapter 11. In Chapter 3, Varricchio, who has been writing about measurement issues related to fatigue since the mid 1980s, acknowledges the limitations inherent in all our current measurement instruments.

Measurement is the consequence of relevant research built on clinically astute observations. The biggest hindrance to identifying indicators or developing outcome measures in cancer fatigue is that few clinicians are adept at assessing the functional issues relating to

About the Contributor

Marilyn Bookbinder insists she always wanted to be a head nurse. She has done that and far more. She has held managerial positions at Long Island Jewish Hillside Medical Center in New York, was acting director of nursing research and director of nursing research at Memorial Sloan Kettering Cancer Center in New York, and is currently director of nursing education and quality improvement, pain medicine, and

the CRFS. These issues, in turn, must be communicated within a fairly rigid framework of the medicolegal system. Figure 14-1 is a proposed model for logically identifying problems and interventions in clinical oncology, for making the progression from clinic to science, from clinicians' skills to policy.

One of the biggest problems in the United States today is that the rehabilitation/disability system is built on a medicolegal foundation. As such, it is essentially adversarial in nature. Commonly, even severely impaired individuals may have to apply for disability benefits as much as three times before they are granted. This usually takes money, an attorney often becomes necessary, and much energy is required as patients try to negotiate the mysteries of the system. They are faced with demotions or loss of employment because they cannot keep up with the rigors of their daily jobs. In addition, because the medicolegal system does not recognize fatigue as a legitimate cause for disability, it is difficult for patients to express their limitations within the framework of existing protective laws such as the Americans with Disabilities Act. With the post-CRFS, or postcancer fatigue, these problems are complicated by the skepticism and disbelief exhibited by many clinicians and bureaucrats, particularly when the cancer survivor appears healthy.

One of our greatest barriers in this whole process has been the lack of criteria on which to identify patients. In a recent publication, Cella and colleagues (1998) took a major step in gaining medicolegal recognition for patients with the CRFS. This publication (and subsequent revisions) should be in the hands of every clinician and researcher interested in cancer fatigue. Among the significant presentations in the article are (1) proposed ICD-10 (International Classification of Diseases) criteria for cancer-related fatigue (1998 draft), and (2) a brief (one-page with a maximum of 14 questions) interview guide entitled "Diagnostic Interview Guide for Cancer-Related Fatigue (1998 Draft)." Use of the diagnostic interview is sufficiently brief so as not to exhaust the patient (a major problem with some fatigue inventories). It incorporates an algorithmic approach for screening clinical patients and could be used to create more homogeneous groups for testing interventions. These documents are included in Chapter 11. Readers should consult the original article for details. Although not everyone may agree on everything included in the diagnostic interview or ICD-10 criteria, it is essential that we finally "nail pudding to the wall" and use some common grounds from which to proceed. We suggest this may be a good beginning, that we

palliative care at Beth Israel Medical Center in New York. Her research focus has been in quality control, pain, and fatigue management. She has had numerous funded research grants and is a well-known national speaker. One of her favorite topics is the relationship between research, standardization, and quality improvement. For relaxation, she enjoys cooking and teaming up with her husband in doubles tennis.

Table 14.1	Select Proposed Interventions for the Cancer-Related Fatigue Syndrome: Quality of Life Versus the Medicolegal System?			
Problem	Existing Intervention Based on Other Populations	Significance	Medicolegal System	Quality of Life Benefit
Cognitive loss related to disease and treatments: memory impairment and cognitive *slowing*	Cognitive retraining with mild traumatic brain–injured patients such as memory training and improving reaction time	Improved on-the-job performance: maintaining job efficiency and employment	Recognized rehabilitative techniques; professionals with appropriate training (can be adapted to cancer); recognized outcome measures including reduced costs to society	Improved feelings of self-worth through maintaining independence and self-confidence
Cognitive loss related to disease and treatments: memory impairment and cognitive *confusion*	Cognitive facilitation with ADHD such as organization, recognizing and carrying out priorities, task completion; pharmacological interventions to support cognitive functioning	Improved on-the-job performance: maintaining job efficiency and employment	[Same as above.]	Improved memory about daily activities and ability to plan and carry out tasks in work as well as social role/family setting
Physical loss (endurance, strength, reaction time, balance, coordination) related to bed rest, prolonged illness, and excessive overall functional decline	Appropriate exercise and physical and occupational therapy interventions; pharmacological intervention with biological agents that minimize infections and decreased oxygenation	Reduced incidence of falls and related injuries; able to engage in physical functioning and independence	Recognized rehabilitative techniques; professionals with appropriate training (can be adapted to cancer); recognized outcome measures including reduced costs to society and reduced morbidity and mortality	More rapid return to independent functioning and ability to participate in social and role activities
Depression related to inappropriate sleep-rest and loss of feelings of self-worth resulting in unncessary but related medical disorders and inability to carry out social role	Pharmacological interventions; "sleep therapy"; light therapy; psychotherapy	Reducing depression-related symptomatology; facilitating differentiation between fatigue and depression	Prefers "quick fix" of drugs versus known benefits of psychotherapy and behavioral interventions	Rapid remediation of symptoms in depressed patients who are not genetically predisposed; possible remediation in those who are; rediscovery of life satisfaction

Figure 14.1	Proposed Model for Identifying Problems and Interventions in Clinical Oncology

Observation of Problem → Assessment (R&D) → Screening (R&D) →
Evaluation (R&D) → Measurement (R&D) → Clinical Outcomes (R&D) →
Continuous Quality Improvement (R&D in Patient Satisfaction, Staff Development,
Monitoring of Outcome Measure) →
Observation (Astute Clinical Observation that Something Is Still Missing) →
Assessment (R&D), etc.

set aside professional and individual differences and start using this instrument to identify patients. Currently, this screening is not happening in most research protocols.

The greatest practical barrier has been the lack of clinical assessment skills in physicians, nurses, social workers, and the various therapists, skills needed to identify problems in patients with the CRFS. Prior to reviewing the assessment skills that need to be developed, here are a few tips:

- Check with family members. Sometimes patients are unaware they are altering their lifestyles to accommodate decreased functioning.
- "Anchor" your questions by comparing how patients feel *now* versus before they were diagnosed with cancer–when they were feeling their best. Then follow up by comparing how they feel since they were last seen by the clinician.
- Ask open-ended questions. Let people provide their own descriptors.
- Watch their facial expression when they don't know anyone is watching. A flat, expressionless face can become quite animated when patients interact with staff. Afterward, they are exhausted. The flat, expressionless face probably is closer to reality.
- Remember this is about how they really live, not how they *say* they are doing when they are excited and in the clinic.
- Ask about changes in energy level–how much they are able to do before they are tired.
- Ask about recovery time–how long it takes them to recover from activity now compared with before the cancer.
- Consider follow-up telephone calls two days later. It is remarkable what people forget when they are put on the spot in the clinic. It is quite possibly the worst time to question people!
- Focus on *changes* and their significance.

Table 14.2	Functional Status Interview Guide: Assessing Fatigue Effects on a Quality of Life Framework

I. Background—Lifestyle, Roles, and Functioning

A. *Brief individual history and characteristics*
   1. Age
   2. Gender
   3. Cultural background/lifestyle orientation
   4. Role expectations and demands
      a. At work
      b. At home
      c. Socially
      d. Income? Breadwinner? Insurance?
      e. Living with? Responsible for?
   5. Normal sleep patterns
   6. Normal activity patterns
   7. Preexisting impairments/disability
   8. Diagnosis
   9. Treatment regimens

II. Impairment/Pathology in Physiological Status

A. *Diagnostic and laboratory tests?*
   1. Decreased hemoglobin?
   2. Hydration status?
   3. Electrolyte imbalance (e.g., sodium, calcium, potassium, magnesium)?
B. *Preexisting metabolic abnormalities?*
C. *Physical/mental assessment—look for changes in:*
   1. Mental status
      a. Alertness and focus
      b. Confusion
      c. Irritability
      d. Short-term memory
      e. Short attention span
   2. Posture (slumped or erect)?
   3. Movement
      a. Gait (shuffle? steady pace? moving slowly and deliberately?)
      b. Coordination
      c. Balance (able to recover when bumped? able to turn quickly?)
   4. Ability to rise from seated position?
      a. Needs to use hands?
      b. Able to rise rapidly from seated to standing position and keep balance?
D. *Consider drug side effects*

III. Functional Work Output

A. *Watch for change (family may observe before patient does)*
   1. Are routine tasks becoming more difficult?
   2. Have you slowed down?
   3. Have you stopped doing some things because of fatigue or other symptoms?
   4. Are you able to participate fully in family activities?
   5. Are you making occupation-related changes?
   6. Have you changed social activities?
   7. Have you changed your eating habits? Drinking habits?
   8. Do you have any other health problems? Anything that affects your activities or ability to work? (Consider need for referrals.)

IV. Feelings Related to Fatigue

A. *Describe sensations related to fatigue. (Do not suggest the word fatigue unless they use it.)*
   1. Encourage the use of metaphors/pictures, to describe the feeling.
   2. Ask about energy levels, tiredness, exhaustion.
   3. Ask how they feel the day after clinic visits.
   4. Establish symptom burden.
      a. Monitor intensity of fatigue and related symptoms.
      b. Get rating on fatigue and other prominent symptoms such as dyspnea, depression, weakness, pain. Use "smiley faces," color scales, or a simple 0 to 10 scale to assess their fatigue-like manifestations, as well as other symptoms.

   0 —— 1 —— 2 —— 3 —— 4 —— 5 —— 6 —— 7 —— 8 —— 9 —— 10

   5. Determine patterns of fatigue (include sleep at night and naps) (patient or family chart/diary).
   6. Evaluate meaning/significance of symptom burden.
   7. How do any of the above affect quality of life?

V. Key Questions to Understanding Quality of Life

A. *What has been lost?*

B. *What is the significance of that loss to patients?*

C. *What can be done to restore or adjust to that loss?*

D. *How acceptable is the outcome?*

The following outline, with clarification, is offered as a guide for interviewing and documenting specific functional changes and losses in the CRFS.[1] It is provided in Table 14-2 in condensed format for use as a clinical resource and to facilitate developing clinical assessment skills.

There is not time to ask all the questions at once. Besides, if we did, we would just exhaust patients and their families. Start with a few questions or a section at a time. As part of continual professional improvement, exchange your observations with others for feedback. This is a whole new area, so no one has to feel shy or inferior! As we hone our observational skills, we start identifying patterns. Pattern recognition is a significant step toward developing the intuition that makes a good clinician, and intuition helps us hone in on one or two things that are really important. It is also the basis on which we can begin to identify more precise research issues and intervention prescriptions. If the whole health care team uses this guide, they will become increasingly aware of patients who fall through the cracks and anticipate possible ways to avoid it. Oncology team members are urged to hold in-service workshops for other members, to show what each discipline can do for patients with the appropriate referrals and how the referrals can be made. This improves quality control in patient care and increases understanding of the concept of teamwork.

Functional Status Interview Guide: A Quality of Life Approach

Note: Watch for Changes!

I. **Background–Lifestyle, Roles, and Functioning**

   A. *Brief individual history and characteristics.* The various functional domains of quality of life differ with each individual. One of the problems in the current health care environment lies in trying to lump everyone into the same box. Since no two people are alike, there will be an infinite variety in the interaction between each of these domains. Cancer makes it particularly difficult because no two people respond the same to disease and treatment. Having said that, we know there are trends or tendencies in groups of people; otherwise health care would be entirely unpredictable. This first section helps us understand the context in which the rest of the domains can be evaluated and explained.

   1. *Age.* Since decreased functioning is–independent of anything else–related to age, consider age as a possible aggravating factor. Every organ system of the body responds to the entropic processes of life (see Chapter 2) from birth to death and deteriorates accordingly.

   2. *Gender.* Only recently has there been recognition of the profound physiological differences between men and women. From the time of conception, the bodies and minds of men and women are shaped by powerful chemical and

genetic influences. For example, one method of determining drug doses is based on body mass index values, which were normed on men not women. Yet, women have smaller livers for metabolizing drugs, metabolize less energy every day, and have less lean body weight and less fluid volume than do men at the same age. Therefore, we can expect more problems with women and medications when body mass index is used for dosing. The myth of the "70-kg male" (see Chapter 2) has dominated the teaching of physiology and pathophysiology to medical students, and most drug studies have focused on the responses and dosing in men. Cyclic menstrual variations throughout much of a woman's life span affect hormonal shifts, drug metabolism, and immunological status.

3. *Cultural background/lifestyle orientation.* Much depends on an individual's cultural background and lifestyle orientation. What are patients' perceived expectations for themselves? What are their fears? For example, do they perceive cancer as a "go to bed and die" experience, or a "get up and fight it" experience? This has less to do with strength of character and more to do with cultural expectations than we might expect. Is their lifestyle one that lends itself to openness or do they feel that revealing their personal, intimate preferences, such as with homosexuals, may lead to rejection by health care professionals?

4. *Role expectations and demands.* Whether people perceive themselves as fulfilling their roles in life has much to do with their satisfaction and quality of life. (Chapter 21 discusses this in a most insightful way.)

   a. *At work.* Can patients keep up with their workload? Obviously this depends on the type of employment or vocation they are in. Even slight cognitive impairment can be crippling to people who are normally high functioning in a role with great expectations. Do they have to cut back on work? Change positions or hours?

   b. *At home.* Once again, gender plays an important role. Many women feel if they aren't in a "nurturing" role, they are failing. Conversely, men may feel they are failures if they are not working to support the family financially.

   c. *Socially.* What are the favorite social activities or expectations? This is usually one of the first areas in which loss appears because it is seen as something that can be given up without jeopardizing income or family roles.

   d. *Income? Breadwinner? Insurance?* Do the patients have a regular income? Are they able to afford medications, supportive child care, housekeeping, etc? Are they the family breadwinner? Does their medical insurance depend on a job that is becoming too much? Are they being faced with loss of income as well as insurance?

e. *Living with? Responsible for?* Are they living with someone who can provide supportive care and function as a reliable reporter?

5. *Normal sleep patterns.* (Figures 11-5 and 11-6 can be used to evaluate sleep disorders.) What time do they arise? Go to bed? What is the quality of their sleep? Do they nap? How long do they sleep at night and how long are their naps? What has changed since their illness began?

6. *Normal activity patterns.* What are their normal activity patterns? Have they changed? Often, friends and family members may notice subtle changes before patients do.

7. *Preexisting impairments/disability.* Does the person have preexisting impairments or disabilities that already affect functioning? When an impairment already exists, the person is at risk of more rapid functional losses.

8. *Diagnosis.* What is the diagnosis, the prognosis, and the normal course of that particular kind of cancer? What kind of functional impairment might be anticipated?

9. *Treatment regimens.* It is commonly recognized that some treatments are more rigorous than others. What functional losses are associated with a particular treatment? It is now becoming clear that some functional losses, such as cognitive losses, are unanticipated and long term.

II. **Impairment/Pathology in Physiological Status.**
Clearly, some functional losses can be clarified from a physiological perspective. This is important, especially if medical treatments can address these pathologies.
A. *Diagnostic and laboratory tests.* Most cancer treatments and monitoring involve a significant number of laboratory and diagnostic tests. Does the performance of these tests impose functional limitations on patients? Prolonged periods of nothing by mouth, inadequate nutritional and fluid intake, and gastrointestinal disturbances can relate to treatments. Frequent monitoring is essential.

1. *Decreased hemoglobin.* The degree to which hemoglobin values are permitted to plummet prior to medical intervention in cancer patients would be intolerable in any other medical field. Patients, having already made subtle compromises in life's activities, often go on to experience profound decrements in activity that are treated as "normal and expected."

2. *Hydration status.* Dehydration is probably one of the most overlooked causes of weakness. Bed rest, vasoconstriction as a result of exposure to cold in radiation rooms and clinic suites, and nausea, vomiting, and diarrhea all contribute to muscular weakness (loss of muscle turgor) and dehydration.

3. *Electrolyte imbalance.* Electrolyte imbalances can impose functional limitations when they impose muscular weakness and similar disorders on daily func-

tioning. While sodium, calcium, and potassium concentrations are usually monitored, electrolytes critical to energetic functioning like magnesium are more difficult to monitor and rarely supplemented.

B. *Preexisting metabolic abnormalities.* Diabetes, pulmonary disease, hepatic dysfunction, and renal disease have a powerful impact on outcomes. They present with metabolic impairments that affect treatment and the ability to process drugs. Surprisingly, critical information related to metabolic abnormalities often is not included on patients' charts in the oncology clinic!

C. *Physical/mental assessment*–look for changes in:

1. *Mental status.* Use of established instruments such as the Folstein Mini-Mental Status can be helpful in screening. Keep in mind that the most common cause of acute change in mental status is not neurological but *hypoxia.* Probably the second most common cause of acute change seen in oncology settings is *dehydration,* which often also presents with nausea. Medication *side effects* and *substance abuse* are also possible significant factors.

   a. *Alertness and focus.* Decrements are a common consequence of acute fatigue, sleep deprivation, and some depressive states. It can also be a side effect of medications.

   b. *Confusion.* This common consequence of acute fatigue, sleep deprivation, and some depressive states can also be a side effect of medications. In unpublished work with breast cancer patients by Winningham (1993), confusion/bewilderment was a far more significant characteristic of breast cancer patients than depression as measured by the Profile of Mood States–Short Form.

   c. *Irritability.* This common consequence of acute fatigue, sleep deprivation, and some depressive states can also be a side effect of medications.

   d. *Short-term memory.* This is a long-term consequence of select treatment and acute fatigue, as well as a common consequence of chronic fatigue, sleep disorders and depression (see Olders's screening guide in Figure 11-5). In unpublished work by Preusser and Winningham (1992), this was the most common loss in patients with preexisting chronic obstructive pulmonary disease.

   e. *Short attention span.* This is a long-term consequence of select treatment and acute fatigue, as well as a common consequence of chronic fatigue, sleep deprivation, and depression (see Olders's screening guide in Chapter 11).

2. *Posture* (slumped or erect). As proprioception and muscle tone decrease in response to decreased activity, muscles of posture are among the first to be affected. Watch for a progressive change in posture over time as well as in the following.

　　3. *Movement*
　　　　a. *Gait* (shuffle, steady pace, moving slowly and deliberately). Vestibular dysfunction as a result of bed rest (which contributes to dehydration) is clearly seen when patients turn: They move slowly, turning the whole body. Sudden movements or turns of the head often lead to dizziness. Hydration and ambulation should be assessed frequently, especially in the very ill and elderly. Gait also changes, from firm planting of feet to a shuffle; again the elderly are at highest risk.
　　　　b. *Coordination.* Coordination is also affected by decreased activity and bed rest. Are patients on a chemotherapeutic protocol that affects peripheral nerves and therefore coordination?
　　　　c. *Balance* (able to recover when bumped, able to turn quickly). Balance also becomes impaired with decreased activity and bed rest. This is critical to assess the risk from falls. Look for bruising: ask about falls or unsteadiness at home. Are patients able to recover when bumped? Can they turn quickly?
　　4. *Ability to rise from seated position.* Consider the "get up and go" screen often used in the geriatric setting.[2]
　　　　a. *Needs to use hands.* The need to use hands to stand up is a significant sign of loss of tone in the erector muscles, and is characteristic of debilitated elderly.
　　　　b. *Able to rise rapidly from seated to standing position and keep balance.* Do patients need to place their hands on their knees or grab bars? Do they "rock" forward prior to standing? Need to bend forward prior to bringing themselves erect? When they return to a seated position, do they plop back down?
　D. *Consider drug side effects.* For example, patients may have a pathophysiological manifestation such as impaired vision, hearing, or proprioception.

III. Functional Work Output.

Subtle changes in work output may occur long before patients notice them. One of the most significant is the trend to short-term bursts of activity interspersed by exhaustion and the need to take a breather. Since patients may consider this embarrassing, they may find ways to hide it. Family members or a significant other can be of particular help in this.

A. *Watch for change* (family members may observe before patients do). These are specific questions that you can ask to help focus on the problem.
　　1. Are routine tasks becoming more difficult?
　　2. Have you slowed down?
　　3. Have you stopped doing some things because of fatigue or other symptoms?

4. Are you able to participate fully in family activities?

5. Are you making occupation-related changes?

6. Have you changed social activities? This may be the first area that becomes obvious. If patients engage in social activities, they may feel fine, even excited, that day, but may be puzzled by the good-day, bad-day phenomenon. Often the excitement of the good day guarantees subsequent bad days.

7. Have you changed your eating habits? Drinking habits? Patients may drastically reduce their caloric and fluid intake as a result of sheer exhaustion. "I'm too tired to eat." Or "Just leave it there–I'll drink it later."

8. Do you have any other health problems? Anything that affects your activities or ability to work? (Consider need for referrals.) Prior accidents, injuries, and especially a history of polio may not be on the chart. Many postpolio patients are not aware of the cause for their symptoms. When it becomes clear that any of these impair activities or ability to work, consider a referral for physical therapy, occupational therapy, or neuropsychology, or to a social worker for vocational and occupational triage.

IV. **Feelings Related to Fatigue**

A. Describe *sensations* related to fatigue (do not suggest the word *fatigue* unless they use it).

1. Encourage the use of metaphors/pictures, to describe the feeling (see Chapters 1 and 23).

2. Ask about energy levels, tiredness, exhaustion.

3. Ask how they feel the day after clinic visits (see Chapters 1 and 2).

4. Establish symptom burden.

   a. Monitor intensity of fatigue and related symptoms. Symptoms rarely present alone. The presence of one increases the burden of all on quality of life.

   b. Get rating on fatigue and other prominent symptoms such as dyspnea, depression, weakness, pain. Use "smiley faces," color scales, or a simple 0 to 10 presentation (see Figure 14-2) to assess their fatigue-like manifestations, as well as other symptoms.

5. Patterns of fatigue. Include sleep at night and naps. It may be helpful to obtain a patient or family log/diary (see Figure 11-6).

6. Evaluate meaning/significance of symptom burden.

7. How do any of the above affect quality of life? This does not require exotic instruments. In response to the request, "Tell me about how you see your quality of life" or "Rate your quality of life on a scale of 0 to 10," most people can answer quite readily.

V. **Key Questions to Understanding Quality of Life.** Let the patient describe the answers. Don't presume to know the answers.

   A. What has been lost? Sense of loss and grief are important as part of the adjustment process.

   B. What is the significance of that loss to patients? Have they lost something for which they feel they cannot compensate? Also consider the possibility of depression as part of this answer.

   C. What can be done to restore or adjust to that loss? What progress in adjustment (coping) are they making? Is the loss permanent or temporary? In an unpublished study by MacVicar and Winningham (1989), patients' responses to the Symptom Check List-90 indicated that regardless of intervention-nonintervention status, patients seemed to improve and normalize over a 90-day period.

   D. How acceptable is the outcome? Patients tend to evaluate their present quality of life based on how bad it could be. Thus, there is an upward bias often introduced into quality of life measures whereby the clinician may actually judge a patient's quality of life to be worse than a patient perceives it.

Where Do We Go From Here?

1. If we are to develop effective assessment skills, we need to take responsibility for ourselves. In addition, we need to share observations and what we have learned among one another. As we reach a common consensus, we can build a solid base for research.

2. In an organizational setting, we need to focus on desired outcomes across disciplines to develop effective teamwork.

3. Specific outcomes should incorporate values at all levels.

4. To be effective, continuous quality improvement techniques require feedback by administration, staff, patients, and employers who support the health care system.

5. We need to incorporate feedback from patients as well as the cultural community on the significance and value of this work.

6. Staff development and education should be a priority. This is the bridge to success between the patient care environment, administration, and policy development at the national level.

Endnotes

1. I (M.L.W.) would like to acknowledge the valuable contributions Mary G. MacVicar made to my awareness of these issues. She taught me to observe not what people *said* they could do, or what others said they could do, but what people actually *could* do, and encouraged me to find valid and reliable indicators.

2. Incidentally, in an intriguing study involving amyotrophic lateral sclerosis patients, Schields et al (1998) noted that improvement in muscle force may occur independently of patient perception of functioning, thus validating the need for objective as well as subjective measures of functioning.

References

Cella, D., Peterman, A., Passik, S., Jacobsen, P., and Breitbart, W. (1998). Progress toward guidelines for the management of fatigue. *Oncology, 12,* 369–377.

MacVicar, M. G., and Winningham, M. L. (1989). Unpublished research. Ohio State University, Columbus, Ohio.

Preusser, B. A., and Winningham, M. L. (1992). Unpublished research. Ohio State University, Columbus, Ohio.

Schields, R. K., Ruhland, R. L., Ross, M. A., Saehler, M. M., Smith, K. B., and Heffner, M. L. (1998). Analysis of health-related quality of life and muscle impairment in individuals with ALS using the Medical Outcomes Survey and the Tufts Quantitative Neuromuscular Exam. *Archives of Physical Medicine and Rehabilitation, 79,* 855–862.

Winningham, M. L. (1993). Unpublished research. University of Utah, Salt Lake City, Utah.

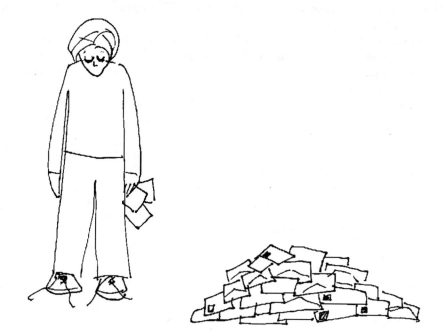

I'll pay my bills . . . tomorrow when I feel better.

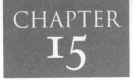

The Role of the Physiatrist

Theresa A. Gillis

It was interesting—my mind just seemed to have these gaps. I forgot to pay my taxes that year; I "lost" several thousand dollars in the checking account; and when the bills came, I threw them in the corner. I just couldn't deal with it. It was like I was aware of them, but I wasn't, you know? Later, I had no memory traces of it. The IRS was really quite patient—not at all what I expected. We were on a first-name basis. I'm still finding errors in my tax papers two to three years later. Sometimes I owe them; sometimes they owe me. . . . And appointments—whole pieces of time disappeared and I couldn't remember day, time, anything. I would look at my appointment book and not link what I was reading with the fact that I had an appointment today. My secretary said I fell asleep at meetings. That's incredible. It's not me. I'm a very responsible person! It's a good thing I own the company or I might have gotten fired!

Non-Hodgkin's lymphoma survivor

Background

Fatigue is a frequent complaint of cancer patients. The problem is that the meaning of the term varies between and among patients and health care team members: No one seems to be certain what it is and what to do about it. Although the fatigue experience in cancer is poorly defined, it *does* appear to be quite different in cancer patients compared to patients with other neuromuscular pathologies such as poliomyelitis and multiple sclerosis. Such patients experience failure at the anterior horn cell, neuromuscular junction, or muscle fiber level, and this is quantifiable on electrodiagnostic testing. Cancer patients with fatigue are not known to have similar findings.

Fatigue may be accompanied by a decline in function or a loss of independence, which may be quantifiable. Conversely, some cancer patients with fatigue manifest no observable limitations or abnormalities, and maintain what appears to be busy, active lives despite this complaint. The heterogeneous experience of fatigue, and the continuum of functional independence on which it is imposed, create difficulties in discussion or communication, research, and treatment.

Physiatry (*not* psychiatry) is a medical specialty that focuses particular attention on patients' functional status and the successful fulfillment of their multifaceted roles in life. As with other physician specialties, the physiatrist has graduate medical training, followed by a residency and often a fellowship. Unfortunately, many patients who could benefit from the practical and unique approach of physical medicine are not considered for referral to a physiatrist. Several characteristics of the specialty have hindered its recognition and widespread involvement in patient care:

1. There are few practicing physiatrists in the world, although recently the numbers of physicians graduating from physical medicine and rehabilitation residencies in the United States has increased dramatically. With so few practitioners, most are fully occupied in the rehabilitation of trauma, birth defects, amputations, cerebrovascular accidents, and similar diagnoses. The physiatric treatment of those with cancer has been comparatively neglected.

2. Many oncologists and other practitioners in cancer care have little knowledge of the functional deficits their patients face, as well as the benefits a physiatric intervention can bring to their patients.

3. Physiatry is not a glamorous field of medicine. Many of the Western-oriented societies, particularly the United States, are fixated on youth and health, as well as the "magic bullet" and glorious cure. Physiatrists, in contrast, care for the disabled or physically challenged, those with chronic disease or disfigurement, and the elderly. The emphasis of the specialty is on recovery or maintenance of function, on adaptation as a means of overcoming disability. Although not as dramatic as some medical disciplines, it focuses on addressing the qualities of daily life and functional independence. As we see more people living longer, and more people surviving cancer, the question of how they shall live makes physiatry relevant to the future of our whole society.

The physiatric assessment includes contrasting patients' *current* level of independence with their most recent period of *maximal* function. Declines may be attributed to fatigue or to more specific pathophysi-

About the Contributor

Originally from western Pennsylvania, Theresa A. Gillis graduated from Northeastern Ohio Universities College of Medicine and completed a residency in physical medicine and rehabilitation at Baylor University College of Medicine in Houston, Texas. In the final year of her residency, she discovered she enjoyed a brand new elective in cancer pain management, at the University of Texas M. D. Anderson Cancer Center under the direction of Richard Payne, Sharon Weinstein, and Stratton Hill. Despite the fact that this was a world-renowned cancer center, there was no physiatric presence and no occupational therapy at that time. She said, "I was impressed by the negative impact cancer pain had upon function; I was even more impressed by the improvement in independence and well-being that effective symptom management and rehabilitative techniques brought to my patients. It was a landmark experience in my

ology with a resulting sense of fatigue. Oncology patients often present with multiple possible etiologies for their experience of fatigue. Broadly, these etiologies may be grouped by categories such as (1) neuromuscular and mechanical; (2) cognitive; and (3) emotional, psychological, and situational. Patients may present with disorders in one or more categories or, frustratingly, with no identifiable contributing factors at all.

Neuromuscular and Mechanical Factors Contributing to Fatigue

Neuromuscular and mechanical problems include pathology of the neuromuscular, cardiovascular, and respiratory systems as well as general metabolic functions. Weakness and poor endurance (i.e., functional capacity) may result from steroid myopathy, paraneoplastic syndromes, chemotherapy-induced polyneuropathies, disuse atrophy, and deconditioning. Limitations in cardiac output from premorbid atherosclerotic disease, doxorubicin-related cardiac toxicity, suboptimal oxygenation resulting from anemia, chronic obstructive pulmonary disease, or other lung pathologies can impede independence and well-being. Cardiopulmonary deficits can improve with the appropriate rehabilitation programs by improving functional capacity without reversing the underlying disease. Restoring adequate levels of hemoglobin and oxygen may also be required. In these cases, improvement in status is a result of improved *efficiency* of functioning.

Advancing age, with the attendant declines in cardiorespiratory reserves, can contribute to the likelihood of fatigue, although age has been disputed as a correlate of fatigue. Other specific biochemical, nutritional, and physiological factors that promote fatigue are discussed elsewhere (see Chapter 2). It is essential that monitoring for treatment-related functional losses contributing to physical impairment be ongoing throughout and following treatment.

life." After completion of that elective, she decided to stay and create a physical medicine and rehabilitation service, now an established section at M. D. Anderson Cancer Center. She continued, "I truly enjoy teaching my colleagues and patients about the value of physiatry in the oncology setting, as I discover new ways to help those facing the dual diagnoses of disability and cancer find symptom relief and optimize their functional independence." When we met Theresa, we immediately decided she should be a contributor to this book. We asked her to tell our readers what she does and how much more could be accomplished in terms of helping people adapt to their fatigue and improve their quality of life if there were more professionals with her preparation and commitment.

Prescriptive exercise can be a successful intervention for muscle weakness and limited endurance. Strengthening specific muscle groups such as the hip abductors and extensors, quadriceps, spine extensors, and trapezius may be beneficial when *weakness* exists. Aerobic exercises (riding a stationary bicycle, running, walking, swimming, etc) and perhaps even vigorous, sustained activities of daily living (gardening, vacuuming, housework, stair climbing) may be effective in improving *endurance* and functional capacity.

Cognitive Factors Contributing to Fatigue

Cognitive fatigue is a common but rarely recognized phenomenon in cancer patients. Contributors to cognitive failure include various chemotherapy agents, biological response modifiers such as interferon alfa, frontal lobe disorders or lesions, and iatrogenic medications such as sedative-hypnotics, narcotics, sedating antidepressants, antiepileptics, and antiemetics.

Sensory deficits, particularly visual or hearing impairments, can interfere with cognitive function. Studies have shown that bed rest alone, independent of any other pathologies, can contribute to visual, auditory, and tactile sensory alterations. Vision may be particularly sensitive to changes in hydration that often accompany bed rest and illness.

Cognitive impairments are easily underestimated. Some patients with near-complete short-term memory dysfunction and loss of executive function discerned only by mini-mental status examinations or formal neuropsychological testing have excellent social interactions.

Interventions to counteract cognitive fatigue include reassessment of medications and the avoidance of polypharmacy, particularly sedating medications. Correction of vision and optimization of hearing aids or pocket talkers may be necessary. Prior to changing prescriptions for expensive corrective lenses, make sure that the problem is not caused by dehydration. In the case of dehydration-related visual changes, the degree of impairment may change on a daily basis! Although as yet unsupported by research, some practitioners employ stimulants or dopaminergic drugs to modulate arousal and alertness in patients with fatigue. Speech and occupational therapy may be prescribed to assist the patient through adaptive techniques for memory and attention.

Emotional, Psychological, and Situational Factors Contributing to Fatigue

Emotional, psychological, and situational factors contributing to fatigue are numerous. Depression, anxiety, and sleep disorders can cause or exacerbate the experience of fatigue. Personality characteristics may influence volition, response to stress, and ability to benefit from support. Excessive stressors in vocational, financial, or familial realms may create sensations of exhaustion and weariness. The physiatrist may recommend treatment of such problems through appropriate pharmacotherapy, psychiatric and/or supportive therapy, support groups, stress-management counseling, and vocational counseling.

Limited rest periods of 30 to 60 minutes for relaxation and restoration of sleep-wake cycles may be particularly helpful in this population. This intervention could qualify as a "reasonable accommodation" in the workplace, consistent with the Americans with Disabilities Act. The physiatrist may also assist the patient with time management, delegation of tasks and mustering familial support, and simple validation and assurance. In particular, the physiatrist can be a key resource for identifying and assessing patients who could benefit from modes of treatment by other specialties (e.g., physical therapy, occupational therapy, speech therapy, cardiac and pulmonary rehabilitation programs, neuropsychologists).

Pain can create fatigue through both neurophysiological and emotional components. Pain is an emotional experience, through its creation of suffering. Weakness and impaired mobility and function result from neurological inhibition of muscle firing at spinal cord and cerebral levels. Management or alleviation of pain is effected through medications and physical medicine interventions. These may include myofascial release and muscle energy techniques, trigger point injections, massage, stretching, and modalities such as ultrasound, electrical stimulation, heat, and cold. Acupuncture techniques for pain management are also within the armamentarium of some physiatrists.

The history and symptom review for the patient experiencing fatigue can be extremely time-consuming. The patient's own perception of contributing factors cannot be minimized, and may have the greatest insight and accuracy when psychosocial factors predominate. Screening forms, completed in the waiting room or at home prior to the patient's visit, may speed the evaluation. Assessment tools, some with visual analogue scales, are being developed and validated, and may one day prove useful in clinical settings. (This is also discussed in Chapters 3 and 14.) Referrals to a physical medicine and rehabilitation specialist are appropriate at initial evaluation; they are essential in patients with weakness, poor functional capacity, and pain.

I can still remember that day. I was mowing the lawn. I mow the lawn every week. It's the man's job around the house. Suddenly, I became so exhausted that I couldn't finish. I barely was able to make it over to sit down under the tree. I couldn't believe it–a little thing like mowing the lawn! I don't know how long it was until I could get up again. . . . Maybe an hour. That's when it hit me–it really hit me: "You have cancer!" And then I thought, "You are going to die." Up until then, I went for treatments, I had lab tests, but I hadn't really believed it.

63-year-old colon cancer survivor

Where Do We Go From Here?

The third-party reimbursement system seems to have difficulty in recognizing the overall benefit of the therapies discussed here. There seem to be three main reasons for this: (1) a paucity of clinical trials that aggressively demonstrate the significance of specific interventions (see Table 15-1), (2) the magic-pill orientation of our society as a means of solving problems, and (3) the lack of awareness that physical medicine and rehabilitation programs can be effective in treating chronic problems. This lack of awareness extends to all levels of cancer care from physicians, to patients and families, to insurance companies. There has been a tendency in recent years to reduce payments for the rehabilitation of stroke and car-

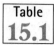

Table 15.1 Interventions for Fatigue

Environmental adaptations

    Activities for daily living (ADL) equipment

    Scheduling/organizing for energy conservation

    Ergonomic evaluation

    Delegation

Exercise

"Judicious rest"

Metabolic corrections

    Potassium

    Calcium

    Magnesium

    Hydration

Hematological corrections

    Transfusions (increase red blood cell count)

    Recombinant human erythropoietin

Nutritional corrections, particularly to prevent muscle wasting

    Supplements

    Dobhoff or Miller-Frederick tube, etc (there are several varieties)

    Gastrostomy

Oxygen (supplemental)

Pain management

    Physiatric/physical therapeutics

    Pharmacological agents

Psychopharmacology

    Antidepressants

    Anxiolytics

    Sedatives for sleep disorders

    Stimulants

Psychosocial

    Support groups

    Counseling

    Vocational counseling

diac patients; most cancer patients who will live longer receive no rehabilitative service provisions at all.

The physiatrist has much to offer the oncology patient with fatigue. Through skills in functional assessment and symptom review, physical medicine and rehabilitation specialists can discern the often multifactorial nature of fatigue and employ appropriate strategies to overcome it. We need to familiarize patients, family members, other physicians, other health care providers, and the reimbursement system about the specialty of physiatry and what physiatrists can do. In addition, we need to increase the number of professionals training in this and related allied health care fields to ensure that every patient has access to services on a nationwide basis.

We need to demonstrate that by keeping people active, independent, and as comfortable as possible we are going to contribute to tremendous savings to the health care system of the future.

Resources

Felsenthal, G., Garrison, S. J., and Steinberg, F. U. (Eds.) (1994). *Rehabilitation of the aging and elderly patient.* Baltimore: Williams & Wilkins.

Garden, F. H., and Gillis, T. G. (1996). Principles of cancer rehabilitation. In R. L. Braddom (Ed.), *Physical medicine and rehabilitation* (pp. 1199–1214). Philadelphia: W. B. Saunders.

Garden, F. H., and Grabois, M. (Eds.) (1994). Cancer rehabilitation. *Physical Medicine and Rehabilitation: State of the Art Reviews, 8*(2).

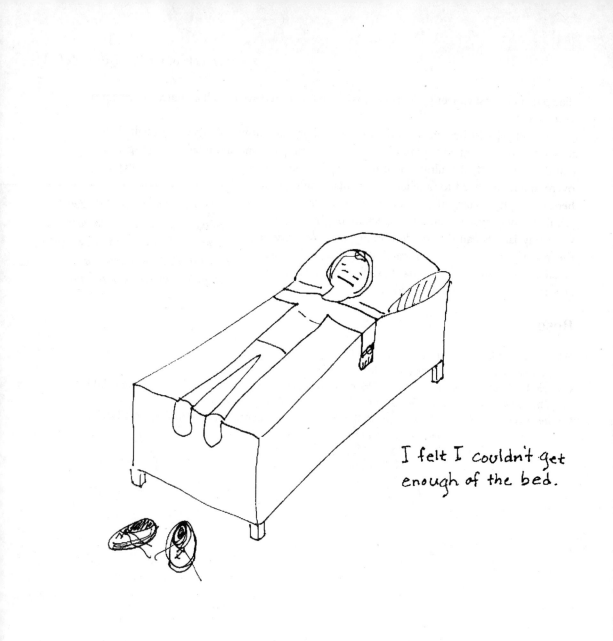

I felt I couldn't get
enough of the bed.

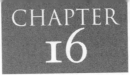

CHAPTER 16

What the Rehabilitation Therapies Can Do

Eileen S. Donovan
and the University of Texas M. D. Anderson
Cancer Center Rehabilitation Services Team

I used to be surprised to see dying patients brighten up when they saw the physical therapist come. I thought maybe it was just because they were bored. Now I realize—it's because they associate moving with living.

Hospice physician

Background

This chapter builds on Chapter 15, and is intended to explain some of the physical issues related to fatigue in cancer. A lot has been written about the phenomenon of fatigue—how to assess, measure, and evaluate it and how to manage it. In the fatigue literature, less attention has been paid to some of the physical factors that contribute to fatigue. This is significant, because many of these factors in the life of anyone—even someone without cancer—would be fatiguing!

Many patients come to the rehabilitation department complaining of being too tired to do the things that they would like to do. After evaluating their physical performance and questioning them to develop a picture of how they manage their days, rehabilitation professionals are frequently surprised that patients manage to do as much as they do. Often, correcting a gait problem, modifying an activity, or providing equipment produces noticeable improvement in both the amount of work that patients can perform and patients' satisfaction with their perception of energy.

Rehabilitation Philosophy in Cancer Management

While the health care community sometimes thinks of rehabilitation in terms of recovery from or adaptation to neurological and musculoskeletal deficits, we must broaden that view to consider rehabilitation in the management of any impairment that interferes with optimal physical or social function. We must implement rehabilitation principles of *prevention*, *restoration, adaptation,* and *palliation* at the time of cancer diagnosis, and continue to include rehabilitation in the ongoing management of patients with cancer. Rehabilitation of persons with cancer also requires that the rehabilitation specialists have a good understanding of issues related to cancer and its treatment in order to appreciate the unique challenges in managing this particular patient population (Healey, 1972).

World Health Organization's Definition of Disabilities

In 1980, the World Health Organization published the *International Classification of Impairments, Disabilities, and Handicaps* (ICIDH). This classification is still in use internationally. Three key definitions must be considered, particularly because these terms have critical medicolegal significance:

- *Impairment*–any loss or abnormality of psychological, physiological, or anatomical structure or function. Examples include limited range of motion, weakness, and fatigue. Usually, this is considered to be at the organ level, that is, dependent on injuries to joints or limbs, neuromuscular paralysis or impairment, defective heart or lungs, and loss of vision or hearing (organ level). Since cancer-related fatigue (CRF) is invisible and multifactoral in nature, the medicolegal system has had difficulty understanding how it fits into this context.

> *Everything you do in a patient's room, after he is "put up" for the night, increases tenfold the risk of his having a bad night. But, if you rouse him up after he has fallen asleep, you do not risk, you secure him a bad night.*
>
> Florence Nightingale, *Notes on Nursing*

- *Disability*–any restriction or lack of ability (resulting from an impairment) to perform an activity in the manner or within the range considered normal for a human being and necessary for some part of everyday functioning (person level). Examples include inability to walk, inability to drive if it is necessary and considered normal, sexual dysfunction, and inability to dress oneself. If CRF impairment contributes to difficulty functioning socially or occupationally, it can be considered a disability. This is important because if fatigue can be clarified to be a disability, patients or survivors may be able to benefit from the Americans with Disabilities Act and apply for "reasonable accommodations" in their workplace.

- *Handicap*–a disadvantage for a given individual, resulting from an impairment or disability that limits or prevents the fulfillment of a role that is normal, depending on age, sex, and social and cultural factors for that individual. In other words, the individual is unable to do something normal people can do. This usually involves a dependency on someone or something else for needs related to normal existence. Examples include inability to work, to care for a child, and to handle money. This is considered to be at the societal level (e.g., the level of the person's functional relationship within society).

Definition of Rehabilitation

The United Nations World Programme of Actions concerning Disabled Persons in 1983 defined *rehabilitation* as a goal-oriented and time-limited process aimed at enabling an impaired person to reach an optimum mental, physical, and/or social functional level, thus providing her or him with the tools to change her or his own life.

Fatigue in Other Chronic Diseases

Fatigue is an impairment common in many chronic diseases (e.g., multiple sclerosis, post-polio syndrome, cardiovascular disease, lupus, rheumatoid arthritis). Fatigue is often experienced as a loss of or lack of energy regardless of the diagnosis. While there are certainly unique problems and considerations in each of these chronic diseases, they share many problems and considerations. Common clinical solutions and techniques used with other patient populations can be applied to cancer patients. In addition, many patients with CRF are already contending with other chronic disease processes as well, placing an additional burden on them. There is a wealth of information to be obtained from the support organizations and individual professionals who specialize in these other chronic diseases. Unfortunately, most cancer patients who could benefit from existing services are not referred for evaluation and treatment.

The following rehabilitation principles should be implemented at the time of cancer diagnosis: prevention, restoration, adaptation, and palliation.

Fatigue in Cancer

Fatigue is the most commonly reported symptom in persons receiving treatment for cancer (Winningham et al, 1994; Vogelzang et al, 1997). It certainly is disruptive to more cancer patients for a longer period than any other cancer-related symptom. The reasons are usually multifactorial. Because this population frequently has multiple-system problems, either due to the disease itself or the treatment of the disease, effective management of the fatigue must include consideration of all those factors.

Fatigue as *Impairment*

Fatigue (as an impairment) results in diminished functional performance (ability to carry out basic and advanced activities of daily living [ADLs]), which is a *disability*. This in turn results in the inability to carry out life roles (e.g., parent, homemaker, breadwinner, and caretaker), which is a handicap. This has rarely been recognized by the cancer treatment or the reimbursement system.

ADLs are commonly divided into basic and advanced activities. *Basic* activities include feeding, dressing, bathing, grooming, hygiene, and mobility. Individuals who are limited to these activities require assisted living (they are often only able to carry them out because

Figure 16.1 Comparison of Energy Costs for Select Activities

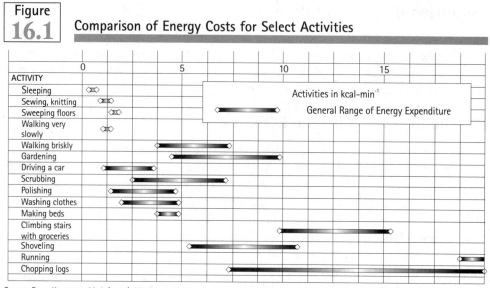

Source: From Karvonen, M. J. (1974). Work and activity classifications. In L. A. Larson (Ed.), *Fitness, Health and Work Capacity* (p. 38). New York: Macmillan. Used with permission.

they are able to pace themselves or benefit from assistive personnel or equipment). *Advanced* ADLs include such things as child care, housework, leisure activities, meal preparation, occupational activities, and shopping. These require considerably higher demands of strength and endurance and are required for independent living. Those who can perform the advanced ADLs still may be extremely limited by CRF. They may have no energy left over for social activities and may collapse after pushing themselves to accomplish even these basic tasks. Obviously an individual able to perform only the basic ADLs and none of the advanced activities is very limited, but this is where many rehabilitation programs stop. Rarely are patients who have difficulty with the advanced activities referred for rehabilitation, even though they may benefit from it the most. See Figure 16-1 for a comparison of energy costs for select activities.

Rationale for Rehabilitation and Fatigue Management in Cancer

The role of rehabilitation in managing persons with fatigue is significant because rehabilitation professionals are experienced in analyzing movement, physical performance, and function and know how to formulate a plan to correct the correctable and teach adaptation or modification when required. Exercise prescription, gait training, correction of impairments, and selection of ambulatory aids and other adaptive equipment are within the scope of practice of physical and occupational therapists.

Overview of Function and Energy Costs

Gordon (1952), who studied the energy cost of various basic and advanced ADLs in a predominantly healthy subject group, presented a table describing a range of energy costs expressed as percentage rise over basal metabolic rate (BMR). He also included data from experiments reported in the literature. He found that the cost of showering was 242% to 377% higher than the BMR, that of walking slowly was 160% greater, descending steps was 320% greater, and ascending stairs was a whopping 1,330% greater or, in his words, "climbing stairs is an extremely arduous activity." Weiss and Karpovich (1947), in developing a graded exercise program, noted that there was a significant difference in the amount of energy cost for different individuals doing the exact same exercise. Similarly, Dean (1991) noted that using tables based on the evaluation of healthy individuals to predict the energy cost of activities in the impaired population was not valid because the impairment itself contributed to the energy cost of the activity. O'Sullivan and Schmitz (1994, p. 787) discussed the problems associated with using normative tables to predict energy cost in a population (patients with pulmonary disease) that "does not respond to exercise in a normative fashion."

Energy Leaks

In order to effectively conserve energy, identification of how energy is being spent and the "leaks" or inefficiencies that occur is helpful. Each person's experience is different depending on the disease, its treatment, lifestyle, occupational demands, and preexisting conditions. The most common energy leaks are pain, poor body mechanics, altered posture, altered gait, altered breathing patterns, and poorly designed tasks or workspace. Increased energy cost of activities leads to increased metabolic fatigue. Inefficiency of function leads to increased metabolic costs. If metabolic energy is wasting because of inefficiency, that energy is not available for purposeful activity. (Refer to Chapter 2 for more on energetics and efficiency.)

Rehabilitation is defined as a goal-oriented and time-limited process aimed at enabling an impaired person to reach an optimum mental, physical, and/or social functional level, thus providing her or him with the tools to change her or his own life.

Pain

Pain as an energy leak causes alterations in posture, movement patterns, sleep patterns, and breathing patterns. Because it takes a given amount of energy to maintain a muscle in spasm, to continually guard against pain, or to maintain an altered posture or gait, pain leads to increased energy cost of activities. It also contributes to more pain because the body is functioning inefficiently and placing forces and imbalances on parts of the body that are then overworked.

Altered Posture

In ideal posture, when a person is viewed from the side, there is a straight line from the ear to the tip of the shoulder, to the trochanter, to the malleolus. This straight line should also equally bisect the body when the subject is viewed from front or back. In poor posture, some of the more common deviations are

- forward head and rounded shoulders;
- increase of the normal thoracic kyphotic curve;
- lateral curve of the spine (e.g., scoliosis), either primary (arising in the vertebral column itself) or secondary (e.g., leg-length discrepancies, pelvic rotation); and
- increased lumbar lordosis.

Any change in the alignment of the body parts produces compensatory changes in other body parts, which increases the overall work of standing, sitting, and moving. For instance, a middle-aged woman with breast cancer who has had a mastectomy will frequently demonstrate forward rounding of the shoulders, which is usually more pronounced on the side of the surgery. This can result in an increase in the kyphotic curve of the thoracic region of the spine, which contributes to an increase in the lordotic curve of the cervical spinal region in order to maintain an eyes-forward position. These postural changes increase the forces acting on the thoracic vertebrae and can increase the likelihood of an osteoporotic fracture. In addition, these alterations in posture can produce impingement of the nerve roots exiting the spinal cord between the vertebrae, causing pain. The relation of the ribs to the spine and sternum is altered, which alters the woman's ability to fully expand the thorax, therefore altering breathing. Maintaining this abnormal posture requires an increase in the amount of work done by the extensors of the spine, which alters the normal alignment of the shoulder joints, which in turn alters the relationships of the muscles of the shoulder girdle. Because she is not respiring with adequate and relaxed depth, she is at higher risk for pneumonia should she acquire a garden-variety upper respiratory tract infection. The complications are nearly endless (O'Sullivan and Schmitz, 1994; Weiss and Karpovich, 1947).

Poor Body Mechanics

Body mechanics simply refers to how humans move and stand, how they lift and carry objects, how they change position, and so on. It involves both static and dynamic balance. One aim of postural integration in man is to keep the line of gravity between plus or minus 7% of the geometric center of gravity (Rasch and Burke, 1971). Everyone's center of gravity (COG) or mass (COM) (while standing in an anatomical position) is not in the same place, but it is roughly 5 centimeters anterior to the body of the second sacral vertebra. The COG changes with any change in position or with additional loading. Pregnancy moves the COG forward; carrying a heavy load in one hand moves the COG toward that side.

<table>
<tr><td>Figure
16.2</td><td>Center of Gravity for Sumo Wrestler and Ballerina</td></tr>
</table>

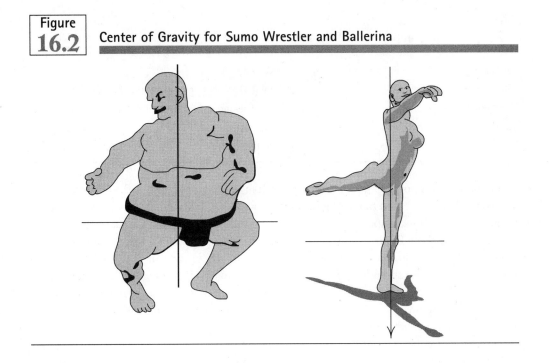

The base of support changes as well, with change in position, addition of support, and so on (Rasch and Burke, 1971).

The neuromusculoskeletal systems integrate balance, responding to changes in COG by increasing or decreasing muscle tone, moving body parts, changing joint positions, and so on, to keep the COG over the base of support. In a pregnant woman (or a patient with hepatomegaly or ascites), as the abdomen enlarges, the COG moves anteriorly. The back extensors tighten, pulling the trunk backward to maintain balance. When carrying a heavy load in one hand, an individual's trunk will shift away from the side of the load to compensate for the shift in COG toward the load. When a person stands unsupported on one foot, the pelvis shifts to one side and the spine curves to maintain the head over the stance foot. The relationship of COG to base of support in a sumo wrestler, crouching with feet apart and arms in waiting position, is very different from that of a ballerina standing on one foot with the other leg extended behind (see Figure 16-2)(Rasch and Burke, 1971).

Alterations in Gait

Gait is the way a person walks. Some of the basic components of gait are stride length, stride width, step length, cadence, velocity, and joint alignment (see Table 16-1). Studies have shown than any alteration in normal gait pattern results in increased energy cost for ambu-

Table 16.1	Basic Components of Gait	
Stride length		Velocity
Stride width		Joint alignment and movement
Step length		Trunk alignment and movement
Cadence		Arm swing
		Weight shift

lation. Just as with posture, gait patterns may change for many reasons. Leg-length differences, limb loss, decreased range of joint motion, joint instability due to weakness or hypermobility, sensory loss, impaired coordination or balance, and pain are just a few of the potential causes (see Table 16-2) (Lehmann and DeLatour, 1990; O'Sullivan and Schmitz, 1994). Inman (1967) found that immobilization of subjects in casts or braces (this included immobilization of the shoulders) produced an approximate 15% increase in the energy cost of gait. Think of the patient who has undergone replacement of the proximal end of the tibia for osteosarcoma, who is required to wear a Bledsoe brace, walk with crutches, and is now resuming chemotherapy.

Waters and colleagues (1983) compared young and older walkers in terms of energy cost. Mean oxygen consumption was comparable; however, the net cost per meter traveled was higher in the seniors owing to slower speeds (73 vs 80 meters per minute), and heart rate in the seniors increased significantly. Changes in velocity of gait can increase energy cost: Increasing the speed of walking increases the energy used on propelling the body forward; decreasing the speed increases the energy used to maintain balance during single stance phase (Inman, 1967). Winter and colleagues, in 1990, demonstrated that the normal, healthy, aged population has a significant reduction in walking velocity due to a shorter step length and an increase in double support stance time. They postulated that this was due to an adaptation by the elderly to increase stability in gait.

Various assistive devices and weight-bearing restrictions will also impact the energy cost of walking. Kathrins and O'Sullivan (1994) studied the physiological responses of non-weight-bearing (designated foot off the ground at all times) versus touch-down (weight on designated leg restricted to 10% of body weight) ambulation. Although they found oxygen demands to be similar, the non-weight-bearing gait resulted in a significantly higher heart rate and rate pressure product, indicating higher stress on the cardiovascular system. In addition, subjects perceived the non-weight-bearing gait to be more strenuous. Baruch and Mossberg (1983) studied healthy elderly (60–80 years old) performing non-weight-bearing gait with a walker. The average heart rate increased 49 ± 14 beats per minute, with the group heart rate rising to an average of 89% of the age-predicted maximum heart rate, leading the researchers to the conclusion that non-weight-bearing gait may require excessive cardiac work, even in the healthy aged. Pagliarulo and colleagues (1979) compared other-

Table 16.2	Some Possible Reasons for Gait Alterations	
Leg-length discrepancies	Joint instability due to weakness or hypermobility	
Limb loss	Casts, braces	
Muscle shortening	Sensory loss	
Limited joint range of motion	Impaired balance or coordination	
	Disturbances of tone	

wise healthy men who had had a below-knee amputation walking with crutches and those walking with prosthesis and cane. Heart rate rise and energy cost were significantly higher in the crutch-walking group. In both groups, energy cost rose when subjects walked either faster or slower than their "free cadence."

Altered Breathing Patterns

Abnormal breathing patterns, although they can be significantly stressful, are not often thought of as energy leaks. As health professionals, we all note breathing patterns in patients with respiratory symptoms, but sometimes do not pay such close attention to the pattern in patients who do not have symptoms. Many cancer patients have poor or inefficient breathing patterns due to postural changes, muscle weakness or tightness, pain and guarding, or simply habit. Persons with kyphosis or scoliosis, persons who have had a thoracotomy or who have pleural effusions or ascites, and persons with tight chest-wall or abdominal muscles (e.g., after transverse rectus abdominal muscular [TRAM] or other abdominal surgery) demonstrate restrictions in their ability to fully expand the thorax. Persons with pain will also alter their breathing pattern to avoid expansion of the painful area. Altered breathing patterns for any of the above reasons can result in a loss of energy by altering the work of breathing and by restricting the ability of the body to keep up with oxygen demands (inefficiency) (Massery and Baldwin, 1998).

Poorly Designed Tasks or Workspace

The term *workspace* as used here includes the environment for performing both basic and advanced ADLs. Poorly designed workspaces or tasks increase the energy required to perform any task. For example, in a poorly designed computer workstation, it takes more energy to hold the arms in the air in order to position hands over a keyboard than it does to support the wrist or forearm to allow the hands to do their work. In the home, storing all frequently used kitchen items on the topmost shelf is inefficient. For the workplace, industries or environmental engineers often analyze tasks to improve productivity, reduce risk of injury, and so on (Ostrom, 1993). For persons with cancer, therapists analyze their basic and advanced daily living tasks, and the environment in which they are carried out, and modify them for the same reasons. The following are some questions used to evaluate tasks and workspaces:

- Are tools and equipment within functional reach?
- Can steps be eliminated or combined to simplify tasks?
- Can the way the task is performed be modified?
- Would the use of adaptive equipment assist in the performance of the task?

Impaired Cognition

Changes in cognition can contribute to or be manifestations of fatigue. Inability to think clearly, remember, and plan can contribute to inefficiencies of function. Many of the drugs used in the cancer population have cognitive side effects. Patients with primary or metastatic brain disease, as well as those who have received radiation to the brain, frequently exhibit changes in cognition that may be readily apparent or very subtle. Stress can also affect cognition. Deficits may be exhibited as subtle changes in memory, organizational ability, reasoning, judgment, or learning ability. They may also present as a dangerous lack of insight or judgment, inability to learn, or poor impulse control (Meyers and Weitzner, 1995; Pavol et al, 1995). Strategies employed in the cognitive rehabilitation of brain injured populations can be applicable in this population as well (Fralish and Guercio, 1998).

Special Patient Populations

Given that a high percentage of patients who undergo treatment for cancer experience fatigue, there are few populations who present a more complex challenge to the health professionals caring for them. Because many cancer patients are elderly, they present a special challenge, and rehabilitation evaluation in this population should be required to prevent further complications.

Patients who are receiving steroids often develop steroid myopathy, which usually presents as proximal muscle weakness, resulting in difficulty performing simple tasks such as getting up from a chair or from the commode (Grant, 1994). In the bone marrow transplant population, fatigue is particularly severe and debilitating as a result of treatment. Add to that the weakness of steroid myopathy, and perhaps motor and sensory changes secondary to neurotoxic chemotherapy, and functional deficits will be the rule rather than the exception.

Patients with bone metastases often have pain with movement. If they are at risk of fracture, they may require bracing or use of ambulatory aids or a wheelchair. Their movement patterns may be altered and inefficient due to the need to protect the area or because of pain. Their risk of injury is thus doubled, from the disease and from the inefficiency. Finally, persons who have postpolio syndrome, rheumatoid arthritis, cardiovascular disease, or any of the myriad other health problems that affect physical, cognitive, or emotional performance require careful evaluation and planning to avoid solving one problem at the cost of causing another.

Management of Cancer-Related Fatigue

Management of CRF must begin with an evaluation of patients, including determining physical sources of energy leaks and environmental, social, cognitive, and emotional factors that may contribute to the problem (see Table 16-3). How do patients move, stand, walk, or sit? Do they wear a brace or prosthesis? Does it fit? Do they use an ambulatory aid? Is it fitted properly? How far can they walk? Can they manage steps and ramps? Do they have pain? What kind of pain and where? What makes it worse? What helps reduce it? Are they able to sleep? Do they have weakness? Is it affecting function? What is the breathing pattern?

Can patients feed, dress, and bathe themselves? Can they move in bed? Get out of bed unattended? Can they get to the bathroom alone? Can they get to the kitchen, get out of the house, drive to the grocery store, and perform other essential activities related to self-care? Who comprises their support system? Do they have family or friends who are willing and able to help them or are they alone? Are there small children?

What is the home environment like? The five-level dream house becomes a trap when it is not accessible! Do patients live in a one-step-entry home or third-floor apartment? How far do they have to walk to get to the bathroom? Is the lighting good? What is the layout of the bathroom? Are the doorways wide enough to get a walker or wheelchair through if they are needed? Do patients work? What is their work environment?

What is the cognitive condition? Do patients have problems with memory or new learning? Can they process instructions? Do they demonstrate impaired judgment or insight? What about their willingness to participate? Are there any cultural barriers to participation? Can they still handle basic finances? Instructions about medications?

Once the evaluation is completed, identified energy leaks and other contributing factors can be addressed. Some of the interventions that may be employed are therapeutic exercise, posture correction, gait training (with or without assistive devices), joint mobilization or stabilization, safety training, modification of ADLs (by changing the way they are done or by using adaptive equipment), cognitive retraining, and so on. Breathing exercises and respiratory muscle strengthening or reeducation can improve ventilatory function. Improved mobility of the thorax and decreased pain can improve ventilatory function as well.

Addressing physical function, correcting gait impairments, and providing appropriate assistive devices can significantly reduce the risk of falls in patients who are at risk. All of these interventions can help to maximize function and contribute to improved independence and quality of daily life. Patient education regarding fatigue management can allow patients to manage themselves. The Arthritis Foundation developed a self-care course for

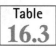

Table 16.3	Barriers to Fatigue Management in Everyday Life

- Failure to view fatigue as a real symptom or problem
- Patients' inability to solve problems themselves, owing to stress, illness, or lack of knowledge
- Patients' unwillingness to admit need for or accept help (e.g., assistive device, wheelchair, change in method) because of culture or values
- Patients' view of intervention as weakness or loss of control
- Lack of any alternatives for some patients because of lack of resources, lack of support, or other obstacles
- Delay of health professionals in recognizing and addressing correctable sources of energy leaks
- Failure to relate the impairment of fatigue to the resulting disabilities and handicaps that third-party payers can better understand the importance of rehabilitation interventions and consequently pay for those interventions
- Lack of awareness in some health professionals regarding current concepts of fatigue management

persons with rheumatoid arthritis that can be useful. Studies have shown that attendees experienced significant health benefits as well as reduced medical costs (Lorig, Mazonson, and Holman, 1993).

Energy Conservation

Energy conservation is one way to promote adaptation to the impairment of fatigue, to facilitate abilities and the resumption of roles. *Energy conservation* is, simply, the budgeting of available energy stores to allow the attainment of goals. This is done in much the same way that many of us budget our financial resources through anticipation of expenses, prioritization, elimination, modification, deferment, or delegation. Some suggest there is a dearth of hard scientific data supporting this intervention, probably because it is so obvious and commonsensical. How many people need to drown to prove that humans need oxygen to live? Energy conservation is a well-known and practiced intervention in many other chronic diseases including heart failure, arthritis, multiple sclerosis, postpolio syndrome, systemic lupus, chronic fatigue, fibromyalgia, and chronic lung disease (Pedretti and Zoltan, 1990; Trombly and Scott, 1977). Studies that would be of value should address the most cost-effective and efficient way of delivering this kind of care in the cancer population.

Principles of Energy Conservation

The fundamental principles of energy conservation are prioritizing, planning, eliminating, delegating, modifying, and pacing. For practical energy conservation tips, see Table 16-4.

Prioritizing

This step entails deciding what has to be done and then, once patients have an idea of the tasks that they consider necessary, deciding which items on their list are most essential and which are less essential. For instance, today a patient has a clinic appointment, she is scheduled for a test at the hospital, and she has laundry that needs to be done, bills to be paid, and groceries to be bought. She is unlikely to be able to accomplish all of this. If she does not get to the test at the hospital, it may not be possible to reschedule until much later in the month. That will be her first priority. She will go on down the list until all tasks are prioritized. We all do this in some form or fashion when faced with too much to do and not enough resources (e.g., time, money, energy) to do it.

When persons are fatigued, they sometimes cannot solve problems effectively, so putting structure around the task can help. Priorities are highly individualized. They may change from day to day. For a person with small children, child care responsibilities will usually be a top priority. If the bills are overdue and the gas company is coming to pull the meter, bill paying will have a higher priority than if there is time before the bill is due. People may need help with solving problems related to the apparently simple tasks in life.

Planning

Planning may be as simple as just taking a look at everything that needs to be done. It can also involve careful planning of the sequencing of tasks, the timing of tasks, and so on. When is the best time to do the task? (Obviously grocery shopping the evening before Thanksgiving will take more energy than doing it early on a Saturday morning and using the store scooter.) We can help patients with this, for example, by focusing their attention on the required task and providing suggestions for planning meals and shopping for what is necessary.

Eliminating

If a task is not necessary, maybe it does not have to be done. Or at least it does not have to be done today. Perhaps part of the task is necessary, but part can be eliminated. Washing the floor may be necessary, but if the patient uses a no-rinse cleaner, the rinse step can be eliminated. Choosing wash-and-wear clothing can eliminate the task of ironing.

Unfortunately, people with cognitive fatigue struggle with these things that formerly required no thought at all. There has been little sensitivity to the widespread presence of this problem in the cancer population; even worse, helpful resources are available but few patients have access to them.

Delegating

Delegating tasks is not always an option, but many persons simply do not take advantage of the help that is available because they do not want to be perceived as weak, they do not want to be a bother, or they do not want to relinquish control. Helping them to look

Table 16.4	Tips for Energy Conservation

BASIC ACTIVITIES OF DAILY LIVING:

Bathing
- Wash hair in shower, not over sink.
- Sit to dry off.
- Use a terry robe instead of drying off.
- Use a shower organizer over the shower head to avoid leaning and reaching.
- Use safety strips on the floor of the tub.
- Install a grab rail.
- Use a shower bench or lawn chair to sit while showering.
- Use a hand-held shower while sitting.
- Use moderate temperature water, rather than hot.
- Use a long-handled sponge or brush to reach feet and back.
- Sponges are easier to handle than a wash cloth.

Grooming / Hygiene
- Sit.
- Don't lean forward unsupported.
- Rest elbows on counter or dressing table.
- Use long-handled brushes or combs to avoid holding arms overhead.
- Use elevated commode seat.

Dressing
- Loose-fitting clothes allow you to breathe more easily.
- Organize early so you won't have to rush.
- Lay out clothes before starting, to avoid extra steps.
- Bring your foot to your knee to apply shoes and socks so you won't have to lean over.
- Lie down to put on pants, socks, and shoes.
- Wear slip-on shoes.
- Use a long-handled shoe horn and a sock aid.
- Fasten bra in front, then turn to back.
- Wear button-front shirts rather than pullovers.
- Use a reacher and/or a dressing stick.
- Use Velcro fasteners instead of buttons or shoelaces.

Mobility
- Wear low-heeled shoes.
- Wear shoes with a shock-absorbent sole or insole.
- Use a wheelchair for long trips (the mall, etc).
- Maintain good posture when driving.
- Use cruise control if possible.
- Install hand rails and use them.
- Install ramps.
- Place chairs strategically to allow rest stops (e.g., along a long hallway).
- Disconnect automatic door-closing mechanisms.
- Ride the elevator.

ADVANCED ACTIVITIES OF DAILY LIVING:

Housekeeping
- Spread tasks out over the week.
- Do a little bit each day.
- Delegate heavy work.
- Hire help.
- Use a wheeled cart or carpenter's apron to carry supplies.
- Sit to do whatever you can.
- Use long-handled dusters, mops, etc.
- Use a long-handled dust pan.

Shopping
- Explore eligibility for handicap parking permit.
- Make a list first.
- Organize the grocery list by store aisle.
- Use the grocery cart for support.
- Use a power scooter if the store has one.
- Request store assistance with shopping and getting to the car.
- Shop at less busy times.
- Shop with a friend.
- Delegate shopping.

Meal Preparation
- Assemble all ingredients before you start.
- Use mixes or prepackaged foods.
- Use cookwear you can serve from.
- Use smaller appliances (mixers, toaster oven, microwave).
- Use electric knife and can opener.
- Buy ergonomically designed utensils (Good Grips, etc).
- Transport items on a rolling cart.
- Store frequently used items at chest level to avoid bending and stretching.

Table 16.4 (continued)

- Line ovens and burner drip pans with aluminum foil.
- Sit while preparing food.
- Rest elbows on table or counter.
- Let dishes soak rather than scrubbing.
- Let dishes air dry.
- Use a dishwasher.
- Delegate dishwashing.
- Use a jar opener.
- Use a rubber mat or wet towel under mixing bowls to help steady them while stirring or mixing.
- Don't lift heavy pans off the stove. Ladle the food out at the stove.
- Use mitten potholders to take advantage of the entire hand to lift.
- Use placemats instead of tablecloths. They are easier to place on the table and easier to clean.
- Use lightweight utensils.
- Prepare double portions and freeze half for later.
- Leave heavy containers where they can be accessed without lifting (on the countertop, etc).
- Drag garbage bags instead of lifting (or use a wheeled garbage can).
- Use a lazy Susan.
- Use a cutting board that fits over the sink.
- Use the garbage disposal.
- Eat in the kitchen.
- Use vegetable spray to cut down on the scrubbing needed after cooking.

Laundry

- Use an automatic washer and dryer if possible.
- Use a laundry cart on wheels.
- Sit to transfer clothes to the dryer, if possible.
- Use commercial prewash instead of scrubbing.
- Wash bras and socks in a lingerie bag to avoid tangling.
- Drain hand washables and press the water out instead of wringing.
- Sit to iron.

- Adjust the ironing board height.
- Use an iron with a spray attachment.
- Slide the iron onto an asbestos pad between items to avoid lifting.
- Use a lightweight iron.
- Wear wash-and-wear or drip-dry clothes.
- Hang clothes on the doorknob instead of the top of the door.

Child Care

- Plan activities around the table or in the living room to allow sitting.
- Instead of going to the zoo, go to the beach or a park where you can sit or lie down.
- Delegate some of the child care responsibilities if possible.
- Take advantage of programs like "Mother's day out."
- Teach smaller children to climb up on lap instead of being lifted.
- Teach children to make a game of some of the household chores.

Workplace

- Plan workload around your best times of the day.
- Arrange workspace ergonomically.
- Take periodic rest breaks.
- Lie down during lunch.
- Request modified duty if necessary.
- Look into eligibility for handicapped license plates.

Leisure

- Wear comfortable clothing.
- Use adaptive equipment.
- Select less strenuous activities.
- Go with a friend.
- Use a wheelchair or golf cart.
- Request wheelchair assistance in terminal.
- Preboard when traveling by air.
- Use wheeled luggage.
- Use cart or skycap.

at this in different ways can sometimes help them to accept help. Many people want to be supportive of their ill friends and family members, but do not know what to do. Allowing them to help gives them a feeling of having contributed. Delegation can also be viewed as a tool in the control of available energy. It is important that the cancer health care system validate the reality of this kind of fatigue and the real need for help. Guidance to the family and friends should be practical and specific if it is going to be effective.

Modifying

Can the task be done differently? Can it be simplified? Are there tools or products that would make it easier or decrease the time needed to do the task? Just because one can cook a huge meal from scratch, without using any appliances, doesn't mean that is the only way or the best way to cook. One can use mixes, appliances, prepared foods, and the microwave. They are called labor-saving devices for a reason–they save labor (energy).

Pacing

Does all of the task have to be done at once? Can it be broken down into subtasks? How can adequate opportunity for rest be planned (Pedretti and Zoltan, 1990; Trombly and Scott, 1977)? There is no doubt that learning to pace requires education, practice, and reinforcement. It is all too easy for cancer patients who are exhausted to overdo it and not realize it until they are on the verge of collapse.

Workplace Modifications

Changes in the workplace will vary widely depending on the type of workplace and the nature of the work itself. In some cases, it may be impossible for individuals with CRF to return to their previous occupation. These persons may require referral to vocational rehabilitation for evaluation, counseling, and retraining (other important areas for research). There has been very little testing of the Americans with Disabilities Act's "reasonable accommodations" and appropriate types of vocational retraining in the cancer population. For persons who can return to work if reasonable accommodation is made, the following workplace modifications may work, as they have worked for patients in the past:

- Being able to sit to do a job instead of standing can mean the difference between capability and incapability. Many jobs are performed standing out of habit or workspace design, not out of necessity.
- Use of a telephone headset (for a person who spends much time on the telephone) reduces the number of times one has to pick up and put down the receiver. It also facilitates a more normal posture than holding a phone against the ear does.
- A well-fitted chair that provides support to the back and arms can reduce the amount of energy it takes to sit, as well as prevent discomfort from sitting for long periods in an unsupported position.

- Motorized scooters may not work for everyone, but for someone whose job requires walking long distances throughout the day, they can be a godsend.
- The workspace can be reconfigured to reduce noise and distraction.
- Parking closer to buildings can minimize the long walk from remote parking lots.
- The workday can be broken up with rest periods or naps.
- Flexible scheduling is helpful.

Patients With Special Problems

Patients who are on high-dose or long-term steroids need close monitoring for functional losses. Strengthening, adaptive equipment, ADL retraining, safety teaching, and energy conservation may all be indicated, but the underlying disease for which the steroids were prescribed must always be considered in designing a program. Prevention of loss might be possible with very early intervention (Grant, 1994).

Bone marrow transplant patients, because of the dosages of drugs (often including steroids), the prolonged treatment course, the high incidence of complications, and the severity of their fatigue and weakness, require careful and constant monitoring and program modification to avoid overdoing.

Patients with multiple bony lesions should be evaluated for the potential for fractures at each location, and a plan devised to maximize mobility and function, hopefully without causing a worsening of the problems. Selection of ambulatory aids and other devices is complicated. A standard walker to relieve weight on a femoral lesion may increase stress on a lumbar vertebral or a humeral lesion. Bracing for spinal stability may interfere with pulmonary function.

Patients with comorbidities require programs that incorporate understanding of their other chronic diseases as well as their cancer.

Where Do We Go From Here?

Persons with CRF should be referred to a rehabilitation professional when they are experiencing difficulty in carrying out any of the basic or advanced ADLs. Recognizing that many patients experience decline in function over the course of treatment, more attention needs to be given to early identification of high-risk persons and the development of prevention programs. A rehabilitation professional is the most appropriate person to evaluate the impairments that affect ADLs and to institute interventions to address those impairments.

References

Baruch, I., and Mossberg, K. (1983). Heart rate response of elderly women to non-weight bearing ambulation with a walker. *Physical Therapy, 63*, 1782–1787.

Dean, E. (1991). Clinical decision making in the management of the late sequelae of poliomyelitis. *Physical Therapy, 71*, 752–761.

Fralish, K., and Guercio, A. (1998). Integrative approaches to cognitive rehabilitation. *Brain Injury Source, 2*(3), 18–20, 40.

Gordon, E. (1952). Energy costs of various physical activities in relation to pulmonary tuberculosis. *Archives of Physical Medicine, 33,* 201–209.

Grant, J. (1994). Corticosteroid side effects: Implications for PT. *PT Magazine, 2*(3), 56–60.

Healey, J. (1972). The quality of success in the treatment of cancer. *Journal of the Oklahoma State Medical Association, 65*(4), 147–151.

Inman, V. (1967). Conservation of energy in ambulation. *Archives of Physical Medicine and Rehabilitation, 47,* 484–488.

Karvonen, M. J. (1974). Work and activity classifications. In L. A. Larson (Ed.), *Fitness, health and work capacity* (p. 38). New York: Macmillan.

Kathrins, B., and O'Sullivan, S. (1994). Cardiovascular responses during nonweight bearing and touchdown ambulation. *Physical Therapy, 64,* 14–18.

Lehmann, J., and DeLatour, B. (1990). Gait analysis: Diagnosis and management. In F. Kottke and J. Lehmann (Eds.), *Krusen's handbook of physical medicine and rehabilitation* (pp. 108–124). 4th ed. Philadelphia: W.B. Saunders.

Lorig, K., Mazonson, P., and Holman, R. (1993). Evidence suggesting that health education for self-management in patients with chronic arthritis has sustained health benefits while reducing costs. *Arthritis and Rheumatism, 36*(4), 439–446.

Massery, M., and Baldwin, B. (1998). *Shoulders and breathing: More linked than you think.* Presentation at the American Physical Therapy Association Combined Sections meeting, Boston, MA, February.

Meyers, C., and Weitzner, M. (1995). Neurobehavioral functioning and quality of life in patients treated for cancer of the nervous system. *Current Opinion in Oncology, 7*(3), 197–200.

Ostrom, L. (1993). *Creating the ergonomically sound workplace.* San Francisco: Jossey-Bass.

O'Sullivan, S., and Schmitz, T. (1994). *Physical rehabilitation: Assessment and treatment.* 3rd ed. Philadelphia: F.A. Davis.

Pagliarulo, M., Waters, R., and Hislop, H. (1979). Energy cost of walking of below knee amputees having no vascular disease. *Physical Therapy, 59,* 538–543.

Pavol, M., Meyers, C., Rexer, J., Valentine, A., Mattis, P., Talpaz, M. (1995). Patterns of neurobehavioral deficits associated with interferon alpha therapy for leukemia. *Neurology 45*(4), 947–950.

Pedretti, L., and Zoltan, B. (1990). *Occupational therapy: Practice skills for physical dysfunction.* 3rd ed. St. Louis: C.V. Mosby.

Rasch, P., and Burke, R. (1971). *Kinesiology and applied anatomy: The science of human movement.* 4th ed. Philadelphia: Lea & Febiger.

Trombly, C., and Scott, A. (1977). *Occupational therapy for physical dysfunction.* Baltimore: Williams & Wilkins.

Vogelzang, N. J., Breitbart, W., Cella, D., Curt, G. A., Groopman, J. E., and Horning, S. J. (1997). Patient, caregiver, and oncologist perceptions of cancer-related fatigue: Results of a tripart assessment survey. *Seminars in Hematology, 34,* 4–12.

Waters, R., Hislop, H., Perry, J., Thomas, L., and Campbell, J. (1983). Comparative cost of walking in young and old. *Journal of Orthopedic Research, 1,* 73–76.

Weiss, R., and Karpovich P., (1947). Energy cost for convalescents. *Archives of Physical Medicine, 28,* 447–454.

Winningham, M. L., Nail, L. M., Barton-Burke, M. B., Brophy, L., Cimprich, B., Jones, L. S., Pickard-Holley, S., Rhodes, V., St. Pierre, B., Beck, S., Glass, E. C., Mock, V. L., Mooney, K. H., and Piper, B. (1994). Fatigue and the cancer experience: The state of the knowledge. *Oncology Nursing Forum, 23*(1), 23–36.

Winter, D., Patla, A., Frank, J., and Walt, S. (1990). Biomechanical walking pattern changes in the fit and healthy elderly. *Physical Therapy, 70,* 340–355.

World Health Organization. (1980). *International classification of impairments, disabilities, and handicaps: A manual of classification relating to the consequences of disease.* Geneva: World Health Organization.

Resources

American College of Sports Medicine (1976). *Guidelines for graded exercise testing and exercise prescription.* Philadelphia: Lea & Febiger.

Astrand, P. O. (1992). J. B. Wolffe Memorial Lecture: Why exercise. *Medicine and Science in Sports and Exercise, 24,* 153–162.

Astrand, P. O., and Rodahl, K. (1977). *Textbook of work physiology.* 2nd ed. New York: McGraw-Hill.

Barry, M. A., Purser J., Hazleman R., McClean, A., and Hazleman, B. (1994). Effect of energy conservation and joint protection education in rheumatoid arthritis. *British Journal of Rheumatology, 33,* 1171–1174.

Basmajian, J. (1990). Crutch and cane exercises and use. In J. Basmajian and S. Wolf (Eds.), *Therapeutic exercise,* (pp. 125–138). 5th ed. Baltimore: Williams & Wilkins.

Berlly, M., Strauser, W., and Hall, K. (1991). Fatigue in post-polio syndrome. *Archives of Physical Medicine and Rehabilitation, 72,* 115–118.

Chavalitskulchai, P., and Houshang, S. (1991). Musculoskeletal discomfort and feelings of fatigue among female professional workers: The need for ergonomics consideration. *Journal of Human Ergology, 20,* 257–264.

Christiansen, C. (Ed.) (1994). *Ways of living: Self care strategies for special needs.* Rockville, MD: American Occupational Therapy Association.

Dean, E., and Ross, J. (1991). Effect of modified aerobic training on movement energetics in polio survivors. *Orthopedics, 14,* 1243–1246.

Hicks, J. (1990). Exercise for cancer patients. In J. Basmajian and S. Wolf, (Eds.), *Therapeutic exercise,* (pp. 351–370). 5th ed. Baltimore: Williams & Wilkins.

Otis, J., Lane, J., and Kroll, M. (1985). Energy cost during gait in osteosarcoma patients after resection and knee replacement and after above the knee amputation. *Journal of Bone and Joint Surgery [American], 67,* 606–611.

Romsaas, E., and Rosa, S. A. (1985). Occupational therapy intervention for cancer patients with metastatic disease. *American Journal of Occupational Therapy, 39*(2), 79–83.

Stewart, A., Hays, R., Wells, K., Rogers, W., Spritzer, K., and Greenfield, S. (1994). Long term functioning and well being outcomes associated with physical activity and exercise in patients with chronic conditions in the medical outcomes study. *Journal of Clinical Epidemiology, 47,* 719–730.

Vallbona, C. (1982). Bodily responses to immobilization. In F. Kottke, G. Stillwell, and J. Lehmann (Eds.), *Krusen's handbook of physical medicine and rehabilitation* (pp. 963–976). 3rd ed. Philadelphia: W.B. Saunders.

Waters, R., Campbell, J., and Perry, J. (1987). Energy cost of three point ambulation in fracture patients. *Journal of Orthopedic Trauma, 1,* 170–173.

Woodward, C., Ucovich, R., Perry, J., and Walker, J. (1985). Rising from a chair: Influence of age and chair design. *Physical Therapy, 65,* 22–26.

Ylvisaker, M., and Feeney, T. (1998). Integrating functional approaches to cognition, communication and behavior after TBI. *Brain Injury Source, 2*(3), 12–16, 48–49.

Young, G. (1991). Energy conservation, occupational therapy, and the treatment of post-polio sequelae. *Orthopedics, 14,* 1233–1239.

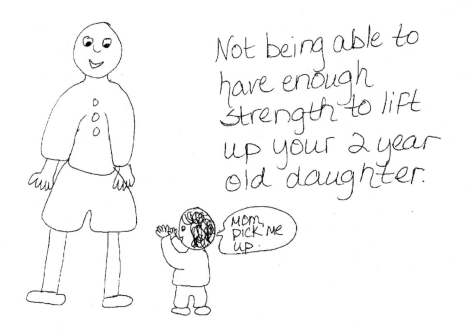

Brenda Heil, 33 years old, 9-year survivor

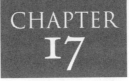

Cognitive Deficits

Christina A. Meyers
As interviewed by
Maryl L. Winningham

You know why you don't understand anything? You don't ask the right questions. Or you ask questions in front of my family when I don't feel free to answer. Or you put words in my mouth. You just don't understand—you don't have a clue. And you know what? I don't think you want to know. Knowing means sitting down and listening to me and listening takes time. I think you're afraid of what you might hear.

Breast cancer survivor about her fatigue

Background

There has been a great deal of difficulty in achieving even a basic understanding of issues related to cancer-related fatigue (CRF) and cognitive impairment. While there are not many answers, this interview with Christina A. Meyers may provide some ideas to help us formulate the questions in a more meaningful way.

Dr. Winningham: Dr. Meyers, can you explain what an oncology neuropsychologist is?

Dr. Meyers: An oncology neuropsychologist has a Ph.D. in clinical psychology with specialty training in neuropsychology who specializes in working with cancer patients. Board certification means someone has passed a specialty exam by the American Board of Professional Psychology (ABPP) with a diploma in clinical neuropsychology.

Dr. Winningham: What do oncology neuropsychologists do?

Dr. Meyers: They practice in an oncology setting and do neuropsychological assessments, testing, therapy, and other interventions. Some are engaged in research on cognitive and neurobehavioral problems in cancer patients; others conduct therapy.

Dr. Winningham: Do you do research or therapy?

Dr. Meyers: My main focus is research, but I also do some therapy. We do a lot of self-hypnosis and relaxation therapy for pain and other types of symptom management.

Dr. Winningham: There is a lot of hype today about self-hypnosis, imagery, and relaxation therapy. In your opinion, and based on your experience, do you think they work?

Dr. Meyers: Well, the technique seems to work best with people who have a high sense of control, people who are self-directed and know what they want. It seems to help reduce the noxiousness of chronic pain, for instance, but it doesn't usually obliterate it. That's one of the problems: People are sometimes disappointed and angry when pain doesn't disappear 100%. They may have unrealistic expectations. The key to living with chronic pain is adaptation, not trying to find some magic that will make it go away. It would be nice, but that probably won't happen. We have to be careful we do not raise unreasonable expectations.

Visualization is another highly promoted technique, but there is not a shred of evidence that it helps control cancer either. People often come to us because they have heard about this magic technique in a book and they have high hopes of a cure. There is no magic; there is no panacea.

Dr. Winningham: The self-help books say a lot of positive things about self-hypnosis and relaxation therapy, about visualization. Is there a downside?

Dr. Meyers: People for whom it could be hazardous either do not understand how the techniques work or have a fear or avoidance of things that might mean overwhelming loss of control. This is usually because they have experienced a traumatizing loss of control at some time in their past. Fortunately, they tend to self-select away from it; in other words, they avoid it or find some excuse not to participate. We should respect that and not try to force them into participation. They have a sense of what is best for them.

About the Contributor

Christina A. Meyers specializes in oncology neuropsychology. She has her PhD in clinical neuropsychology from the University of Houston and is board certified in clinical neuropsychology by the American Board of Professional Psychology. Early educational experiences in biology and psychology contributed to her fascination with how the brain works. She found her experience working as a graduate student in the psychology service with Muriel D. Lezak of the Veterans Administration Medical Center (VAMC) in Portland, Oregon, to have been one of the most formative experiences of her career. At the VAMC, she was exposed to a broader range of neuropsychological problems–head injuries, war wounds, long-term substance abuse–than could be gathered in many years of experience elsewhere.

Dr. Winningham: How about people who have dissociative disorders (i.e., posttraumatic stress disorder or dissociative identity disorder)? Are these techniques safe for them?

Dr. Meyers: That's a good question. Probably some of these patients are the very ones already identified in the last question. With dissociative disorders, there is often a psychiatric history already. These folks are highly vulnerable. Wherever there is a history of something like this, or other psychiatric problems, or substance abuse, there should be a referral for appropriate psychiatric evaluation and treatment.

Dr. Winningham: Cognitive fatigue is a common complaint among patients in general–the "I feel my mind is in a fog" feeling. Can these techniques you mentioned earlier, self-hypnosis and relaxation, also be used for cognitive fatigue?

Dr. Meyers: It's worth trying. Some people benefit from learning relaxation techniques as a means of calming their mind. It may be diversionary.

Dr. Winningham: Can we change the subject? Differentiating between impairment, disability, and handicap presents a special problem in our medicolegal system. Cognitive fatigue is invisible. I know several people undergoing treatment who lost jobs because they couldn't focus. They were high-functioning individuals with demanding jobs. The mental fatigue was more threatening to them than the physical fatigue. They were at a loss how to explain or manage this. It was very humiliating. I know a number of individuals who have lost jobs or suffered broken families because they did not know what was happening to them or why they were behaving the way they did.

Cancer patients often report they have a cognitive problem that is short term or temporary. There may be many temporally related problems; yet, these patients don't seem to qualify for disability help, are rarely viewed in terms of having a legitimate disability or handicap, and are not likely to evoke sympathy. People may appear to be irresponsible and irritable. It may help to warn them about this fatigue and let them know that with most

Neuropsychologists who specialize in oncology are rare. Most psychologists in cancer centers do therapy. She says she "fell into" working at M. D. Anderson: They had a new department opening up and the department chair wanted a neuropsychologist. She is currently considered one of the national leaders in examining the effects of pharmacological agents on cognitive fatigue and in exploring means of rehabilitating cancer patients with cognitive deficits. What she shares with us is remarkable and, in places, unexpected. We knew she had important things to share, but the only way to pin her down was by doing a telephone interview. That's how this chapter was written.

therapies, they will recover. Unfortunately, the damage–the impaired relationships or lost employment–may be irreparable. What I find remarkable is that people often don't even know what to call this–this thing that has happened to them. There are no words that adequately describe the experience. No wonder they are bewildered!

There are the World Health Organization classifications of impairment, disability, and handicap. These classifications are important because of their medicolegal significance, yet I have rarely seen these words used with reference to CRF. Could you please clarify CRF in the context of these definitions? For instance, fatigue, regardless of the definition, is a commonly reported aspect of cognitive impairment. What is cognitive impairment? How do you see it expressed in cancer patients? What is characteristic of short-term impairment versus long-term impairment? Which types of individuals can be reassured that their cognitive abilities will recover? What populations are particularly vulnerable?

Dr. Meyers: This may sound simplistic, but with respect to *impairment,* "dysfunction of the brain or thought processes" for whatever reason is probably the most straightforward definition. The expression, the way it manifests itself, depends on the cancer, the treatment, and the uniqueness of the individual.

Patients on biotherapy usually get better, but it is important to consider that this phenomenon also can affect mood. Interferon produces organic depression. This is not just limited to cancer patients; it is also seen in patients being treated for hepatitis. For example, consider some of the profound changes that are taking place in the body where there are so many biochemical interactions: Interferon induces changes in the cytokines. Interleukin-1 and tumor necrosis factor are toxic to the brain. There is an increase in functioning in the stress cascade: With increased cortisol you get a disturbance in the hypothalamic-pituitary axis (HPA). All this has an effect on mood states. Not only should mood state be monitored, but also periodic cognitive assessments should be made.

Treatment-related cognitive effects, such as occur with radiation and interferon, exhibit as a slowing in mental processing. Patients often describe it as "I feel like I'm in a fog," "I can't think as sharply," "I can't get motivated," "I just don't seem to care," "I poop out fast." It is descriptive of a general perceived inefficiency compared with their usual expectations. They can definitely differentiate between mental and physical fatigue phenomena. These are some of the same characteristics you would find with postconcussion syndrome. There is a difference between inefficiency or slowing of brain functioning and actually having a hole or gap in memory or abilities. Regardless, any time you have to make adjustments in functioning or in how you are interacting with life, you are likely to experience unusual fatigue.

You know, it's unfortunate, but patients are often stuck with long-term cognitive deficits, emotional struggles, and the resulting exhaustion from trying to negotiate everyday life. It adds to their burden when they have to fight a health care system to try to get the care they need, when that system doesn't believe they have a problem. There is not much long-term follow-up. They're just stuck. These are not the glowing outcomes the health care system likes. Of course, the most obvious are those with injury such as those with a primary or metastatic brain tumor. How it is expressed, or how severely, depends on the location. Biotherapy can also produce permanent changes.

Obviously, anatomical damage from tumors is permanent, but some functional recovery may occur even in the presence of anatomical lesions. Remember, the treatment also harms surrounding normal tissue. With brain tumors, you find focal neurological symptoms, language disorders, or spatial disorders. It all depends on the size of the lesion and where it is.

Now back to the problems of disability and handicap. It all depends on patients, what they normally do, and their occupation. High-functioning people are hit hardest. Not only do people expect more of them, but they expect more of themselves. After all, they look okay, but they can't do what they normally do. Often, they don't even know why because no one has ever explained it to them.

Dr. Winningham: You spoke of similarities with the postconcussion syndrome. Do cancer patients also get the severe headaches and irritability you might find with postconcussion syndrome?

Dr. Meyers: Well, you get irritability, overall aching, and miserable flu-like symptoms—including joint pain—with interferon. In general, headache is not a major complaint.

Dr. Winningham: How difficult is it to get a "quick and dirty" or "eyeball" clinical assessment of this? With excitement such as patients often experience in the presence of their physician, are they likely to look better than they are, worse than they are, or present realistically?

Dr. Meyers: With excitement, they may appear better than they are. In addition, they may be unwilling to complain in the cancer setting because they don't want to go off a drug that may be effective against their cancer. Often cancer clinicians are not aware of other options.

Treatment-related cognitive effects, such as occur with radiation and interferon, exhibit as a slowing in mental processing. Patients often describe it as "I feel like I'm in a fog," "I can't think as sharply," "I can't get motivated," "I just don't seem to care," "I poop out fast." It is descriptive of a general perceived inefficiency compared with their usual expectations. They can definitely differentiate between mental and physical fatigue phenomena. These are some of the same characteristics you would find with postconcussion syndrome. There is a difference between inefficiency or slowing of brain functioning, and actually having a hole or gap in memory or abilities. Regardless, any time you have to make adjustments in functioning or in how you are interacting with life, you are likely to experience unusual fatigue.

With forced performance, however, they may become agitated and fall apart, depending on the environment and the degree of perceived threat. Again, they may exhibit characteristics such as inability to do multiple tasks, slowed cognitive processing, and rapid fatigue with mental tasks. There is an *apathy syndrome* that is quite separate from a depressive mood. Again, there is no doubt that physical fatigue and cognitive fatigue are perceived by patients to be very different phenomena.

Before we go back to the disability and handicap issue, I would like to talk about some of the clinical phenomena I am currently seeing that relate to this. I am often seeing well-educated, highly functional professional people. Interferon alfa treatment in leukemia may go on for as long as ten years. There is a need for support systems and accommodations in the workplace. Patients with chronic myelogenous leukemia (CML) tend to be older and, prior to the development of their disease, functional. As with other types of cancer, a select number of them receive bone marrow transplants (BMTs). With BMT, all the problems come together: the interventricular therapies can make them deathly sick. With the total body irradiation, immunocompromised state, high-dose chemotherapy, repeated complications, and profound lifestyle alterations, we are now seeing long-term effects we never anticipated.

Dr. Winningham: Like what?

Dr. Meyers: Even a few years ago, people who developed viral encephalitis died. Now they are living, but they are demonstrating complete anterograde amnesia. This is because in viral attacks, the virus has the tendency to go to the temporal lobes. They are emotionally aware, characteristically irritable, and angry. Their insight is damaged and variable. They are often professionals or used to have their own business. It seems the last place problems show up is in the brain. With these individuals, the reasoning may be intact, their prior education and training is intact, but they have no memory from several weeks after the onset of the viral encephalitis.

Dr. Winningham: Can you elaborate on what that means for patients and families?

Dr. Meyers: Let me explain it like this. Beginning at a point several weeks after their acute episode, these patients become stuck in time, as it were. They require full-time supervision; many end up in nursing homes. They can't dress themselves because they can't figure out the sleeve from the pant leg. They can still drive a car because that is a skill, but they would have no idea where they are or where they are going from one moment to the next, so they wouldn't be safe. They could read the same magazine over and over and not remember having just read it. They can learn new skills, but wouldn't remember how they learned them or be able to rationalize how to apply them. They have no memory for

---

The KGB used to call on Friday and say, "You must come down to the police station Monday morning. We have some questions for you." I panicked all weekend while I racked my brain trying to figure out what they might want. Had my wife betrayed me? One of my children? My neighbor? My best friend? I couldn't sleep, I couldn't eat, I developed bleeding ulcers. I packed a small bag of supplies to take along. Who knew when I would ever return home. When I finally arrived on Monday morning, I would have to wait in a line for several hours to be seen. Finally, I would get to the desk. The officer would look in his book. "No, no, your name isn't here. It must have been a mistake, comrade." This happened for many years until I had no more will to fight. You don't have to put a mark on a man to torture him.

Political dissident, Moscow, 1967

life episodes. You can imagine the disastrous social and financial problems this presents for families!

The problem is in the survival. I can't overestimate this. Many of these people were highly functioning professionals. Externally, they may appear quite normal. They are left with devastating impairments and we have no idea what to do about this. There are no interventions. The health care system is not prepared to handle any of this, and neither are the families. Because of the high degree in which this affects their everyday life and functioning, they are totally disabled. A detailed assessment will confirm that these problems are very real (Meyers et al, 1994).

Now let's return to the concepts of impairment, disability, and handicap. An impairment becomes a disability when it affects one or more of life's major activities. For example, if fatigue bothers you somewhat, but it isn't a big deal and doesn't really interfere with your life, it's an impairment. It's not normal, but it is not a hindrance. Now, if fatigue impairs your ability to focus at work or limits your ability to engage in social activities, it becomes a disability. If the employee can perform the essentials of the job with "reasonable accommodations," according to the Americans with Disabilities Act, the employee may be able to keep on working. A nap, for instance, or a less distracting environment may help. I frequently help patients develop guidelines for this. If the person is unable to work, even with accommodations, they may be candidates for disability. This is difficult, however, because in the disability system, physicians do not know how to handle this kind of problem, this invisible problem.

Dr. Winningham: In my experience, the disability system is difficult enough to negotiate, let alone when you're dealing with a cognitive/fatigue problem. There appears to be no sympathy or understanding for something like this. So how do you assess or test for cognitive impairment?

Dr. Meyers: Tests typically include formal psychometrically tested assessments for memory, word recognition over time, spatial awareness (e.g., block construction, manual manipulation tests)–there is a whole battery of tests. It is important to emphasize that the person may have a significant cognitive deficit that will *not* show up on various scans or traditional medical diagnostic tests. The neuropsychological tests, however, may be more sensitive. Again, whether an impairment exists depends on what the person normally does.

Unfortunately, physicians have generally been taught that if they can't see the problem on a medical exam or reflected in laboratory tests, it's not a real problem. If patients are talking and walking, they are considered a medical or surgical success. You often hear about "eloquent" and "noneloquent" parts of the brain, as if parts of the brain were superfluous! The outcome of this kind of thinking and practice has been disastrous for patients and families. Patients are denied resources and benefits they need. They may even be inappropriately labeled as malingering or lazy. What is interesting is that neurosurgeons seem to understand these issues least! They are used to dealing with definitive lesions. If they don't see them, they must not exist! It inappropriately conveys the message that nothing is wrong when there is something wrong.

Dr. Winningham: This reflects what Tricia Corbett relates in Chapter 23. In fact, in her case, she still has a very obvious abnormal brain scan, but tested very well on the neuro-psychological tests. Obviously, we have not even begun to ask the right questions about this, let alone find answers. But I interrupted you—go ahead.

Dr. Meyers: I have had breast cancer patients on chemotherapy tell me they became so tired and confused they threw bills in the corner and forgot them because they couldn't deal with them. They are working harder than ever in their lives and no one is acknowledging it. They complain they are forgetting things, but others laugh it off saying, "Yea, we're all getting older." They may exhibit bad judgment and show deficits in functioning that are unpredictable and quite diverse. This may lead to loss of employment and health care benefits. Not only are the patients bewildered, but families are frustrated and health care providers may consider complaining patients to be a pain. So the blame game continues. And third-party payers aren't about to pay for helping someone who looks lazy or crazy. There is a broad range of symptom dismissal by professionals.

Dr. Winningham: When I explain to patients about fatigue—including the mental aspects—I often hear patients say, "You mean this is real? I thought I was going crazy!" What simple signs of temporary cognitive impairment might patients notice in their everyday activities that will improve with time?

Dr. Meyers: Ability to concentrate, short-term memory, less irritability, normalized sleeping patterns, and ability to handle money and appointments (time) are some of the things that seem to recover with time.

Dr. Winningham: Earlier, you spoke about the types of conditions that can be permanent and irreversible. Is there anything, right now, that can help in terms of retraining and rehabilitation?

Dr. Meyers: There are several possibilities:

1. In 1997 we published a study (Sherer, Meyers, and Bergloff, 1997) where we tried adapting a posttraumatic brain injury program to cancer patients with brain tumors. Note that the word *adapting* is important here. We tried to identify what specific components of this kind of program would be useful. We found there is potential for success in a well-designed program, but it must be in the context of the type of cancer. We did a survey: Most rehabilitation centers see only about five cancer patients per year, and they treat them traditionally, like head trauma and stroke patients. In addition, there are several problems. Many rehabilitation centers are afraid to take cancer patients. And, most cancer specialists don't think to refer

their patients. Don't forget, survival from these kinds of cancers is relatively new. For this reason, it is difficult to conduct good clinical trials.

In adapting a posttraumatic brain injury program for cancer patients, it is essential to use careful preliminary testing to select the patients wisely and to establish appropriate goals. Actually, given targeted interventions, cancer patients do better than many other patient populations receiving rehabilitation. There is potential that a well-done head injury program can be successful for cancer centers. Unfortunately, since most cancer centers don't see more than a half a dozen patients like this per year, it is difficult to gather a lot of information and just as difficult to teach students and staff in these techniques. There would be tremendous benefit in having an electronically based rehabilitation registry.

2. We have examined the potential for using pharmacological interventions to improve the slowed cognitive processing associated with brain injury, interferon, and the like. We just published an article on the use of methylphenidate (Ritalin) (Meyers et al, 1998). Methylphenidate therapy improved cognition, mood, and function in a group of brain tumor patients. It seemed to work especially well on patients who had received brain irradiation. There was a dramatic improvement. The drug has a fast half-life so if patients develop difficulties, you can take them off it immediately. The benefit is also immediately evident: You can vary the doses according to the individual and see a rapid response. It seemed to work at all ends of the spectrum from patients with mild to those with severe limitations. This was just a beginning. We need to examine other drugs, as well.

Dr. Winningham: I have heard some people suggest there is abuse potential for methylphenidate. It is being prescribed as an off-label use to other groups of cancer patients.

Dr. Meyers: Well, it is not abuse if it is the appropriate use of the drug, and if it's been shown to be safe. I think of it as being equivalent to the potential for abuse of opioids for pain management in cancer patients. If they need it, it's indicated and appropriate, and it can help normalize life. Period. However, it soon became obvious to us that the positive effects of methylphenidate were not universal. For instance, we also tried using it in patients suffering from neurocognitive slowing from interferon treatment and got some paradoxical reactions. In this case, the results were not good, and we stopped the clinical trial after fewer than ten patients. We have to be cautious about generalizing from one group to others.

Dr. Winningham: Did you ever publish these findings?

Dr. Meyers: No; editors usually don't want to hear about negative outcomes on small numbers of subjects.

Dr. Winningham: I know that is true; however, this is really valuable information—perhaps worth at least a letter to the editor of an oncology or medical journal. It can serve as a warning that we need to test these drugs on specific groups of patients before we make broad assumptions and sweeping generalizations.

There is little research on the significance of cognitive issues on quality of life in cancer. In this chapter, it is obvious that it is a big problem. Patricia Buchsel, who contributed to Chapter 8 in this book, told me she knows of patients demanding methylphenidate or other drugs from their physicians based on palliation and quality of life issues. They are desperate and willing to take the risk because they find the fatigue so distressing. I find this a little alarming, particularly in view of what you just shared. Perhaps I am overreacting. I can understand the desire of clinicians to respond to the desperation of their patients. Currently, the National Cancer Institute's (NCI's) Physician's Data Query (PDQ) lists recommended doses of psychotropic medications for symptom relief, and methylphenidate is among them. What are your thoughts on this? (The current NCI-PDQ recommendations related to this are discussed in Chapter 11.)

Dr. Meyers: There is, as yet, no rationale behind the use or recommendations for use of any pharmacological agent for cognitive issues in other populations. When I say "rationale," I mean based on double-blind clinical trials. That's different from a physician individually prescribing something based on clinical judgment. Without controlled clinical trials to examine these issues, we have to be very careful. As I pointed out earlier, sometimes we may get paradoxical effects. A number of centers are doing prophylactic antidepressant therapy, but we'll have to wait to see what the results are. Drugs are not without side effects and we have no idea what the interactive effects are between these drugs, drugs for other conditions patients may have, and drugs being used to treat the cancer. Again, we have to be very careful about generalizing from one study on one group of patients to all people with cancer.

Dr. Winningham: Earlier you referred to the research article you published in 1997 in which you and your colleagues tried applying postacute brain injury rehabilitation to brain tumor survivors (Sherer, Meyers, and Bergloff, 1997). You talked about the generally bleak survival potential with respect to independent functioning. I really appreciated how you presented individualized data on each patient so the reader could evaluate individual history, status, and goals. I think the way you categorized status could serve as a model for other studies. Could you share a brief review of what techniques you applied that were helpful?

Dr. Meyers: Our study had 13 patients, all of whom had had surgery and radiation therapy; in addition, all but one had chemotherapy. In postacute brain injury, cognitive, behavioral, affective, and social functioning are usually affected to some degree. In addition, each person has individual differences depending on the location of the injury, so individualization of the rehabilitation intervention is critical. Therapy was provided by psychologists, speech-language pathologists, occupational therapists, and vocational specialists. The use of a daily organizer to help keep track of time, particularly for pill taking and to support memory tasks, was critical. Therapy was focused toward the level of restored functioning that was desired. Sometimes this involved help in preparing resumes, evaluating appropriate vocational potential, and organizing a job search. The therapist would visit the job site and evaluate it for appropriateness and need for compensation strategies, and recommend alterations in site or job duties required to ensure optimal performance. Periodic follow-up contacts were made to ensure maintenance of therapeutic gain.

Dr. Winningham: I especially noted your opinion that with cognitive improvement, by whatever mechanism, there appeared to be an improvement in mood and perception of quality of life.

Dr. Meyers: Yes. The mechanism for this is unknown, just as with postacute head injury, but it does appear to happen. I want to emphasize that this was a pilot study—we need to find out much more about this.

Dr. Winningham: What do you see for the future?

Dr. Meyers: We are desperately in need of well-designed, strategic, step-by-step, controlled intervention clinical trials. Then, based on these outcomes, we need to develop decision trees based on symptoms as well as the results of tests. We need pharmacological as well as behavioral rehabilitation interventions. Right now, we don't even know where to start. As mentioned earlier, my colleagues and I published an article where we demonstrated that postacute brain injury rehabilitation programs may be *modified* to serve patients with primary malignant brain tumors (Sherer, Meyers, and Bergloff, 1997). The data indicated this to be a cost-effective intervention. That was only a beginning, but it showed promise. We need an influx of qualified professionals who can work in this field. There aren't nearly enough, and there is very little funding. This area of study hasn't been taken seriously.

Dr. Winningham: It's at least helpful for us to start becoming more aware of the problems. Perhaps we can start being more proactive in searching for solutions. What suggestions would you make to patients and families who have to live with this?

Dr. Meyers: To patients I would suggest: Learn what you've got, be your own advocate, and ask for what you need. The type of help you need probably is not available on a routine basis. The more knowledge you can acquire, the better. Reimbursement and disability issues in fatigue and cognitive impairment are not clear and are not easy to access. You have to make a big case that the person is medically stable. Although patients who have had a cerebrovascular accident (stroke) often don't live as long as cancer patients, reimbursement and rehabilitation follow-up are more routine. We have to make the case that rehabilitation in cancer is cost-effective. Right now, we don't have parameters to go by. It's pretty difficult to fight for these things when patients are already suffering from the everyday exhaustion resulting from trying to adapt to cognitive deficits.

To families I would say: Get support for yourselves. The caregiver or caregivers are at high risk for burnout. Quality of life is not just an important issue for the person who has cancer, it is also critical for caregivers. That part is often ignored. To the extent that patients are unable, whether from cognitive deficits or fatigue, to advocate for themselves, it is necessary to advocate for them. Ask about support groups and organizations where information and support may be shared.

Dr. Winningham: I think much of what you shared applies to patients with other CRF issues as well, particularly individuals who continue to suffer from long-term fatigue. Thank you for sharing your expertise with us. I hope our readers have learned as much as I have.

References

Meyers, C. A., Weitzner, M., Byrne, K., Valentine, A., Champlin, R. E., and Przepiorka, D. (1994). Evaluation of the neurobehavioral functioning of patients before, during, and after bone marrow transplantation. *Journal of Clinical Oncology, 12,* 820–826.

Meyers, C. A., Weitzner, M. A., Valentine, A. D., and Levin, V. A. (1998). Methylphenidate therapy improves cognition, mood, and function of brain tumor patients. *Journal of Clinical Oncology, 16,* 2522–2527.

Sherer, M., Meyers, C. A., and Bergloff, P. (1997). Efficacy of post acute brain injury rehabilitation for patients with primary brain tumors. *Cancer, 80,* 250–257.

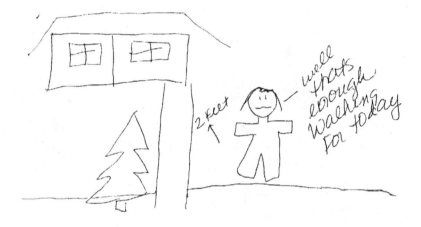

Brenda Heil, 33 years old, 9-year survivor

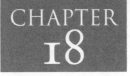

Therapeutic Exercise:
Guidelines and Precautions

Maryl L. Winningham

I like to exercise and keep busy. Every day while recovering from chemo treatments, I would have all these wonderful ideas of how to keep busy. I would get all ready to walk around the block, about a half mile, and some days by the time I got to the end of the driveway, I would just about collapse from exhaustion.

Brenda Heil, 33 years old, 9-year survivor

Background

There is no doubt that diminished activity is, in and of itself, a malignant process that contributes to proportional deterioration of every organ system of the human body (Greenleaf and Kozlowski, 1982; Greenleaf et al, 1982; Luu et al, 1990). This observation dates back to the time of Hippocrates (Chadwick and Mann, 1950); research over the last 50 years has established it beyond a doubt. Remarkably, although Karnofsky and associates noted this problem to be a clinical by-product of cancer treatment as early as 1948 (Karnofsky et al, 1948) and 1949 (Karnofsky and Burchenal, 1949), it was over 30 years before a clinical trial applied the use of therapeutic exercise to a group of cancer patients undergoing chemotherapy treatments.

Energy is the concept most associated with health and well-being (Dixon, Dixon, and Hickey, 1993). Hence, it is logical to propose positive physical as well as psychological benefits from an intervention that mechanistically promotes energetic potential. Rehabilitative exercise is the only intervention with the potential to directly affect the body's ability to combine fuel with oxygen, over a matrix of oxidative enzymes, to enhance energy production. The questions about the use of exercise in people with cancer were: How do you put energy into the body? How do you put energy into cells? How do you maintain the energy for everyday functioning? How do you give people the energy they need so they can do what they

---

Precautionary Note: Information in this chapter is not meant to represent a standard of practice. It is meant to present select, minimal guidelines and recommendations for the safe use of therapeutic, rehabilitative exercise for people with cancer. General health risks, specific cancer- and treatment-related complications, and motivational issues should be taken into account when developing individualized exercise protocols.

need or want in the face of cancer and its treatment? Can you minimize loss? Can you maintain what they have? Can they improve in spite of cancer and treatment? Can you safely apply traditional cardiopulmonary rehabilitation techniques to this population?

Energy cannot be put into cells by incision, by ingestion, or by injections. A certain amount of activity is a homeostatic imperative for maintaining independent organic functioning. Although the biochemical pathways are clear, and the techniques have been established in other populations, there have been several significant barriers to applying therapeutic exercise to cancer patients:

1. *Attitudes.* Through to the mid 1980s, the attitude of health care professionals, patients, and families was that cancer patients needed rest; in fact, complaints of fatigue were met with, "What do you expect? You have cancer. Get more rest!" Attitude still constitutes a major barrier to rehabilitative, energetic exercise. The power of prescriptive therapeutic exercise to affect all dimensions of quality of life has been grossly underestimated.

2. *Understanding metabolic mechanisms.* The metabolic relationships of exercise to rest often are misunderstood. Despite frequent references to "activity-rest," few understand the acute versus chronic biokinetic processes of metabolism with sufficient insight to be able to make prescriptive recommendations and predict associated outcomes. Understanding the dose-response relationship between various elements of the exercise prescription also requires an understanding of the catabolic mechanisms of the stimulus and the anabolic mechanisms of the outcomes.

3. *The problem of treatments.* Standard medical interventions associated with other illnesses work with the body to facilitate systemic health and balance. Nutrients used by genetic mechanisms to support the growth of healthy cells also support the growth of cancerous cells. In contrast, treat-

---

The least little excitement or disturbance–an argument, a disruption by a phone call, or a knock on the door–was enough to keep me awake all night. I would lie awake–waiting–and wanting so desperately to sleep. I was beyond exhaustion. Where was the healthy, vigorous person I once knew? I watched the clock: Midnight, one o'clock, two o'clock...I put off getting up to go to the bathroom as long as I could–I was so exhausted. Finally, I had to. After I washed my hands, I leaned on the sink to recover. I looked up and I saw my face in the mirror: It puzzled me every time. Who was that? Was that me? That couldn't be me. That was an old lady in the mirror. Haggard. A stranger.

I slowly shuffled back to bed and dropped myself down, my heart pounding. The sheets were tangled. I didn't even try to get underneath–I didn't have the energy. I reached over to take my pulse, but it was so fast I couldn't even count it. It was always worse when I was anemic. My heart was skipping beats. I could feel the adrenaline surge just from this little bit of exertion. I tried to take a deep breath, but my chest felt as if there were a dead weight on it. Just breathing was laborious. My arms fell back in exhaustion.

I tried to calm my thoughts. I used to pray, to recite poems, to write poems in my mind to amuse myself, to sing. I couldn't think of anything. Everything seemed too laborious. My mind was flying around. Is this how I am going to meet my Adversary? He seemed to haunt me, to stalk me, to torment me when I needed

ments for cancer work against the body to destroy or control malignant processes. Hence, treatments for malignant cells also affect healthy cells. Untested side effects and interactions of cancer treatments present potential problems that should not be taken lightly.

4. *The need for guidelines, precautions, and protocols.* As mentioned in Chapter 2, the essential question is not whether therapeutic exercise is beneficial for people with cancer; the real point is that *lack* of activity is devastating. The question then became, What kind of exercise (therapeutic activity) would yield the best response, in the shortest amount of time, without harming the individual, and what measures had to be taken to ensure optimal *safety?* In 1981, there were few animal studies (some dating back to early in the century), and there was no national database to help identify exercise-related potential risks and safety problems. There was one final problem to consider: While doing nothing meant leaving many cancer survivors to deterioration, the maxim "first do the patient no harm" had to be the overriding rule.

History of Exercise and Cancer

Few interventions have the potential to address the collective physical, psychological, behavioral, and social problems associated with cancer. Although cardiovascular conditioning began to be a significant component of cardiac rehabilitation in the 1950s, these techniques were not applied to the oncology rehabilitation arsenal until the early 1980s. The actual testing of the efficacy and safety of aerobic exercise in breast cancer patients

---

rest more than anything. Restlessness seemed to overwhelm me. Was this the face of death? Or was it some other enemy? It was as if the memories of the past and fears for the future conspired to mock me. Maybe this was all a nightmare. When would it be over?

I would have given anything for a few minutes of restful sleep. The clock ticked. With horror I could see the faintly breaking rays of day–but then, somewhere I finally drifted off into an exhausted, tormented sleep.

My alarm rang. I awoke with a start. I'd had less than two hours' sleep. I had to quickly shower, clean my port, dress, and go to work. It wasn't much, but it was the only way I could keep any kind of medical insurance. I had no savings to fall back on.

I almost fell asleep three times before I reached work. I couldn't focus. I would have given anything to go lie down. The thought of doing anything filled me with dread.

"How are you doing?" said Doug, over his shoulder, as he passed me on his way to the coffee machine.

"Fine," I answered back in as chipper a tone of voice as I could muster. He wouldn't understand; besides, it would take too much energy to even explain it. If I said fine, at least he would leave me alone.

42-year-old breast cancer survivor, now deceased

receiving chemotherapy was pioneered in 1983 (Winningham, 1983), and involved a comparison group of breast cancer patients as well as normal, healthy women. This study also examined mood states (Profile of Mood States) and the Levinson Locus of Control. Cancer patients who exercised showed a similar physiological response to the exercise stimulus as did healthy women. Since there was no precedence, this study required development of a variety of instruments and techniques to monitor patients' response and medical status. Most significant of these was the Symptom Activity Checklist, which associated symptom occurrence and severity with activity. From this study, and subsequent studies using the Winningham Aerobic Interval Training (WAIT) protocol (1983), evidence began to accumulate that therapeutic aerobic exercise could have a powerfully positive effect on reduction of fatigue and negative mood states, and could promote development of the body's energetic resources. This, in turn, had a positive effect on multiple variables associated with quality of life (MacVicar and Winningham, 1986; Winningham, 1983). As part of ongoing research, a group of master's degree students in the oncology program at Ohio State University's College of Nursing, under the advisement of Mary G. MacVicar and my direction, examined a variety of different aspects of quality of life in response to participation in the exercise program. Much of what is being called "new" now was studied by them a decade ago or more (see Table 18-1). There was a great deal of skepticism about the possibility of exercising cancer patients at this time. To ensure optimal safety, these programs required a protocol with individualized, laboratory-condition monitoring, costly equipment, and supervisory personnel. This work has been described elsewhere (MacVicar, Winningham, and Nickel, 1989; Winningham, 1983). Especially noteworthy in these studies was the use of oxygen uptake during peak exertion to obtain objective measures of energetic capacity. The advantages of these studies, including the tight controls, also limited the generalizability of research results as well as the practical application of this kind of exercise to cancer patients in general. However, they demonstrated that given appropriate guidelines and precautionary screening, cancer patients receiving treatment (usually chemotherapy, sometimes chemotherapy and radiation) could exercise safely. All aspects of quality of life seemed to be positively influenced. Guidelines and precautions for exercising cancer patients have been published elsewhere (Winningham, 1992; Winningham, 1994; Winningham, MacVicar, and Burke, 1986).

The question about the use of exercise in people with cancer was, How do you put energy into cells?

Prescriptive Exercise Versus Recreational Activity Versus Activity

There is a distinction between therapeutic prescriptive exercise, activity in general and nonspecific recreational activity. The development of therapeutic prescriptive exercise, as historically discussed in Chapter 13, was an essential component of the rehabilitation model

Table 18.1	Master's Theses in Cancer and Exercise, Ohio State University College of Nursing, 1984–1988*	

Name	Year Completed	Topic
L. Hartkopf	1984	Participation in exercise and reports of fatigue and weakness in individuals with cancer
S. Ezzone	1985	The relationship between functional capacity and perceived exertion in women with breast cancer
M. Knuth	1985	Effects of aerobic exercise on psychosocial adjustment to illness of women receiving adjuvant chemotherapy for stage II breast cancer
B. Westercamp	1986	The effect of aerobic training on functional capacity and perception of select symptoms in women with breast cancer
D. Henderson	1986	Effect of exercise on frequency of nausea in women with breast cancer
L. Foor	1987	The effects of therapeutic aerobic exercise on nausea in women with breast cancer
P. Luetkemeier	1988	The effects of aerobic training on functional capacity in healthy women and in women with stage II breast cancer receiving adjuvant chemotherapy

* From 1982 through 1984, the data on dissertation and postdoctoral clinical trials were collected by Maryl L. Winningham. From 1984 through 1988, the data were collected on various clinical trials, with Mary G. MacVicar as principal investigator and Maryl L. Winningham as project director.

and was intended to enhance functional capacity (cellular energetic potential) in cancer patients. While relatively few cancer patients qualify for a traditional rehabilitation program, nearly all could benefit from energetic rehabilitation.

Therapeutic prescriptive exercise relates the stimulus of training to the response of predictable functional outcomes. Although nonprescriptive recreational exercise may provide relief, physical challenge, enjoyment, or even a spiritual experience, its outcomes are not clinically predictable, nor is it likely to lead to acceptable standards of practice or third-party reimbursement. There is no way to demonstrate a direct cause-effect, stimulus-response, or process-outcome link. Therapeutic prescriptive activity results in what is known as the "training effect," that is, an improvement in enzymatic functioning at the cellular level in muscles that permits an individual to physically perform in a more efficient manner.

Exercise is a powerful and effective intervention; in fact, it is the most powerful intervention developed to date, with multiple benefits touching nearly every aspect of quality of life. Every powerful intervention carries concomitant risks. Since the mid 1950s, when the therapeutic benefits of exercise began to be widely recognized, there were two trends toward developing safety parameters for exercise research and programs. The formulation of American Heart Association (AHA) guidelines, dominated by cardiologists, followed the medical model and focused on clinical populations. On the other hand, the American College of Sports Medicine (ACSM) developed a more interdisciplinary, diverse, fitness-oriented model with certification standards and published guidelines for the safe conduct of exercise tests, the development of appropriate exercise prescriptions, and therapeutic programs. More recently, the American Association for Cardiovascular and Pulmonary Rehabilitation (AACVPR) has focused on exercise rehabilitation in clinical populations from a multidisciplinary perspective. While AHA guidelines are mentioned in this chapter, they are more limited in scope. ACSM guidelines are widely acknowledged as a minimal standard for safety for research and clinical practice and exercise programs with all individuals. As such, they should also provide a basis for screening, testing, and program development for cancer patients. Although the ACSM does not claim to mandate a "standard of practice," observing ACSM guidelines provides a reasonable and prudent approach to clinical practice or research. All individuals involved in exercise counseling, programs, or research in people with cancer would be wise to familiarize themselves with these standards.

The ACSM has a number of published references. Their most well known is a book, *ACSM's Guidelines for Exercise Testing and Prescription*. This book, now in its fifth edition, features more quantitative clinical data than earlier editions. According to the preface, the purpose of this book is "to present state-of-the-art information in a usable form for both the fitness and clinical exercise professional." The intent is to "limit the book's focus to exercise testing in its broadest sense and exercise prescription in all of its forms" (American College of Sports Medicine, 1995). Additional precautions for cancer patients are based on the premise that cancer patients should also be screened for other preexisting or coexisting limitations from occult or known cardiovascular, pulmonary, or metabolic conditions. In addition, treatment-related conditions or after-effects may place cancer patients of any age group at higher risk than the general population, independent of other risk factors.

The Exercise Prescription

There has been a tendency to use self-paced exercise interventions in research and then to draw conclusions based on outcome measures. This is misguided. How can predictive information be obtained and understood without appropriate monitoring and quantification of the process? The answer is, it can't. Exercise functions as an endogenous drug and stimulates a wide variety of biochemical changes at all levels in the body. As with medications, safe and effective exercise programs for cancer patients should be based on an exercise *prescription*. Unless there is a therapeutic prescription, we are looking at recreational activity, not therapeutic exercise. The conclusions that can be drawn from self-paced programs are far less generalizable than those from prescriptive exercise programs. At this point, the efficacy of exercise for cancer patients in general has been established. What need to be established are (1) the potential for community acceptance of such programs, (2) safety parameters for patients at risk or with special needs, (3) how to take the patients at greatest risk for functional loss and apply space-program science to minimize functional losses during treatment, (4) predictive safety and efficacy of multiple treatment-exercise interactions, and (5) the cost-benefit ratio that would help justify reimbursement for such programs. All of the cancer exercise programs in the United States successfully receiving third-party payer reimbursement with which I am familiar are based on a *traditional, prescriptive, cardiac rehabilitation model.*

Following work by the Ohio State University team, others have taken up the study of various aspects of exercise as rehabilitation in cancer. Victoria Mock and associates (1994), currently of Johns Hopkins Hospital, Baltimore, Maryland, examined the effects of a comprehensive exercise intervention program on multiple outcome measures in breast cancer patients. Bernadine Pinto of the Miriam Hospital, in Providence, Rhode Island, is focusing on certain psychological aspects of patient responses to exercise (Pinto et al, in press). A research team in Alberta, Canada has conducted several studies examining community cancer-exercise program participation (Courneya and Friedenreich, 1997; Fredenreich and Courneya, 1996; Fredenreich et al, 1998). Fernando Dimeo, in Germany, a sports medicine specialist doing impressive work on higher-risk patients, is examining safety as well as outcome issues using biological markers in cancer patients (Dimeo et al 1997a; Dimeo et al 1997b; Dimeo Rumberger and Keul, 1998). Exercise as an intervention in cancer patients is also being investigated in Korea, Sweden, and Norway, as well as other countries.

Energy cannot be put into cells by incision, by ingestion, or by injections.

Research on reimbursement issues is lacking but essential if people are going to gain access to a much broader scope of oncology rehabilitation. Cardiac rehabilitation facilities in North America sit empty for hours a day when they could be available for cancer patients. These are missed opportunities! There also is a need for the few, well-credentialed professionals who currently are leaders in developing energetic exercise training to "cross train" exercise physiologists, physical therapists, nurses, and physicians in prescriptive exercise rehabilitation oncology techniques.

One of the biggest problems from the beginning has been the difficulty anticipating the possible interactive or negative effects of cancer treatments. This problem does not exist to the same extent in other patient populations. In 1982, I was shocked to discover that cancer drugs underwent neither human nor animal studies on the interactive effects of cancer treatment and exercise. With other chronic illnesses, the Food and Drug Administration requires extensive drug testing that includes exercise effects. Well-intended health professionals who would never tell a diabetic "take some insulin" think nothing of telling patients to "get some exercise." The aerobic/endurance exercise prescription must specify mode, intensity, frequency, duration, and rate of progression (Heyward, 1991). In addition to guidelines developed by the AHA, ACSM, and AACVPR, exercise prescriptions for cancer patients must take into account the effects of the cancer, the stage of disease, and its treatment protocols (Winningham, 1994).

The following paragraphs provide an explanation of exercise prescription as it applies to people with cancer. For more details, refer to the chapter by Winningham (1994) in Goldberg and Elliot's book, *Exercise for Prevention and Treatment of Illness*. This book is particularly useful because it includes exercise issues pertinent to other disease states, conditions that may also account for comorbidity in cancer patients.

There are six basic considerations in designing an exercise prescription. Each has to be tailored to the individual for optimal benefit and to minimize potential harm.

1. *Status of the patient.* It is essential to determine the background of the patient in terms of common risk factors. Cancer does not preclude heart disease. Please refer to ACSM resources for a discussion of screening issues. Occasionally, one discovers long-term, undiagnosed neurological, cardiac, or pulmonary disorders that probably came from earlier cancer treatment. In my experience, I found patients who had a history of uncontrolled diabetes, heart failure, thyroid disease, hypertension, and valvular disease for which special care was required. Yet, their charts in the oncology clinic said nothing about these conditions. It would be foolhardy as well as unsafe to place such individuals in an unmonitored exercise program; yet, one frequently hears well-meaning health care professionals tell patients to get some exercise with no guidelines.

   Specific screening should include the following:
   a. Perform a background check for risk factors, cardiovascular and pulmonary disease, and family history of heart disease or sudden death.
   b. Get individual clearance by the physician most responsible for the treatment.
   c. Obtain knowledge of the effects and side effects of the treatment protocols.
   d. Obtain knowledge of the effects of exercise protocols in general.
   e. Determine which of the exercise protocols would be best for that individual.
   f. Consider use of a Prescriptive Rehabilitative Energy Promotion (PREP) protocol such as the WAIT (Winningham, 1983) or a basic walking program. Any program should be used and developed based on knowledge of functioning and recovery of all three energy systems (adenosine triphosphate-phosphocreatine (ATP-PC), lactic acid, and aerobic) as well as the conditioning status of the patient.
   g. Determine what monitoring requirements are necessary for the safe conduct of the program. Telephone calls can be effective for monitoring as well as motivators in walking programs.
   h. Use monitoring instruments specific to the task. In home programs, a journal of heart rate and perceived exertion response can be kept. Heart rate can be monitored using an inexpensive watch with a second hand.
   i. Monitor regularly for changes in clinical status, especially acute changes such as dehydration, anemia, nutritional and fluid deficiencies, and damage in neurological, cardiac, and pulmonary systems.

j. To monitor clinical symptom status, the Symptom Activity Checklist (Winningham, 1983, 1993) is an excellent instrument. While most symptom checklists were developed for data collection, this was developed with the primary objectives of clinical validity, usefulness, and safety.

k. Especially monitor for changes in exercise tolerance and fatigability.

l. Make patients aware of contraindications to unsupervised exercise:
   - bone or joint pain of recent origin
   - muscular weakness of recent onset
   - intravenous chemotherapy
   - onset of nausea during exercise (may be a sign of dehydration)
   - sudden shortness of breath
   - severe nausea, vomiting, or diarrhea during previous 24 hours
   - unusual fatigability
   - fever or chilling
   - cachexia

In addition, patients should be warned about exercising during periods of acute anemia, low platelet count, or low absolute granulocyte count. *Drinking fluids* should be encouraged prior to, during, and after exercise.

2. *Type or mode of exercise.* This refers to the type of activity and specifies an activity that is rhythmic and repetitive in nature and involves large muscle groups. Obviously gum chewing, horseback riding, and bowling do not qualify. The best exercise to use for community, unmonitored programs is walking. *Walking* is easy, is the mainstay of activities of daily living, is not associated with special costs, and can be pursued under a variety of conditions. Those who do not live in safe neighborhoods can consider a group program in an unused part of a park or parking garage. Malls are also good places to exercise, particularly in the morning. Malls often open their doors early so people can exercise before the crowds arrive. With walking, one can easily monitor response and modulate activity accordingly. Bicycling is also a good sport; however, one should be aware of the risk of falls when bruising is a risk. In addition, swimming should be avoided where there is potential for slips at the poolside and risk of opportunistic infection from fungi. Low-impact types of exercise are best. Additional advantages to a home-based walking program include flexibility in scheduling, convenience, lower risk, and lower cost.

3. *Intensity.* This refers to the degree of exertion and is usually monitored by heart rate. Of all the variables involved in the exercise prescription, intensity probably is the most critical and the least understood. High intensity is not necessary for exercise to be beneficial; on the contrary, it is probably healthier to engage in moderate-intensity exercise. A heart rate range as low as 50% to 60% of maximum yields benefits over time; in addition, participants in lower-intensity exercise have a lower incidence of injuries.

4. *Frequency.* This refers to how often the exercise should be conducted. It is best to start with three days a week, allowing for a rest day in between, then gradually increase to six days per week. If the person is able to tolerate heart rates of 60% to 85% of maximum, three days should be sufficient (Heyward, 1991). For very deconditioned patients, even walking down the hallway two or three times daily, with rest between, may be more than they have done previously.

5. *Duration.* This is the length of time the individual engages in the activity at the recommended intensity. For instance, a walking protocol may start at 10 to15 minutes each time and progress to 45 minutes per day, several days per week. With deconditioned individuals, two to three minutes may be a good beginning.

6. *Rate of progression.* This is an important factor: Cancer survivors should increase what they are doing, gradually, alternating variables. For example, if patients increase the duration of exercise this week, they should not try to increase intensity. Increasing at the rate of two minutes per week (same time during each session of the week) is quite acceptable. *At no point should the person be stiff, sore, or fatigued as a result of the exercise!* The most significant improvement occurs during the first weeks of a program. In my experience, the first two weeks are critical in deconditioned or sedentary individuals. After that, the benefits of the exercise make it self-reinforcing.

Use of the Symptom Activity Checklist has made it possible, even through telephone calls, to monitor home programs, to discover developing problems before a crisis point is reached. It has been noted that as increased symptoms contribute to sudden, decreased activity, patients are actually experiencing prodromal indications of an impending crisis. Examples of disease- or treatment-related problems, picked up at an early point through use of this instrument, include a pulmonary fibrosis reaction to cyclophosphamide (Cytoxan), thrombophlebitis, and port infections, all unrelated to the exercise program. Patients developing problems are not permitted to exercise but are immediately referred to the physician for care. Further, patients are not permitted to return to the exercise program until the condition is addressed, and a clearance from the physician is obtained.

Where Do We Go From Here?

The efficacy of exercise as a powerful intervention affecting all dimensions of quality of life has been demonstrated for several varieties and stages of cancer and treatment. If a medication were discovered to have so many benefits, no side effects (if conducted properly), and low cost, it would be heralded as a wonder drug. Even more than research on drug interactions and the use of exercise with higher-risk cancer populations, we need to find out why this is not recommended for every appropriate patient. Why has cancer exercise rehabilitation therapy, something with such powerful potential benefits, been so slow to catch on? As someone once said, "Probably because it makes such sense!"

References

American College of Sports Medicine (1995). *ACSM's guidelines for exercise testing and prescription.* 5th ed. Baltimore: Williams & Wilkins.

Chadwick, J., and Mann, W. N. (1950). *The Medical Works of Hippocrates* (p. 140). Oxford: Blackwell.

Courneya, K. S., and Friedenreich, C. M. (1997). Relationship between exercise pattern across the cancer experience and current quality of life in colorectal cancer survivors. *Journal of Alternative and Complementary Medicine, 3,* 215–226.

Dimeo, F. C., Fetscher, S., Lange, W., Mertelsmann, R., and Keul, J. (1997). Effects of aerobic exercise on the physical performance and incidence of treatment-related complications after high-dose chemotherapy. *Blood, 90,* 3390–3394.

Dimeo, F. C., Rumberger, B. G., and Keul, J. (1998). Aerobic exercise as therapy for cancer fatigue. *Medicine and Science in Sports and Exercise, 30,* 475–478.

Dimeo, F. C., Tilmann, M. H., Bertz, H., Kanz, L., Mertelsmann, R., and Keul, J. (1997). Aerobic exercise in the rehabilitation of cancer patients after high dose chemotherapy and autologous peripheral stem cell transplantation. *Cancer, 79,* 1717–1722.

Dixon, J. K., Dixon, J. P., and Hickey, M. (1993). Energy as a central factor in the self-assessment of health. *Advances in Nursing Science, 15*(4), 1–12.

Friedenreich, C. M., and Courneya, K. S. (1996). Exercise as rehabilitation for cancer patients. *Clinical Journal of Sports Medicine, 6,* 237–244.

Friedenreich, C. M., Courneya, K. S., Bryant, H. E. (1998). The lifetime total physical activity questionnaire: development and reliability. *Medicine and Science in Sports and Exercise, 30,* 266–274.

Greenleaf, J. E., and Kozlowski, S. (1982). Physiological consequences of reduced physical activity during bed rest. *Exercise and Sport Sciences Reviews, 10,* 84–119.

Greenleaf, J. E., Silverstein, L., Bliss, J., Langenheim, V., Rossow, H., and Chao, C. (1982). Physiological responses to prolonged bed rest and fluid immersion in man: A compendium of research (1974–1980). NASA technical memorandum 81324. Washington, DC: National Aeronautics and Space Administration.

Heyward, V. H. (1991). *Advanced fitness assessment and exercise prescription.* 2nd ed. Champaign, IL: Human Kinetics.

Karnofsky, D. A., Abelmann, W. H., Craver, L. F., and Burchenal, J. H. (1948). The use of the nitrogen mustards in the palliative treatment of carcinoma. *Cancer 1,* 634–656.

Karnofsky, D. A., and Burchenal, J. H. (1949). The clinical evaluation of chemotherapeutic agents in cancer. In C. M. MacLeod (Ed.), *Evaluation of chemotherapeutic agents* (pp. 191–205). New York: Columbia University Press.

Luu, P. B., Ortiz, V., Barnes, P. R., and Greenleaf, J. E. (1990). Physiological responses to prolonged bed rest in humans: A compendium of research (1981–1988). NASA technical memorandum 102249. Washington, DC: National Aeronautics and Space Administration.

MacVicar, M. G., and Winningham, M. L. (1986). Promoting the functional capacity of cancer patients. *Cancer Bulletin, 38,* 235–239.

MacVicar, M. G., Winningham, M. L., and Nickel, J. L. (1989). Effects of aerobic interval training on cancer patients' functional capacity. *Nursing Research, 38,* 348–351

Mock, V., Barton-Burke, M., Sheehan, P., Creator, E., Winningham, M., McKinney-Tedder, S., Powel, L., and Liebman, M. (1994). A nursing rehabilitation program for women with breast cancer on adjuvant chemotherapy. *Oncology Nursing Forum, 21,* 899–907.

Pinto, B. M., Maruyana, N. C., Engebretson, T. O., and Thebarge, R. W. (in press). Exercise participation: Mood and coping in early state breast cancer survivors. *Journal of Psychosocial Oncology.*

Winningham, M. L. (1983). "Effects of bicycle ergometry on functional capacity and feelings of control in women with breast cancer." Doctoral dissertation, Ohio State University, Columbus, OH.

Winningham, M. L. (1992). The role of exercise in cancer therapy. In R. W. Watson and M. Eisinger (Eds.), *Exercise and disease* (pp. 63–70*)*. Boca Raton, FL: CRC Press.

Winningham, M. L. (1993). Developing the symptom/activity 27: An instrument to evaluate perception of symptom effects on activity. Presented at the Oncology Nursing Society 18th Annual Congress, Orlando, FL.

Winningham, M. L. (1994). Exercise and cancer. In L. Goldberg and D. L. Elliot (Eds.), *Exercise for prevention and treatment of illness* (pp. 301–315). Philadelphia: F. A. Davis.

Winningham, M. L., MacVicar, M. G., and Burke, C. (1986). Exercise for cancer patients: Guidelines and precautions. *Physician Sportsmedicine, 14,* 125.

Resources

American College of Sports Medicine (1991). *Guidelines for exercise testing and prescription.* 4th ed. Philadelphia: Lea & Febiger. (Pages 178–180 specifically address cancer.)

American College of Sports Medicine (1995). *ACSM's guidelines for exercise testing and prescription.* 5th ed. Baltimore: Williams & Wilkins.

Astrand, P-O., and Rodahl, K. (1986). *Textbook of work physiology: Physiological bases of exercise.* 3rd ed. New York: McGraw-Hill. (This classic text is on the shelf of every exercise scholar; however, few have read it from cover to cover. It is heavy reading but good for classic references.)

Clarke, D. H., and Eckert, H. M. (Eds.) (1985). *Limits of human performance: American Academy of Physical Education paper no. 18.* Champaign, IL: Human Kinetics.

Hargreaves, M. (Ed.) (1995). *Exercise metabolism.* Champaign, IL: Human Kinetics. (Excellent book on lipid, protein, and carbohydrate metabolism during muscular exercise and fatigue.)

Houston, M. E. (1995). *Biochemistry primer for exercise science.* Champaign, IL: Human Kinetics. (Good for general review; includes an overview of basic chemistry.)

McArdle, W. D., and Katch, F. I. (1995). *Essentials of exercise physiology.* Philadelphia: Lea & Febiger. (Streamlined, earlier version of the McArdle, Katch, and Katch book.)

McArdle, W. D., Katch, F. I., and Katch, V. L. (1996). *Exercise physiology: Energy, nutrition, and human performance.* 4th ed. Philadelphia: Lea & Febiger.

Mellerowicz, H., and Smodlaka, V. (1981). *Ergometry: Basics of medical exercise testing.* Baltimore and Munich: Urban & Schwarzenberg.

PART
IV

Personal
Issues

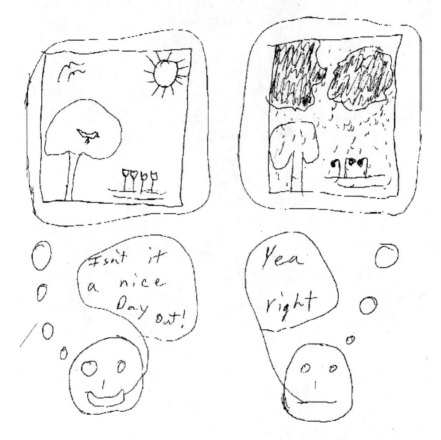

It seemed to me that when my wife was in her chemotherapy treatments, everything seemed kind of *blah* to her.
Robert Heil, spouse of breast cancer survivor

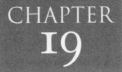

CHAPTER 19

Fatigue and Quality of Life With Cancer

Marcia Grant

I appreciate the fact that you acknowledge fatigue because most of the time it's like, well, it's all in your head. And you really begin to worry that maybe it is in your head. And I did not have chemotherapy but I had three surgeries. So, it took me, I'd say a year, before I felt normal, whatever normal is. And, I was young and healthy and exercising. And, it scared me. And so I do a lot of comforting of women who call me ... friends from all over the United States. And one of the things they always ask me about is the fatigue. And as soon as I tell them, it's okay, it's normal, it seems to be fine. If the doctors ..., I don't know if they really address fatigue. They can't treat it. They can't give you a pill and they can't cut it out. It's such a vague thing and yet it impacts the quality of your life. It's very important that you ask. It's just very important.

Ferrell et al, (1996) "Bone Tired"

Background

While it is clear from the patients' viewpoint that fatigue in cancer is common and affects quality of life (QOL), the occurrence of fatigue in cancer patients and its relationship to QOL are relatively unexplored areas of research. Discussion of these concepts includes some background information on QOL research in cancer, a view of fatigue through a QOL framework, an identification of issues that remain, and the needs and opportunities for further research and for changes in clinical practice. Previous chapters have thoroughly developed definitions, theoretical perspectives, measurement issues, and known interventions for fatigue. Therefore these will not be repeated here.

Quality of Life Research

QOL is an important concept for those of us who work with cancer patients. Through work by a variety of health-related disciplines over the last 20 years, some agreement has developed in relation to definitions, models, and approaches appropriate to research on

QOL. Important characteristics of this concept are that it is health related, subjective, and multidimensional. The focus of QOL in cancer populations includes aspects of life quality that are affected by a medical condition and the treatment of that condition. The attributes of QOL may be either negative (unwanted symptoms such as nausea) or positive (a second chance to live) (Grant et al, 1990). The subjective characteristic of QOL means that patients are the accepted authorities on their QOL. Asking a health professional, friend, or family member to rate an individual's QOL may produce very different results from those identified by the patient.

Current definitions of QOL emphasize the need for inclusion of multiple dimensions. For example, Spilker (1996) recommended that QOL be viewed from several levels: a global perspective that is described as an overall measurement of QOL, a second level that includes broad domains or dimensions, and a third level composed of specific items under each of the domains or dimensions.

In the report of the Workshop on Quality of Life Research in Cancer Clinical Trials cosponsored by the National Cancer Institute (NCI) and the Office of Medical Applications of Research, National Institutes of Health, QOL was identified again as a multidimensional concept. "Health-related quality of life is the value assigned to duration of life as modified by impairments, functional states, perceptions, and social opportunities, and as influenced by disease, injury, treatment, or policy" (U.S. Department of Health and Human Services, 1990).

QOL research has been conducted with many cancer populations. In some studies the major focus was studying QOL as an outcome of disease or treatment (Grant et al, 1992). Other studies combined QOL measurements with other outcome measurements to evaluate specific cancer therapies or disease patterns (Sarna, 1993).

Research methods used in QOL studies have included both qualitative and quantitative approaches as illustrated by reports published in peer-reviewed journals. However, some researchers argue that only qualitative data are valid and that reducing QOL descriptions to a number omits the very nature of the concept of QOL (Leplege and Hunt, 1997). This position, however, makes it difficult to measure QOL in large populations of cancer patients. To negate the value of a quantitative description of QOL in large studies omits providing information to augment such outcomes as morbidity, mortality, and tumor response. A compromise position takes advantage of both research methods and can provide fairly extensive information on patients' QOL. One method that combines the best of both research methods is to include an open-ended question when using quantitative ques-

About the Contributor

Marcia Grant is a highly respected researcher in several areas related to quality of life in cancer. Pain, nutrition, and fatigue management have comprised a significant part of her scientific pursuit. She received her doctorate from the University of California, San Francisco, and has been active in clinical nursing

tionnaires to describe QOL. This provides a way for individual responders to identify QOL issues that are especially relevant to their particular situation but not evaluated in the quantitative questionnaire.

Colleagues and I have combined both research approaches in our studies. We use in-depth interviews of patients and/or families to identify QOL concerns. Then we use this information to develop population-specific QOL quantitative questionnaires that can be used subsequently in descriptive, correlation, and experimental studies. The interview data have provided a rich source of actual patient comments about QOL issues and concerns, and the information used in building a four-dimensional model of QOL now used in all of our studies. The City of Hope–Quality of Life (COH-QOL) model in Figure 19-1 provides a way of organizing information about QOL, analyzing results of in-depth interview data, identifying potential interventions that may improve QOL, and contributing valuable information for building multidisciplinary clinical interventions for improving patient care.

Fatigue Viewed Through a Quality of Life Framework

The relationship of the QOL concept to cancer-related fatigue has only recently become apparent. In our QOL studies, the bone marrow transplant survivor population has been a model (1) for studying extreme fatigue during an acute and toxic treatment and (2) for following a symptom that persists throughout life for many patients. While the relationship between QOL and fatigue has been a recent focus of cancer research, some beginning evidence of the nature of the relationship is available. This is reviewed below using dimensions of QOL.

The COH-QOL model consists of four dimensions: physical well-being, psychological well-being, social well-being, and spiritual well-being. The *physical well-being* dimension includes both physical symptoms and functional ability. Maintaining control over symptoms and independence are included in this functional perspective.

The relationship of fatigue and physical well-being is relatively obvious. Fatigue is frequently described by patients as a decrease in the ability to carry out daily activities, a decrease in normal function. Patients may report that they are limited in their ability to carry out their usual daily activities, have difficulty completing usual tasks, and are generally dissatisfied with these changes (Stewart and Ware, 1992). Changes in fatigue levels are also reported. For example, the amount of fatigue experienced may be increased when other symptoms such as pain are present.

reseearch since the mid-1970s. Grant has received local and national funding for her research and has authored over 100 publications. She has been a member of many national as well as international committees and is always sharing her knowledge and support with others.

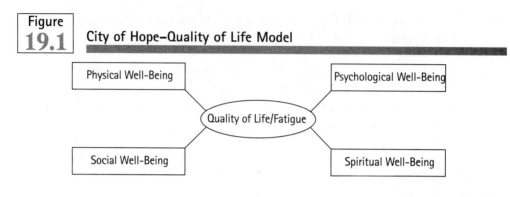

Figure 19.1   City of Hope–Quality of Life Model

My husband Don was diagnosed with bone cancer in October 1996, and began his treatment at that time. Before you have time to deal with the initial diagnosis, they are already undergoing treatment, and then reality sets in. Your whole world turns upside down. Nobody is ever prepared for the devastation that cancer does to your life.

We were luckier than most. As an RN, I was already familiar with dealing with cancer treatments, side effects, dressing changes, flushes, etc. Working with cancer patients and their families and actually living with it–having cancer invade your home–are two totally different entities. I was prepared to handle a lot of the side effects and deal with them as they came up. I was not prepared for the fatigue that goes along with the diagnosis. Sure I knew that the patients were fatigued; it all sounds so simple. Well it isn't that easy. I believe that the fatigue that goes along with cancer and its treatment is the most crippling side effect that cancer brings your way. Most people think of nausea and vomiting or pain when they hear the words cancer *and* chemotherapy. *That was the least of our concerns; there are numerous and effective drugs out there to treat these side effects. There is not a miracle drug to treat fatigue.*

I used to sit and watch my husband as he lay totally wiped out and wonder if the treatment was going to kill him–I was no longer afraid of the cancer killing him, but the treatment. I knew that his body and mind couldn't take much more; there was no quality of life left. He would get up mid to late morning, eat, and hit the couch. He would be out like a light–that was his energy level. He, at that point, no longer feared death. He just wanted to feel alive for a couple of months. After that he said he didn't care anymore. As a family member you are totally at a loss in dealing with this. It is especially difficult for children in the family to understand and comprehend. Their father, who once worked seven days a week, now couldn't do a thing with them or for them. They learn to understand the hospitalizations altogether too well, but they cannot comprehend that the side effects carry over from those hospitalizations until it is time to go back to the hospital–it's a vicious cycle. It's like being on a roller-coaster ride that you did not want to get on in the first place, but nevertheless you are on it for the scariest ride of your life, never knowing if you are going to get off or if one of the curves is going to do you in.

In my experience with a local multidisciplinary, multiinstitutional team of nurses and a physician where multicultural aspects of fatigue and QOL in cancer patients were being explored, some pilot data on interviews with patients revealed valuable information on the nature of fatigue (Grant et al, 1998). In one particular instance, the decreases in daily activity were extensive. A physician coinvestigator explored the nature of fatigue during clinic visits with patients. One patient undergoing radiation therapy denied having fatigue to the physician. However, he was interrupted by his wife who discounted her husband's reply, claiming that the only thing her husband did was go to radiation therapy and then spend the rest of the day, evening, and part of the night in the recliner chair at home. Two interpretations of this episode are important. First of all, the patient denied having fatigue. This may mean that some patients may not recognize their fatigue or use the term *fatigue*.

I believe there are many variables that contribute to the fatigue in cancer-the actual treatment and its side effects, the havoc that the treatment plays on your body, the ever-changing lab values, the ups and downs, the treatment for these changes, the psychological effects of cancer, nutritional needs that are now at a maximum, and so on and so on. Therefore, the treatment should be aimed at treating all of these aspects. Treatment should be a holistic approach–the mind-body connection. A lot more emphasis can be placed on treating the mind–the depression, anxiety, fear, anger, etc. Counseling should not be an option but mandatory–people listen to healthcare professionals and if explained that this is part of the treatment plan, most would accept it, and most insurance companies cover counseling at 90% versus 80%!!! Can you imagine the fatigue caused by the feeling that mentally death is always chasing you, and you are constantly on the run from it?

Support groups should be readily accessible. More could be done right at the hospital: Start a buddy-type system, or hook up two or possibly more people to talk to people in similar circumstances–like having those who have lived through it come into the hospital and talk to people just starting. It doesn't have to be people who have survived; it can be people who may be close to or in the same phase of treatment. I do believe my husband would be more than willing to talk with others in the same circumstances–like Mr. H with osteosarcoma who is undergoing the same protocol. But they need a specific time to talk rather than the hit and miss of a doctor's waiting room.

Also physical therapy or an exercise physiologist could establish some type of a program for patients at the start of treatment, when their energy level is at the highest that it will be for a long time–a short walking program or something. As I said, patients listen to their healthcare providers, but they don't take these suggestions well from a family member–I speak from experience here!!! Not only does this aspect of care assist them physically, but it is also a boost to them mentally.

There are numerous aspects of care than can assist patients and their families in dealing with cancer fatigue that do not involve pills or injections, and I sincerely hope that they will be more utilized in the future.

Debra Whitman

These patients may need education to become aware of their own fatigue and to begin to assess their own fatigue level on a daily basis. Second, fatigue may be insidious, increasing gradually so that patients are not aware of the level of fatigue present. In this instance, fatigue may first become apparent only when a significant activity can no longer be completed. These examples provide some beginning description of the physical aspects of fatigue.

The *psychological well-being* dimension consists of both positive and negative aspects, and includes the sense of control in life-threatening illness, emotional distress, and fears of the unknown. Because fatigue affects mental, emotional, and physical activity, it can have a profound impact on psychological well-being (Cimprich, 1992; Nail and Winningham, 1993; Piper, 1993). The inabilities to focus attention (Cimprich, 1992) and to meet activity expectations (Nail and Winningham, 1993) cause stress for the individual. Prolonged stress can be a principal cause of fatigue (Aistairs, 1987), which in turn influences perceived well-being. The fatigue-inertia spiral illustrated by Winningham and colleagues (1994) depicts the lose-lose condition resulting from decreased activity in response to fatigue. It is easy to visualize this downward spiral being applied to the relationship between fatigue and psychological well-being (Winningham et al, 1994). Cancer-related fatigue exerts a negative effect on psychological well-being. The psychological well-being dimension of QOL provides sufficient evidence to warrant additional study aimed at determining nursing interventions that interrupt and reverse the downward spiral of increasing fatigue and decreasing psychological well-being.

The *social well-being* dimension of QOL includes the roles and relationships that define an individual's life (Ferrell, 1996). Fatigue research has been designed primarily to examine individual patient responses, but studies have also revealed the strong impact of fatigue on family roles and relationships and on family caregivers (Winningham et al, 1994). Patients with cancer who are experiencing fatigue may be unable to perform self-care, maintain usual function, and participate in leisure activities (Rhodes, Watson, and Hanson, 1998). Patients describe having insufficient energy to work, yet being forced to continue employment in order to meet the financial demands of illness or to maintain health insurance. Changes in work and delays in completing school are not uncommon experiences of cancer survivors and may be related to persistent fatigue.

The *spiritual well-being* dimension of QOL includes both religious aspects and existential concerns. Specific aspects include the ability to maintain hope and to derive meaning when faced with uncertainty. In a recent study (Ferrell et al, 1996), patients described the existential impact of fatigue in terms of how this symptom made them feel "mortal." Some patients reported feeling abandoned by their bodies because of overwhelming fatigue. Others were able to report positive coping and seeking meaning through the contemplation and quiet time imposed by the fatigue. Many patients describe altered priorities imposed as a result of having diminished energy. For example, they eliminated some activities and saved energy for only the most essential activities.

This brief description of the relationship between QOL and fatigue provides beginning evidence of the importance of fatigue as a symptom associated with cancer and its treatment. Fatigue affects all four dimensions of QOL and interferes with important aspects of life. A recent study of bone marrow transplant survivors is described next. In this group of patients, fatigue during and following the procedure is extensive, and illustrates areas of high priority for future studies. In addition, the data from this study reveal some of the fatigue issues of particular importance to the patient and to the nature of the research that is needed.

Issues of Particular Importance

A cross-sectional study of fatigue in survivors of bone marrow transplantation provides evidence of the frequency, extent, and persistence of fatigue following this procedure (Grant, Rivera, and King, 1997). Toxicities related to bone marrow transplantation are caused by the lethal doses of chemotherapy and radiation therapy, coupled with the impact of the cancer itself. This population can be used as a model of extensive fatigue.

If this is what life is like, it's not worth living.

Fatigued cancer patient

Information on fatigue was collected by a survey mailed to and returned by 311 respondents (66% return rate). Data included patients' comments about fatigue, as well as responses to a single-item 10-point fatigue scale. To participate in this study, respondents had to be at least 18 years old, and were at least 6 months after allogeneic or matched-unrelated-donor (MUD) transplantation or at least 100 days after autologous transplantation. Respondents' median age was 34, and age ranged 18 to 66 years. This population of cancer patients was relatively young. Fifty-five percent of the respondents were men, and 45% were women. Some ethnic diversity existed, with the vast majority being white (78%) and the remainder composed of African Americans, Asians, and Hispanics. Primary diagnoses included acute and chronic leukemias, and Hodgkin's or non-Hodgkin's diagnoses. Only 57% of the survivors had returned to work full-time, with an additional 22% working part-time. This left a relatively high proportion (21%) who were unable to return to work.

When fatigue was examined in relation to time since transplantation, scores illustrate how this symptom persisted even years later (see Table 19-1). These scores compare to fatigue in a well population, where the average fatigue score was 2.8 on the same scale. The data illustrate several issues of fatigue for survivors. First, fatigue, on average, improves only slightly over time and is far greater than the fatigue experienced by a nontransplant patient. In addition, the range of fatigue scores reveals that severe fatigue (as rated as a 10) was experienced in all the groups tested, even those who completed the transplantation five or more years ago. Patients with severe fatigue are undoubtedly unable to carry out full-time work.

Table 19.1 Fatigue Scores* in 311 Survivors of Bone Marrow Transplantation		
Time Since Transplantation	Average Fatigue Score	Range of Fatigue Scores
< 1 year (N = 10)	5.6	2 – 10
1 year (N = 46)	5.2	0 – 10
2 years (N = 60)	4.6	0 – 10
3–4 years (N = 97)	4.9	0 – 10
≥5 years (N = 98)	4.2	0 – 10

*Scale: 0 = no fatigue; 10 = extreme fatigue.

Because respondents were accrued to this study following acute transplantation, they were asked to recall what fatigue was like before the procedure, during the treatment period, and 3 months following the treatment. Table 19-2 illustrates these findings. The average fatigue score prior to the transplant experience was very low (2.3). However, fatigue recalled during the acute phase of treatment was profound, as illustrated by the average score of 8. Also during this time, only 3% of the respondents reported experiencing no fatigue. Three months following the acute phase of the procedure, the levels of recalled fatigue remained high, and only 2% of the respondents reported no fatigue. The final rating for "Now" combines patients who had transplantation less than 1 year to over 20 years ago. Fatigue persisted, with an average level of 4.2, well over the average reported by noncancer patients.

My son was diagnosed with acute lymphocytic leukemia during his sophomore year in high school. Although they found a perfect donor, he had so many complications. He was sick again and again. Then he had a recurrence. Then he went into septic shock–he almost died. He seemed to be in a coma for nearly six weeks. He just lay in bed–barely responsive–he was so weak. Two days after he went home, he was back again with pneumonia. It went on and on like that. . . . And he was always exhausted.

He's sick every three to four months–severe colds and bronchitis. As soon as I hear him cough once, I know…that's it: He's getting sick again. And he does. Because he's 23, I have no more control. I can make suggestions and be tactful about it. You can understand why he doesn't want to go to a doctor. …If I keep after him, he may finally pick up the phone and call for an appointment. It tires him out just getting to the clinic. I ask the doctor about it, but my son belongs to an HMO. . . . He's never seen an immunologist or a pulmonologist. It's been difficult enough getting basic care. …If he's in remission, why is he always sick? No one will answer that.

Table 19.2	Fatigue Ratings* Recalled by 311 Survivors of Bone Marrow Transplantation		
Time in Relation to Transplantation	Average Fatigue Score	Range of Fatigue Scores	Percent Reporting No Fatigue
Prior	2.3	0 – 10	33
During	8.0	0 – 10	3
3 months after transplantation	7.9	0 – 10	2
Now	4.2	0 – 10	11

*Scale: 0 = no fatigue; 10 = extreme fatigue.

The recalled levels of fatigue during and three months following the transplant procedure illustrate interesting perceptions of fatigue. When information is recalled or collected retrospectively, the potential validity problem with the answers is that people will not be able to accurately recall what happened in the past. In the current study, recalled fatigue was more profound than that reported in prospective studies. Thus, there is the potential for inaccuracy. This difference between prospective and retrospective fatigue may be interpreted in several ways. It may be that fatigue is extreme during and following the transplant procedure, but during this time, patients are putting up with the fatigue, getting by from day to day, learning what to expect and when to expect it. Changes occurring from day to day may be subtle. Fatigue gradually increases and builds to higher levels. Then when the acute phase is complete, and patients look back on what they went through, they realize how

I have the feeling the doctor doesn't understand. Maybe he doesn't want *to know. He's a good oncologist, but he only sees my son for a few minutes. He has to live with this every day. Why can't they do something about this?*

He works so hard, but he's had no special training. The only work he could find was in a dusty warehouse. I know that's bad for his lungs, but what can I say? He's pretty taciturn, rarely complains. . . . He says he's glad to have a job. He comes home at night and immediately has to take a nap. He has friends, but there is no doubt his exhaustion limits his social activities. I don't know how he makes it at work. How long can he keep this up? He's always tired, barely putting one foot in front of the other.

It's embarrassing for him. His body looks like a battleground from all the surgeries and treatments. And he's always exhausted.

Life has never been the same again. I don't know what's going to happen to him. I'm not sure he thinks much past today. It exhausts him to make plans. . . . After all, he's seen so many of his friends from the hospital and the support groups die.

Mother of 23-year-old bone marrow transplant survivor

Table 19.3	Patients' Comments Related to Fatigue	
QOL Dimension	**Subcategory**	**Illustrative Comments**
Physical well-being	Decreased concentration	I find that I am not able to "keep up" with my colleagues at work. I run out of energy and find it difficult to concentrate on more than a few things at a time.
Psychological well-being	Depression	I thought it would never, never end! I would force myself out of bed (first 3 months after transplantation) and sit in a chair where I'd fall asleep. The weakness was extremely depressing and scary.
Social well-being	Changes in role	I was a professional athlete before cancer. I just don't have the stamina now. Deep breaths are tough to come by.
Spiritual well-being	Changed priorities	I have arrived at my own set of priorities, things that are important to me. I try not to waste mental energy on things I cannot change.

profound their fatigue was. The difference between fatigue ratings in prospective and retrospective studies may also be related to learning what fatigue is and how to rate it. Prior to having the bone marrow transplantation, patients are unlikely to have had experience in rating fatigue. Even during and immediately following the transplant procedure, it would be unusual in most clinical settings for patients to assess their level of fatigue on a regular basis (e.g., daily). As the experience unfolds, patients begin to get comfortable recognizing their fatigue and become more skilled at rating the level of fatigue. Thus, patients are learning to evaluate their fatigue as they experience it.

In addition to the ratings of fatigue, the bone marrow transplant survivors also provided some written comments to open-ended questions about their fatigue. Examples of a typical comment within each of the four QOL dimensions are found in Table 19-3. Comments related to the inability to work were common in the physical well-being dimension, while comments in relation to fatigue and psychological well-being reflected the emotional impact of this symptom. Within the social well-being dimension, typical comments related to changes in the work role and changes in relationships. Finally in the area of spiritual well-being, changed priorities were a typical response.

Where Do We Go From Here?

While the area of fatigue and QOL is relatively unexplored, information currently available has implications both for needed research and for clinical practice. Combining the concepts of QOL and fatigue in clinical nursing research studies can provide valuable information on the care of patients with cancer. In looking back or recalling what fatigue was like, patients were able to describe how profound fatigue can be during acute treatment periods. Retrospective data have resulted in the most extreme ratings of fatigue for bone marrow transplant survivors. This approach needs to be repeated in other cancer populations.

Descriptive studies that compare various patient populations and fatigue trajectories are needed to tailor teaching approaches and identify possible fatigue interventions. These descriptive studies can also be useful in raising the consciousness of all professional staff involved in the care of the cancer patient about fatigue and assisting them to assess and recognize fatigue. Like pain, fatigue needs to become one of the vital signs reported on all cancer patients.

Clinical implications, while not currently based on sufficient research evidence, can nevertheless be made. Certainly, accurate and regular assessment for the intensity of fatigue should be incorporated into the clinical pattern of assessment. Results should be used to identify patients with severe fatigue so that a work-up for causes can be done, as well as evaluation of what impact this severe fatigue is having on their QOL.

Patients should be instructed on how to manage, cope, and prioritize their activities, using the four dimensions of QOL. Prioritization of activities is essential. Teaching should help patients establish realistic expectations about what they can and cannot do. Energy-saving approaches to usual daily tasks are important for patients and staff to learn. The impact of fatigue on the four dimensions can provide information on the need for consultation from multidisciplinary team members in the development and implementation of the patient's plan of care. Chaplains, priests, and other religious support staff can assist patients when fatigue interferes with spiritual well-being. Social workers can assist when fatigue impacts social or psychological well-being. Physicians and dietitians may be able to assist with the physical aspects of fatigue through diet and blood product interventions. Even though many gaps in knowledge about cancer-related fatigue remain, increasing staff awareness of this symptom can bring about more rapid changes in patients' fatigue and improve their QOL.

References

Aisters, J. (1987). Fatigue in the cancer patient: A conceptual approach to a clinical problem. *Oncology Nursing Forum, 14*, 25–30.

Cimprich, B. (1992). A theoretical perspective on attention and patient education. *Advances in Nursing Science, 14*, 39–51.

Ferrell, B. R. (1996). The quality of lives: 1525 voices of cancer. *Oncology Nursing Forum, 23*, 907–916.

Ferrell, B. R., Grant, M., Dean, G. E., Funk, B., and Ly, J. (1996). "Bone tired": The experience of fatigue and impact on quality of life. *Oncology Nursing Forum, 23* 1539–1547.

Grant, M., Anderson, P., Ashley, M., Dean, G., Ferrell, B., Kagawa-Singer, M., Padilla, G., Bradshaw Robinson, S., and Sarna, L. (1998). Developing a team for multicultural, multi-institutional research on fatigue and quality of life. *Oncology Nursing Forum, 25*, 1404–1412.

Grant, M., Ferrell, B., Schmidt, G. M., Fonbuena, P., Niland, J. C. and Forman, S. J. (1992). Measurement of quality of life in bone marrow transplantation survivors. *Quality of Life Research, 1,* 375–384.

Grant, M., Padilla, G. V., Ferrell, B. R., and Rhiner, M. (1990). Assessment of quality of life with a single instrument. *Seminars in Oncology Nursing, 6,* 266–270.

Grant, M., Rivera, L. M. and King, C. (1997). The impact of fatigue on quality of life in bone marrow transplant survivors [abstract 129]. *Quality of Life Research, 6,* 651.

Leplege, A., and Hunt, S. (1997). The problem of quality of life in medicine. *Journal of the American Medical Association, 278,* 47–50.

Nail, L. M., and Winningham, M. L. (1993). Fatigue. In S. L. Groenwald, M. H. Frogge, M. Goodman, and C. H. Yarbo (Eds.), *Cancer nursing principles and practice* (pp. 608–619). 3rd ed. Boston: Jones & Bartlett.

Piper, B. F. (1993). Fatigue. In V. Carrieri-Kohlman, A. M. Lindsey, and C. M. West (Eds.), *Pathophysiological phenomena in nursing: Human responses to illness* (pp. 279–302). 2nd ed. Philadelphia: W. B. Saunders.

Public Health Service, National Institutes of Health (1990). *Quality of life assessment in cancer clinical trials.* Bethesda, MD: U.S. Department of Health and Human Services.

Rhodes, V. A., Watson P. M., and Hanson, B. M. (1998). Patients' descriptions of the influence of tiredness and weakness on self-care abilities. *Cancer Nursing, 11,* 186–194.

Sarna, L. (1993). Fluctuations in physical function. Adults with non-small cell lung cancer. *Journal of Advanced Nursing, 18,* 714–724.

Spilker B. (1996). Introduction. In B. Spilker (Ed.), *Quality of life and pharmacoeconomics in clinical trials* (pp. 1–10). 2nd ed. Philadelphia: Lippincott-Raven.

Stewart, A. L., and Ware, J. E. (1992). *Measuring functioning and well being. The Medical Outcomes Study approach.* Durham, NC: Duke University Press.

Winningham. M. L., Nail L. M., Barton-Burke, M., Brophy, L., Cimprich, B., Jones, L. S., Pickard-Holley, S., Rhodes, V., St. Pierre, B., Beck, S., Glass, E. C., Mock, V. L., Mooney, K. H., and Piper B. (1994). Fatigue and the cancer experience: The state of the knowledge. *Oncology Nursing Forum, 21,* 23–36.

Robert Heil, spouse of breast cancer survivor

The Family Experience

Margaret Barton-Burke

I did not experience the cancer treatments myself, but I did watch and care for my wife as she went through them. I remember asking her to come and sit on the couch for awhile, instead of laying in bed all day.

Cancer patient's husband

Background

Scenario 1. *W. T., a 16-year-old Vietnamese immigrant, was recently diagnosed with non-Hodgkin's lymphoma and currently is undergoing treatment. This adolescent boy lives in an apartment in the inner city with a large multigenerational extended family that includes grandparents, an aunt, an uncle, and several siblings.*

The definition of *family* ranges from a social unit consisting of parents and children to a group of people related by ancestry or marriage, and may even include a group of people living together under one leader. Obviously, cultural traditions determine these relationships. Since the readers of this chapter represent a broad variety of cultures, the picture of family is painted with the broadest brush and these broad definitions are used to characterize families.

The family depicted in Scenario 1 is not unlike a family that may be seen in any cancer treatment facility anywhere there are immigrant populations. This adolescent's cancer has an impact not only on the child but also on the entire family. The cancer, its treatment, and disease sequelae including fatigue can, and probably will, upset the entire household.

Interestingly but not surprisingly, the scientific literature on cancer and the family suggests that family plays a major role in the psychosocial adjustment to the cancer experience (Cordoba, Fobair, and Callan, 1993; Hill and Gallagher, 1996; Jensen and Given, 1991; Stetz, 1998). Each family member is deeply affected by the diagnosis and may experience the same feelings that affect the individual (Hill and Gallagher, 1996). This may be true for most of the psychological responses to cancer, but is it also the case for physical and physiological responses? Cancer-related fatigue (CRF), one of the physical, physiological, and psychological responses to cancer, is a frequently reported symptom of both individuals with cancer and their family caregivers (Jensen and Given, 1991).

There is a notion that CRF in family members is an expected outcome of the cancer experience, yet this reality often is not recognized by health care professionals or legitimized by employers and third-party medical reimbursement systems. In part, this is true because fatigue has only recently been given credence as a bona fide symptom for the individual with cancer. However, the small body of literature on the subject of cancer, CRF, and the family gives us clues as to expectations and what we need to learn.

The experience of a single family can help us understand the experiences of many. Throughout this chapter, examples like the one at the beginning of this chapter will be used to explore the link between cancer and CRF as experienced by the social structure called *family*.

Theoretical Underpinnings

Scenario 2. *K. C., a 30-year-old man of Irish descent, has a four-year history of testicular cancer. A former soldier, he was a construction worker at the time of diagnosis, standing 6 feet 2 inches and weighing over 200 pounds. He lives with both parents and four siblings in a one-family home in a suburban location.*

Scenario 3. *S. B., a 40-year-old African-American woman was diagnosed one year ago with locally advanced breast cancer. She is married with two children, a 14-year-old daughter and a 16-year-old son. Both she and her husband work outside the home, financially requiring both paychecks to make ends meet.*

Each family has rules, regulations, and roles that govern the interactions among the members. After cancer is diagnosed, these rules, regulations, and roles change to a greater or lesser degree as the family attempts to find ways to adjust to a chronic or life-threatening illness. The influence of ethnicity, religion or spiritual identity, and socioeconomic background is closely connected to a family's functioning. Cultural and religious backgrounds

About the Contributor/Editor

Margaret Barton-Burke, a doctoral candidate at the University of Rhode Island and colonel in the U.S. Army Nurse Corps, is still discovering what she wants to be when she grows up. She is a wife and mother, and has over 25 years' experience in nursing with more than 20 of those years spent in oncology nursing. Most of that work has been in such reputed oncology institutions as Massachusetts General Hospital, Pondville Hospital, one of the National Cancer Institute's original Comprehensive Cancer Centers, and Dana Farber Cancer Institute of Boston.

Currently, she is principal of Oncology Consulting Services, a consulting business focusing on assessing, planning, implementing, and evaluating programs related to oncology nursing. As a dynamic speaker, Margaret has lectured extensively locally, regionally, nationally, and internationally on topics related to cancer nursing. In addition, she has written a cancer drug trilogy with her trifeminate team of coauthors. Two of her textbooks have been honored with the American Journal of Nursing *Book of the Year Award (1992, 1997, and 1998).*

Margaret's avocation is as a soldier. A colonel in the U.S. Army Nurse Corps, she has over 19 years of military service as a reservist. She is the deputy commander of Detachment 6 (Medical) and chief nurse

help shape the meaning given to illness and provide a context within which families interpret this meaning. A large amount of emotional energy is directed toward the construction and reconstruction of meaning for all members of the family, thus contributing to family fatigue. As the disease and treatment status change, meaning and relationships have to be redefined.

Some cultures regard cancer as a source of shame and its presence in certain parts of the body may assign specialized meanings of shame. In Scenarios 2 and 3, culture is highlighted as a variable that may potentially influence the manner in which these families deal with cancer and CRF.

Psychologists, sociologists, anthropologists, medical anthropologists, and nurses have developed many theories that explain the family as a social unit. Although a detailed discussion of each of these theories is beyond the scope of this chapter, a list of the most common theories is provided in Table 20-1. These theories help practitioners and researchers reach conclusions about the family by describing, explaining, and predicting reactions to cancer and treatment side effects. They may also provide rationale for scientific and empirical interventions, particularly for the CRF experienced by both patient and family.

While each theory offers a significant contribution to understanding a family's cancer experience, no single theory usually is sufficiently comprehensive to explain all areas under scrutiny. For example, some families operate as closed systems. That is, they rely mostly on their own resources to maintain a balance, thus minimizing stress and fatigue *as they perceive it*. In the face of the enormous stress of cancer on the entire family system, the old coping mechanisms may break down. Instead of reevaluating and developing new options,

for the Massachusetts National Guard (MAARNG). In this role, Margaret has been responsible for reengineering, process redesign, and quality assurance for the medical readiness of the MAARNG. She has authored numerous technical manuals and is project officer for the Women in the Military Memorial, as well as consultant to the Professional Development and Quality of Life Conference planning committees.

As a doctoral candidate, her research interest is in the experiences of women with breast cancer. Her interest in fatigue began in 1991, while in a conversation about the problem of energetics, depression, and fatigue with Maryl L. Winningham. From this dialogue, which culminated in the first Oncology Nursing Society (ONS) State of the Knowledge Conference on Fatigue (November 1992 in Park City, Utah), this think-tank approach contributed to what was to become the ONS Fatigue Initiative and the Fatigue In Research and Education (FIRE) Project. The rest is history.

For relaxation, Margaret enjoys just being Irish, ballet and Irish step dancing, church activities, and studying Bickram's Hatha yoga. In her spare time, she keeps track of her husband, two beautiful daughters, and two golden retrievers.

Table 20.1	Social Theories with Family Components and Implications for Fatigue in Cancer

Type of Theory	Description
Crisis	Examines adequacy of coping repertoire in response to acute stress to determine whether there is a resolution to the stress. Cancer-related fatigue (CRF) presents increased stress with less ability to resolve it through customary coping mechanisms. (Aquilera and Messick, 1974; Fink, 1967; Janosik, 1986; Lubkin and Larsen, 1998)
Adaptation	Examines the dynamic, unending, evolving process by which behavior adapts to meet regular challenges; how organisms modify to suit new conditions. In CRF, organisms may encounter diminished resources for adaptation and modification. (Coehlo, Hamburg, and Adams, 1974; Dimond, 1983; Mechanic, 1983; Roy and Andrews, 1991)
Systems[a]	Focuses on the family as a unit, not on individuals; what influences one family member affects all others in the system. The family unit can support and facilitate the fatigued member. Conversely, the fatigued member can also cause fatigue in the other members as they take over responsibilities. (Parsons, 1951[b]; Broderick and Smith, 1979)
Developmental	Individuals go through various relational processes as they mature. Appropriate maturation can be inhibited by CRF because the person needs to focus on survival and has limited ability to reach out and interact with others in a giving, growing way. Alternatively, the individual with CRF may be forced to reexamine values and goals and focus on priorities. (Erickson, 1950)
Coping and adjustment	Individuals develop a process for managing adjustment threats or demands that are greater than they are able to control. How well they meet those demands has an interactive effect on the social health and well-being of other family members; this, in turn, forces them to adjust in negative or positive ways. (Cohen and Lazarus, 1983; Kiely, 1972; Lyon, 1992)
Role	All individuals have social roles within the social system: Illness is also a role that when legitimized, insulates that individual from usual role expectations. Fatigue does not fit into normal illness roles because it is difficult to define and is often thought to be faked. In this case, society does not sanction relief or respect for time to heal. This model is best suited to acute illnesses. (Parsons, 1951)

[a]Readers with a historical/philosophical bent may find Ludwig von Bertalanffy's *General Systems Theory: Foundations, Development, Applications* (1968) fascinating. He began this work prior to World War II, but the outbreak of the war and communication difficulties kept him from being recognized as the "Father of General Systems Theory" until many decades later. All researchers could profit from reading von Bertalanffy's classic text.

[b]Talcott Parsons's *The Social System*, first published in 1951, was an encyclopedic work. Current scholars owe this work a debt of gratitude whether they agree with it or not. He addressed every major social structure in Western society from a systems perspective.

within the context of their system, they struggle and fight to cope within the old system. This private style of functioning tends to devalue outside help, resist any form of support, and demonstrate what outsiders see as ineffective coping patterns. To further the problem, health care providers tend to hasten judgment on patients' and families' "poor coping" when, in effect, it may reflect a lack of contextual understanding. This may result in unnecessary stress on both sides.

Other families appear to operate as open systems, shown by a readiness to utilize external resources, and may be seen as better able to cope with the cancer and side effects of treatment such as CRF. In either case, both systems and coping theory may be used to understand a family's response to cancer. True open-system families, families that are willing to accept help and renewal from the outside, do much better than closed-system families because the former recognize the limitations of their own emotional and physical resources. Furthermore, open-system families may cope by allowing a volunteer from their church to help with housecleaning or cooking each week. They are more likely to admit to their need for therapeutic interventions such as group support and psychotherapy. Some closed-system families may use superficial communications and friendliness to cover for their fear. Closed-system families are often perceived by health care professionals as rejecting and disinterested in help, a circular perception that is reinforced, as time goes on, by both sides. Because the reimbursement system has usually focused on the individual, there has not been much focus on family dynamics. Much needs to be learned about the various types of coping in the family-cultural context with respect to optimal coping strategies and a view to discovering how to minimize fatigue in the family.

The following two quotations from patients elegantly illustrate the fatigue experience:

> *Fatigue means to be extremely tired. Not having any energy. Wanting to lie down and sleep. It also means I don't have any desire to expend any energy. I do get relief from sleep. I just take naps here and there. I feel helpless to some degree. I feel unable to do for myself. Sometimes I struggle to get up and get something, or do something that actually takes very little effort. I have a lot of frustrations and anger over not feeling like doing ordinary things.*
>
> *It was a mental strain. I was too tired to think. It took all my effort to get out of bed* (Camarillo, 1992).
>
> *The fatigue I have experienced affects physical and emotional, intellectual and spiritual senses. It is difficult to meditate, for example, when weary to the bone. I have said to family, oncologist, and friend alike, "I would gladly trade the fatigue for additional nausea"–not as pleasant for others in the vicinity–but indicative of how bad the fatigue is* (Ferrell et al, 1996).

The fatigue literature has focused on individuals' subjective experience when describing the qualitative nature of the fatigue experience, while the parallel experience of family members has been virtually ignored.

Contributing Factors to Cancer-Related Fatigue in the Family

Scenario 4. *E. G., a 6-year-old girl, was diagnosed with a brain tumor. She lives with both parents, has an older (8 years old) brother, and attends the local day care center regularly. Both her parents work; her mother is a teacher and her father works for a large consulting firm.*

Available literature commonly refers to the family as a caregiving system, but research literature indicates that more typically, one family member assumes the role of primary caregiver (Stetz, 1998, p. 164). The heaviest burden often falls on the mother or on the patient's spouse or partner. He or she must continually manage daily family life and actively support the person with cancer. The energetic burden of duties and responsibilities is shifted to the supportive person. Families often have to focus so much attention on the person with cancer that the well members may be confused about expectations and feel emotionally neglected.

Children are enormously sensitive to changes in the availability of their parents as primary caregivers and it may seem reasonable to expect children to undertake certain responsibilities. Disciplinary problems may arise with regressive behaviors at home (i.e., bed-wetting, tantrums) or at school; in addition, nightmares and somatic complaints such as stomachaches or headaches may occur. Teenagers may engage in risk-taking behavior such as reckless driving, drug or alcohol use, or running away from home.

Jensen and Given (1991) conducted a study to examine the relationship between caregiving and fatigue in families with cancer. Results of the study found that there was a significant relationship between the number of hours of daily care and the severity of fatigue. The authors also reported that there was a positive relationship between the reported fatigue severity score and the impact on the caregiver's schedule. Jensen and Given found no relationship between (1) age of caregiver and severity of fatigue, (2) severity of fatigue and employment status of caregivers of cancer patients, and (3) duration of care and the severity of fatigue.

In a study of ovarian cancer patients, Jamar (1989) described several important aspects of an individual's fatigue. Among their physical problems subjects reported an alteration

---

We just celebrated our thirtieth wedding anniversary. Immediately after we got married, my husband was shipped off to Vietnam. That was a symbolic beginning. There's never been a chance to rest. Life seems to have been one battle after another. Then our child was diagnosed with cancer. It's been a seven-year battle.

We were lucky. My husband and I–our family–grew closer together throughout all this. I've seen families fall apart. My husband and I have tried to take special time with the other children so they didn't feel neglected. As a couple, it's the total exhaustion that's affected both of us.

I have been with our child through it all, through every treatment. I feel like I've had cancer myself. I've had surrogate cancer. It broke my heart to watch it. He's never had the energy to get a driver's license.

in their pattern of sleep and indicated a need for naps during the day and more sleep at night. Most of the women reported that activities had to be given up or changed and that they needed help at home.

One may extrapolate from this study that a parallel experience is occurring for family members. However, since family members are not "sick," they may not be permitted, nor may they permit themselves, to take the same adaptive coping measures as the individual with cancer, such as to sleep more at night, take naps during the day, and give up activities (e.g., going to work and social functions).

Jamar (1989) found that the highest levels of fatigue in patients were among single parents and those without help at home. This finding not only makes sense but also correlates with the findings of Vogelzang and colleagues (1997), which identified the individual at risk for CRF as being younger or female who was going to receive chemotherapy. Practitioners had always suspected this was the case; Vogelzang and colleagues' study confirmed the extent of CRF as a bona fide condition.

Vogelzang and colleagues' research also presented additional findings regarding the primary caregiver's CRF fatigue. They found that the primary caregiver had perceptions of fatigue that were similar to those of the cancer patient, but the caregiver tended to rate the prevalence and impact of fatigue higher. That is, from the primary caregiver's firsthand observations, the CRF fatigue was more realistically assessed by what the individual could and could not do on a daily basis.

These findings are similar to those of Sneeuw, Aaronson, and Spranger (1997) who observed that caregivers reported more impaired levels of patient functioning and lower levels of well-being than did the patients themselves (Vogelzang et al, 1997, p. 10). This is not uncommon in other illnesses such as pulmonary disease.

Finally, an interesting finding in Vogelzang's (1997) article was that individuals with cancer and their primary caregivers did not discuss fatigue with their oncologists because of the belief that fatigue was an inevitable side effect of the treatment or disease; the caregivers felt there was nothing that could be done for the fatigue.

When he has to go to the clinic for checkups, we both suffer through it. We can't sleep several nights prior. I drive to the city to the medical center. We've talked about it: We both have upset stomachs. We're both so exhausted afterwards that we can't sleep for several days. In the midst of all this, my mother became an invalid and I had to take care of her. She just died a few weeks ago. . . . I've recently been diagnosed with depression and fibromyalgia. It's occurred to me it might rather be exhaustion or posttraumatic stress disorder!

Mother of childhood cancer survivor

Interventions for Families

Scenario 5. *C. J., a 65-year-old Latino man was diagnosed with small-cell lung cancer six months ago. He is a certified public accountant with a local insurance company who is nearing retirement. Currently his health insurance covers the costs of his treatment. He is divorced and lives alone in a two-bedroom apartment near a large metropolitan area in the Northeast. He has two adult children, a daughter and son, who are 28 and 31 years old, respectively.*

For the person with cancer, fatigue is often described as the *subjective feeling of tiredness and lack of physical energy*. Fatigue also has several dimensions of expression and multiple influencing factors. These factors may apply to family members, as well as the individual, and include activity, hydration, nutrition, and motivation. Family members bound by the excess or changed role requirements may have little or no time for exercise or social activity. They may not eat or drink sufficiently to reenergize themselves, while the psychological energy drain of a chronic illness can be fatiguing in and of itself.

Changes in sleep patterns, concomitant diseases, and other social situations are known to affect individual fatigue levels. It is highly likely that they affect family members as well.

Concerns about survival, daily activities, family concerns about daily life (e.g., paying bills, maintaining a job and insurance coverage), and the stress of having a cancer diagnosis compound the psychological nature of CRF within a family. In Scenario 5 the individual has many of these concerns, but they are more complex owing to the nature and kind of separateness of all family members. Thus, the CRF that this family experiences is unique and different. Family members who are estranged from one another, or in the face of frequent conflicts, are also likely to experience increased fatigue. Guilt and anger have powerfully debilitating effects and can exacerbate already existing poor coping strategies. Such families are usually perceived as closed systems since the individuals have trouble meeting

Survivorship Problems . . . A Mother's Observation

It's been interesting watching the fatigue issues that pop up in cancer support groups for kids and their parents. Most of the parents comment on fatigue they observe during treatment. But I'm interested in something else I've noticed–maybe they're related.

Even when kids seem to have recovered energy levels, many seem to have lost a sense of direction in their lives. I notice they are not able to hold down jobs or go to school. Maybe they can look normal–is it possible they still have lower internal energy levels?

Many are not able to hold down jobs or go to school–they don't seem to be able to focus. Is that part of that postcancer fatigue? There seems to be some kind of emotional or intellectual inertia. Many of those we know who had cancer when they were teenagers are still living with their parents.

Think about it–when you're a teenager, there's not much realistic thinking about the future. You don't know who you are. But these kids don't seem to be able to get their act together afterward. Then again,

emotional needs in a healthy manner and fear opening up to outsiders. Remarkably, such individuals may be heard to declare emphatically how tough they are and how no one in their family needs counseling or a psychiatrist!

Participation in peer support activities, particularly recreation, and individual or family counseling can help family members. Open and forthright communication is fundamental to dealing with most of the issues related to cancer. One intervention that may help a family's fatigue is for family members to tell each other when they need a rest or some time away from the intense nature of the family situation. Silence or minimal to no communication should be a concern to the health care practitioner. The longer silence continues, the more likely there are serious difficulties between family members

Validating family members' reports of perceived fatigue is the most common way to currently assess fatigue in clinical populations. Helping family members to look at the patterns associated with the fatigue is an intervention that may reduce family fatigue. Additional interventions include teaching family members to identify the time of day they are most vulnerable to fatigue, baseline energy levels of individual family members, changes in fatigue patterns over time, and the influence of circadian rhythms on CRF. It is important that energy levels, livelihood, relationships, roles, and leisure activities be discussed within the context of the family and the impact that CRF will have on all these aspects of family life.

Where Do We Go From Here?

Scenario 6. *A. P., a 35-year-old woman who lives in a rural area of Massachusetts with her lesbian partner, was diagnosed with and treated for breast cancer five years ago. She works as a health care professional in a major teaching hospital. In addition to her partner, she identifies her golden retriever and her Siamese cats as her significant others. She does not discuss her extended or "birth" family.*

there is the constant fear of recurrence: Why study when you might die tomorrow? We've seen many drop out because they could not concentrate enough to study. One of the group just finished his freshman year in college with good grades, but another dropped out in the middle.

. . . Then again, so many of their friends from the hospital didn't survive. They've watched many others die. There seems to be like an emotional regression. They had to face this horrible environment and they don't seem to be able to pop out of it. They never had the chance to be normal teenagers. And now, they're too exhausted and unfocused to do anything to get back on track.

Parent observing support groups and survivorship issues

This chapter closes with Scenario 6, that of an individual who represents a group of disenfranchised members of society who may fail to disclose personal information about lifestyle and possibly other health care or disease-related conditions such as CRF until there is a strong bond of trust established with the health care provider.

As the patient and family adjust to the cancer experience, their normal lives involving jobs, homes, friends, and pursuits of interest, as well as the basic activities of daily living, remain important to them. CRF often disrupts the patient's and the family's ability and desire to maintain viable role functioning. It is critical that health care providers *acknowledge fatigue in order to grant it legitimacy*. This is the first step in eliciting trust and cooperation toward developing effective interventions.

Despite the limited empirical research regarding the scientific underpinnings of CRF within the family, strong clinical evidence suggests that fatigue is a prevalent problem not only among persons with cancer but also within the family structure. By integrating five decades of medical sociological research and the tenets of basic stress theory, a foundation can be laid to anticipate where fatigue will most influence family life. Validating both the patient's and the family's symptoms of fatigue and acknowledging their existence and basis may be valuable in helping the family to cope.

Despite the high incidence and multifactorial nature of fatigue and its impact on the individual with cancer and family members, this symptom remains difficult and illusive to treat for the health care practitioner, but real and constant to the patient. Further investigation is needed on fatigue as an individual experience as well as a family experience. Such studies should examine the occupational, economic, and social costs to the family within the larger societal context.

A significant discrepancy can exist between a health care professional's perception of the fatigue experienced by a particular family and the family's unique perception. Family members at particular risk are those who already have significant health problems. It is important that health care providers not assume the ability of a parent or spouse to provide supportive or home care. The supportive family member may be at greater risk and have worse health than the patient! Taking the time to develop trust and accurately assess a family's fatigue experience can offer valuable information for determining the best therapeutic, prophylactic, and palliative interventions.

References

Aquilera, D. C., and Messick, J. M. (1974). *Crisis intervention theory and methodology*. St. Louis: C. V. Mosby.

Broderick, C., and Smith, J. (1979). The general systems approach to the family. In W. Burr, R. Hill, F. Nye, and I. Reiss (Eds.), *Contemporary theories about the family* (pp. 112–129). New York: Free Press.

Camarillo, M. A. (1992). The oncology patient's experience of fatigue. *Quality of Life: A Nursing Challenge, 1,* 39–44.

Coehlo, G. V., Hamburg, D. A., and Adams, J. E. (1974). *Coping and adaptation.* New York: Basic Books.

Cohen, F., and Lazarus, R. S. (1983). Coping and adaptation in health and illness. In D. Mechanic (Ed.), *Handbook of health, health care, and the health professions* (pp. 608–635). New York: Free Press.

Cordoba, C. S., Fobair, P., and Callan, D. B. (1993). Common issues facing adults with cancer. In N. M. Stearns, M. M. Lauria, J. F. Hermann, and P. R. Fogelberg (Eds.), *Oncology social work: A clinician's guide* (pp. 43–77). Atlanta: American Cancer Society.

Dimond, M. (1983). Social adaptation in the chronically ill. In D. Mechanic (Ed.), *Handbook of health, health care, and the health professions* (pp. 636–649). New York: Free Press.

Erickson, E. H. (1950). *Childhood and society.* New York: W. W. Norton.

Ferrell, B. R., Grant, M., Dean, G. E., Funk, B., and Ly, J. (1996). "Bone tired:" The experience of fatigue and its impact on quality of life. *Oncology Nursing Forum, 23,* 1539.

Fink, S. L. (1967). Crisis and motivation: A theoretical model. *Archives of Physical Medicine and Rehabilitation, 48,* 592–597.

Hill, H. L., and Gallagher, J. (1996). The emotional impact of cancer. In R. T. Osteen (Ed.), *The cancer manual* (pp. 210–221). 9th ed. Framingham, MA: Massachusetts Division of the American Cancer Society.

Jamar, S. (1989). Fatigue in women receiving chemotherapy for ovarian cancer. In S. Funk, E. Tornquist, M. Champagne, L. Archer Copp, and R. Wiese (Eds.), *Key aspects of comfort: Management of pain, fatigue and nausea.* New York: Springer.

Janosik, E. H. (1986). *Crisis counseling: A contemporary approach.* Sudbury, MA: Jones and Bartlett.

Jensen, S., and Given, B. (1991). Fatigue affecting family care givers of cancer patients. *Cancer Nursing, 14,* 181–187.

Kiely, W. F. (1972). Coping with severe illness. *Advances in Psychosomatic Medicine, 1,* 105–118.

Lubkin, I., and Larsen, P. D. (1998). *Chronic illness impact and interventions.* 4th ed. Sudbury, MA: Jones and Bartlett.

Lyon, B. L. (1992). *Stress: Coping and conquering.* Research Triangle Park, NC: Glaxo.

Mechanic, D. (1983). *Handbook of health, health care, and the health professions.* New York: Free Press

Parsons, T. (1951). *The social system.* New York: Free Press.

Roy, C., and Andrews, H. A. (1991). *The Roy adaptation model: The definitive statement.* Norwalk, CT: Appleton & Lange.

Sneeuw, K. C. A., Aaronson, N. K., and Spranger, M. A. G. (1997). Value of caregiver ratings in evaluating the quality of life of persons with cancer. *Journal of Clinical Oncology, 15,* 1874–1880.

Stetz, K. M. (1998). Quality of life in families experiencing cancer. In C. R. King and P. S. Hinds (Eds.), *Quality of life from nursing and patient perspectives* (pp. 157–175). Sudbury, MA: Jones and Bartlett.

Vogelzang, N. J., Breitbart, W., Cella, D., Curt, G. A., Groopman, J. E., Horning, S. J., Itri, L. M., Johnson, D. H., Scherr, S. L., and Portnoy, R. K. (1997). Patient, caregiver, and oncologist perception of cancer-related fatigue: Results of a tripart assessment survey. *Seminars in Hematology, 34*(3 suppl 2), 4–12.

von Bertalanffy, L. (1968). *General systems theory: Foundations, development, applications.* Revised edition. New York: George Braziller.

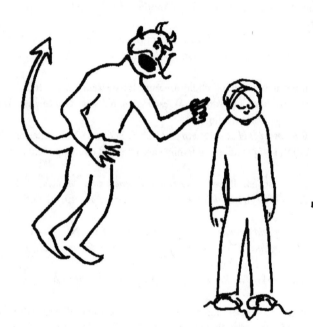

Fatigue as a
Spiritual Crisis

Gerald Kelly

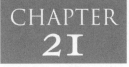

Never make a patient repeat a message or request, especially if it be some time after. Occupied patients are often accused of doing too much of their own business. They are instinctively right. How often you hear the person, charged with the request of giving the message or writing the letter, say half an hour afterwards to the patient, "Did you appoint 12 o'clock?" or, "What did you say was the address?" or ask perhaps some much more agitating question—thus causing the patient the effort of memory, or worse still, of decision, all over again. It is really less exertion to him to write his letters himself. This is the almost universal experience of occupied invalids.

Florence Nightingale, *Notes on Nursing*

Background

The phenomenon of fatigue in cancer, whether part of the disease or as a result of treatment, has been viewed predominantly from psychobiological perspectives. This chapter on fatigue as a spiritual issue suggests the need for another approach to the understanding of fatigue that cannot be ignored by clinicians and researchers. In the end, this spiritual dimension to fatigue may be the most important to each individual as he or she deals with cancer, its attendant therapies, and its outcomes. It suggests a focus on the individual as the final authority on what it means to live with cancer. It is primarily through the reports of cancer survivors themselves that we come to understand the deeper implications of the experience of fatigue. It is only through their personal accounts of fatigue-related suffering that we begin to understand the phenomenon of fatigue as a true spiritual crisis.

I'm just so sick and tired of being sick and tired. If this is what my life is going to be, I'm not sure it's worth it.
Cancer survivor

My strength has already run out. Tell me how much longer I have left.
Psalm 102:23

A review of the literature yields few references that recognize the spiritual aspect of fatigue. Several studies do include spirituality as one dimension of quality of life (QOL) affected by fatigue. Ferrell and colleagues (1996) found that fatigue influenced spiritual well-being because it heightened awareness of illness and resulted in feelings of uncertainty and hopelessness. Dean and Ferrell (1995, p. 25) suggested that fatigue is not just a physical symptom, but ". . . an all-consuming experience that disrupts family and work, creates help-lessness, and results in despair." Winningham (1996, p. 5) observed, "Spirituality is central to cancer patients' struggle to find satisfaction and peace in spite of diminished energy, increased fatigue, and demands of everyday survival. . . . To ignore the pervasive role of spir-ituality in the daily survival of our patients is to insult the human spirit." This same essay went on to explore spirituality as an important link between energy, fatigue, and quality of life. It is striking, in this context, that health care providers know so little about spiritual adjustment to fatigue. Cancer survivors, on the other hand, become well acquainted with the spiritual struggles involved.

> *What makes the fatigue so frustrating is that I don't have time for this. I want my life back, now, before anything more slips away from me.*   Cancer survivor

> *For my days are vanishing like smoke. . . .*   Psalm 102:3

In what sense does fatigue contribute to a spiritual crisis? Why is it that we have been so insensitive and unaware of the seriousness of this conflict? Part of the difficulty in answer-ing this question is that *spirituality* is difficult to define. Research on spirituality has often been limited to the study of religious practices. More recently, the term *spirituality* has been expanded to apply to all humans whether or not they are "religious" in the traditional sense (Post-White et al, 1996). Some such as Brocollo see spirituality as a way of coping with life (Giblin, Wicks, and Parsons, 1993, p. 314). Others, including Schneider, describe it as the experience of constantly striving to integrate one's life in terms of ultimate values (Giblin, Wicks, and Parsons, 1993, p. 314). According to Frankl (1963), a Holocaust con-centration camp survivor, the spiritual is ". . . that which makes us human" and causes us to seek meaning in all facets of experience. In its broadest sense, spirituality is the ". . . process of apprehending, ordering, representing–of ascribing value and meaning to

About the Contributor

With a bachelor's degree in radio and television from Ithaca College, New York, Gerry Kelly set out to work as a Top 40 rock 'n' roll disc jockey for WSRF (Ft. Lauderdale, Florida), WGOW (Chattanooga, Tennessee), WYND (Sarasota, Florida), and WOLF (Syracuse, New York). He explains that the isolation of the entertainment world led him to attend Westminster Theological Seminary in Philadelphia to earn a master's degree in divinity in 1980. He spent several years in the pastorate and found himself drawn to working with people in crisis. During a two-year residency in clinical pastoral education at the Amarillo

experience . . . [it is] the unifying factor in human life," as J. E. Heathcock suggested (personal correspondence, April 1997).

Biblical imagery may help to illustrate. The creation narrative of Genesis describes the Spirit of God bringing "light" (order) out of "darkness" (chaos) (Genesis 1). Similarly, our own spiritual nature is revealed as we attempt to bring order to the diverse as well as the confusing aspects of our life experience. Religious faith facilitates believers' interpretation of their own reality whenever it assures them that there is intrinsic meaning and value to human life. This happens when people see their lives from the perspective of a loving God. Being part of a religious community that cares for and helps its members may aid patients in retaining hope (Mays, 1981).

When an individual's view of life is challenged, a spiritual crisis occurs. If it is found to be inadequate in interpreting or explaining his or her life experience, as Heathcock (1975, p. 120) cautioned, ". . . some measure of disintegration may result." Fatigue may precipitate such a spiritual crisis when survivors don't have the energy to make spiritual adaptations. That is, they are exhausted by the effort involved in overcoming the spiritual hurdle of integrating their experience of fatigue with their world view. As fatigue increasingly limits their ability to function in terms of their own expectations and the expectations of others, their life, as they have known it in the past, appears to lose meaning and grinds to a halt. Unless they are able to find meaning and renewal in their experience of fatigue, they may lose hope and begin to withdraw. They may also feel an increased burden of guilt, perceiving themselves to be a failure and morally weak. If a spiritual resolution is found, Madden (1970) told us, it must provide something beyond mere "positive thinking." It must be able to counteract the feelings of hopelessness, the sense of doom.

Having cancer, in and of itself, often incurs feelings of guilt and shame. Cancer patients frequently ask, "Why has this happened to me? What did I do wrong?" This can lead to an anguished soul searching where the suffering of cancer is attributed to character flaws or wrongdoing. Fatigue presents a special problem: Patients often fear their fatigue is evidence of laziness, moral weakness, or lack of willpower. To make things worse, well-intended friends and relatives reinforce these fears with accusations. In Chapter 1, Albert Schweitzer's definition of *pain* was quoted as ". . . anything that diminishes life." Patients

Hospital District, he became chaplain resident at the psychiatric hospital in Amarillo, Texas. When the Don and Sybil Harrington Cancer Center opened in Amarillo, he became the chaplain, working with cancer survivors and families. In 1994, he became director of supportive care at the Harrington Cancer Center, where he continues to help individuals find meaning in their cancer experiences. He strongly believes that addressing spiritual needs is an integral part of comprehensive cancer care. A number of years ago, he began to identify fatigue as one of the more problematic issues in cancer.

often try to "pull themselves up by their bootstraps" only to fall back into an exacerbated exhaustion. This leads to a despair and hopelessness that is not to be confused with depression.

Whether the person is religious or an atheist, there are several parallel arguments that feature essentially the same logical flaw:

> "If you had the right attitude, your cancer would go away."
> "If you exercise just a little willpower, you could overcome this."
> "Stop being a wimp: Pull it together."
> "If you had enough faith, you could be healed."

Sometimes patients interpret suffering as the price one pays to live. It is as if they have bargained with God, but somehow come out poorly. Having been allowed to live, they seem to feel they must now fend for themselves without God's help, "bearing their cross" of fatigue alone. This undermines their faith in a loving God and becomes an enormous burden. The expectations of performance they place on themselves may be heightened by guilt and shame when reinforced by other people, especially by authority figures. This leads to a vicious, destructive cycle, which results in further fatigue.

There is one central flaw in all of the above arguments: Those who think willpower or self-manufactured faith can produce a cure should remember that everyone, no matter how positive or spiritual, eventually dies. No one can will themselves to live. People with everything to live for still die: That is one of the apparently impenetrable mysteries of life. Indeed, the ability to go on and find peace in the midst of this is a sign of maturity and faith.

Lack of suffering is often interpreted as a sign of goodness; conversely, patients and others may think suffering is a result of guilt or a sign of wrongdoing. One of the most ancient and remarkable stories of all time addressed this problem of unexplained pain with the question, Why do good people suffer? It is the story of Job.

According to the story, Job was a wealthy man who lived an unreproachable life. He was a great and generous benefactor in his community. In addition, he exercised concern in looking after the spiritual well-being of others. Then, in a series of disasters, he lost everything he had—children, wealth, health, and social standing. He was in agony.* The only thing left to him was his sharp-tongued wife who advised him, "Curse God and die" (one wonders whether she was left to torment him).

Now Job had three friends. When they heard of all that happened to him, they came to mourn with him and comfort him. They sat with him in silence for seven days and seven nights, sharing his grief. Finally, Job burst out in the bitterness of spirit and suffering he was experiencing. He started by cursing the day he was born and proceeded to give voice to the

---

Thanks to Wendy S. Harpham and Maryl L. Winningham for their input in this section.

*Although most English Bible translations tell us Job was smitten with "sore boils" from head to foot, the Lamsa translation of the Bible of the Aramaic church of the East states Job had cancer throughout his whole body. (Lamsa, 1957).

depths of his despair. Unfortunately, that opened the opportunity for his friends to give their opinions on why this happened to Job. In different ways, each concluded Job had done something to deserve his metastatic cancer. Job did his best to defend himself, arguing every point, using much energy to try to maintain his innocence, to make sense of his experience. He told them they were saying nothing new, but he also told them they were speaking hurtfully because they had never been in his position. At one point, he tells his friends, "I have heard many such things: miserable comforters are ye all" (Job 16:2).

It is important for cancer patients to know that well-intending people who say hurtful things obviously have never had a personal encounter with suffering. Healthy people seem to have a peculiar compulsion for tormenting the sick with ill-advised lectures and sermons. Psalm 69:20 sums up the resultant feelings, "Reproach hath broken my heart, and I am full of heaviness. I looked for someone to take pity, but there was none, and for comforters, but I found none." What a sorrowful expression of the loneliness experienced in serious illness and suffering!

Beyond the story of accusations and suffering, the ending to the book of Job contains some remarkable observations. God's response to all the human verbiage was this: "Who is this that darkeneth counsel by words without knowledge?" (Job 38:2). Then comes the secret of Job's eventual discovery of peace and healing. First, he humbles himself and acknowledges that he doesn't understand God's ways at all: no more arguing, no more struggling. Beyond that, God expresses his anger with Job's friends for their rash and hurtful words, for presuming to speak for God. In an insightful picture of community healing, we are told that Job is asked to pray for his friends that God's anger may be turned away from them. As Job intercedes for them, he starts to find the way of spiritual healing, as it says ". . . [then] the Lord also accepted Job, . . . and the Lord turned the captivity of Job . . ." This example is mindful of the wisdom in the Lord's prayer, "Forgive us our wrongs, as we forgive those who have wronged us."

It is difficult to forgive those who are judgmental and misguided in their accusations. Their painful accusations make the burden more difficult and come at a time when the person is exceptionally vulnerable. For the well, the lesson of life seems to be, "Be careful what you say if you have never experienced what the patient is experiencing.

You mean this is real? I thought I was losing my mind!

Common comment among cancer survivors

You don't know what you are talking about." For the ill, the lesson of life seems to be, "Forgive them, they don't know what they are saying." A wise person once wrote, "Don't let your peace be in the mouths of men." The way to peace and spiritual growth lies not in self-recrimination and accusations; those things only make things worse and contribute to increased exhaustion. They also lead to increased feelings of alienation and hopelessness.

What is the wise friend to do? Job's friends were much better off as long as they kept their mouths shut, as long as they sat with him to grieve with him. Sometimes, in the face of suffering, it may be best to say nothing. The best thing a friend can do is be there, support, comfort, and gently encourage. Those who have lived through similar suffering have received a gift, a gift of understanding. They are the ones who have the most to offer.

What kind of a mother am I now? I've even had to ask friends to pick up my kids after school. I just can't do it anymore.   Young mother with cancer

Whoever wants to save his life will lose it, but whoever loses his life will find it.
                      Matthew 10:30, Matthew 16:25, Mark 8:35, Luke 9:24, John 12:25

Fatigue involves many experiences of loss. Indeed, the fatigued survivor's experience is one of constant attrition. As more and more connections to the world are severed by the limitations imposed by fatigue, cancer survivors lose important reference points of self-definition (Bridges, 1980). The cry "What kind of mother am I now?" by the young mother with cancer echoes the profound nature of this loss. As Bridges (1980) observed in a similar situation, a significant aspect of identity was disintegrating, and with it the sense of order and meaning in life. Her fatigue precipitated a spiritual crisis because it would not reconcile with her definition of a good mother. Feelings of guilt and failure are a profound source of distress and suffering. Trite and thoughtless suggestions by well-intended health care providers, clergy, or significant others may only intensify this suffering and despair. To make sense of her life and bring order out of crisis, this mother will have to do more than repair dysfunction (i.e., such as ask her friends to help with her children). Such attempts at resolution, though helpful as temporary coping strategies, circumvent the spiritual reality of the crisis and fail to bring peace. Her ability to adjust to changes in her life that are imposed by fatigue depends on her ability to set aside the past. It is only by accepting her present reality that she can experience renewal and "find" her life again (Bridges, 1980).

When Jesus said people would have to surrender their life in order to find it, he identified a paradox often confronted by patients with fatigue. The crisis in their lives presents a critical dilemma (Madden, 1970). Will they attempt to re-create or maintain their past self, expending their already depleted resources of strength and energy, or will they come to terms with themselves in a present that is very different from the life they had been living?

I kept waiting for my strength to rally. I could even picture myself getting back to jogging. Now I realize I was kidding myself. Physically, I don't have the energy to get out of bed. No, this is where I need to be now, and I have peace about that.   Cancer survivor in a hospice

But those who wait upon the Lord will renew their strength. They will soar on wings like eagles. They will run and not grow weary, they will walk and not faint.   Isaiah 40:31

The woman in a hospice who surrendered her wish to return to jogging was not giving in to resignation and despair, nor was she exhibiting spiritual or moral weakness. She was making a courageous choice to move forward to live in her present reality. Rather than remain forever waiting on the past to come again, she demonstrated a true state of spiritual health. In the process, she found a new kind of strength and peace. Her statement reveals something of what it means to find spiritual resolution. As tempting as it is to retreat in the face of crisis, there is no real comfort to be found in dwelling on the past. To do so robs the present of any potential for insight or heightened meaning (Heathcock, 1975). Renewal and resolution are found only through *acceptance of present reality*. As Madden (1970, p. 116) stated, "To see God is essentially to be in the present. This is the action of the Spirit. This is God's power to move a man along the path of reality."

It is painfully difficult to wait in the midst of fatigue that seems to stretch on forever. To the extent that fatigue represents the absence of those experiences which give life purpose and direction, it is natural that cancer survivors will rush to find ways of replacing those missing elements (Bridges, 1980). Seen in this light, the fatigue seems meaningless for individuals and can accentuate feelings of hopelessness and helplessness. Under these circumstances, it is difficult for them and others around them to integrate the fatigue with the rest of their experience. Fatigue is seen simply as an intrusion imposed from outside, something that sends their life, their hopes, and their dreams into crisis. It seems to be a bitter taunt of better days. Remarkably, out of this very circumstance of extremity, "with their backs against the wall," some patients discover another possibility, the experience of "blessing" (Madden, 1970).

The word *blessing* is often associated with superficial forms of religious language and practice (Leon-Dufour, 1973). When correctly defined, the concept of blessing is closely associated with vision and insight. To be blessed is to receive reassurance and direction, even when one is caught in frightening circumstances that make no sense. The cancer survivor who must prioritize activities to save energy for only the essential may come to a heightened awareness of what is truly important (Ferrell et al, 1996). The waiting imposed by fatigue can provide time to think, to bring life, the present crisis, and faith together in a meaningful way (Heathcock, 1975). In Jewish tradition, the concepts of patience and waiting are central to spiritual growth and development. Madden (1970, p. 125) also suggested, "The ability to wait might be the chief Christian virtue. . . . The blessing is promised to the one who can still expectantly wait for new life." Indeed, this value is common to most of the major world religions.

> . . . *this has been hell to live with. Absolute hell. If it wasn't for my wife and a few people who have stood by me, I don't think I could have made it. Well, I just wouldn't be here today.*
>
> Cancer survivor

> *Even though I walk through the valley of the shadow of death, I will fear no evil, for you are with me. . . .*
>
> Psalm 23:4

As important as it is for patients to be encouraged to find meaning in their present reality, it is not always reasonable to expect them to do so by themselves. For many reasons, survivors may come to the point where they are unable to marshal further resources to deal with the many problems fatigue creates. Winningham (1996, p. 4) noted, "This . . . results in ongoing internal conflict, sadness, grief, and hopelessness." At such times, to "walk through the valley" alone is to invite despair. Alone with his fatigue, the cancer survivor quoted above was unable to move beyond the loss and confusion he felt. It is not surprising he said he was stuck in a kind of "hell," ". . . in the lowest pit in the darkest depths" (Psalm 88:6). In these circumstances, one can only hope for deliverance to come from outside. Personal resources are no longer enough.

As this man discovered, it was the people who "stood beside" him who helped him survive his ordeal. Their presence and concern may not have altered the profound sensation of his fatigue, but they clearly changed the meaning of the experience for him. Their support reassured him that his life had purpose and value even when his fatigue disrupted his ability to function normally. In religious language, their blessing was what he needed to pronounce his own benediction and find peace.

This illustration suggests that resolution of spiritual crisis may never be completely divorced from some meaningful social context (Leech, 1992). The belief that grace and blessing are imparted from one person to another has been recognized by many religious groups. For centuries, the religious community was emphasized to be an environment of healing. It was in the community of faith that the means of grace were available to the afflicted. Those who were ill were encouraged to call upon their elders to lay hands upon them, ". . . to pray over them and anoint them with oil. . ." (James 5:14). This ancient tradition reflects a deep appreciation for the important role interpersonal relationships play in both physical and spiritual healing (Madden, 1970).

Those who wish to be a "means of grace" or a bringer of blessing must learn to resist the impulse to rescue survivors in crisis. To do so prematurely may rob persons of important opportunities for finding peace within their crisis. Focusing exclusively on symptoms without giving patients time to talk about the effects and significance of fatigue on their life may actually communicate that one does not take their situation seriously enough to "stand beside" them (Dean and Ferrell, 1995). The result may be an increase in their level of frus-

My fatigue experience began in October 1996 when I was diagnosed with a malignant fibrous histiocytoma bone tumor, at which time I began an intensive regimen of combination chemotherapy, which would go on to last ten months. My first impression was that this stuff made me somewhat sick, but it wasn't as bad as I had heard or was anticipating. It soon became evident that with each treatment the fatigue was becoming increasingly worse.

While it is obvious that the buildup of chemicals caused most of my physical backslide, it is also complicated by the severe mental stress of having a possibly fatal disease. I always went to bed worried and woke up scared, and rarely would I have an uninterrupted night of sleep.

For the first couple of months I would have several good hours in the morning. But as time went on, it got to be less and less, to the point that in the last couple of months it has been a tremendous struggle just to get out of bed. Single tasks seemed to be giant burdens. Taking a shower, answering the phone, or sometimes

tration, leaving them with feelings that are often experienced as isolation, failure, and guilt. Spiritual resolution demands more than technical expertise; it calls for a "laying on of hands" (Madden, 1970). For patients of religious faith, this may involve the appropriation of the rituals and symbols of their religious tradition to help expand meaning and provide comfort. However, just being present, listening, and giving encouragement as people struggle to make sense of their fatigue can be among the most valuable interventions offered (Post-White et al, 1996).

Some cancer survivors fear that treatment for the distress of depression, which may be interactive with fatigue, will rob them of religious growth through their suffering. It is important that survivors, as well as clergy, families, and other care providers, not confuse spiritual suffering with physical or mental torment. In my experience, the appropriate treatment of depression, including medication, in no way interferes with or inhibits spiritual growth and development. On the contrary, treatment for depression can set survivors free to explore their experience of illness and opportunities for spiritual growth during this time of crisis.

Peace I leave with you; my peace I give to you. I do not give as the world gives. Do not let your hearts be troubled and do not be afraid.   John 14:27

By conceptualizing fatigue as a spiritual crisis, we can better understand the profound struggle individuals undergo in adjusting to the changes cancer brings. Fatigue, perhaps more than any other side effect of cancer, is a lingering, unmistakable reminder of the human condition with all its frailty, vulnerability, and lack of control. Limitations imposed by fatigue challenge and confront the assumptions with which the healthy and energetic approach life and the world. It may be that fatigue creates a crisis partly because it is such a collision with reality.

even eating seemed not worth the effort. Just walking, I felt like this little person inside a huge thousand-pound body. Dealing with the everyday medication schedule and chemo side effects seemed like a full-time job. Also as my physical condition worsened, it became harder to fight off the feelings of depression and hopelessness, which in turn was having a negative effect on my already stressed family.

Now that I've finished my chemo and I'm hopefully on the road to recovery, I am feeling better every day. My first advice to someone who is about to go through chemotherapy is to not fight the fatigue, but to "go with the flow" and to view it as a time of healing and rest–allowing your strong medicine to work. You deserve this time and if you fall behind on something else, so what? Your first concern must be to keep your eyes on the light at the end of the tunnel, and get through this. When it is all over, it is worth it!

Daniel T. Whitman

What difference does this awareness make in the care of cancer survivors? The answer is something of a paradox in that it makes all the difference and at the same time, none at all. The symptoms of fatigue are no less troublesome because fatigue is recognized as a spiritual crisis. However, as long as patients perceive their fatigue to be merely a complex of symptoms that constitute an interruption of their lives and something to be fought, it will likely remain a frustrating and essentially meaningless experience for its duration. Attempts to get back to "normal" by trying to repair their lives are not the way to peace. This idea of finding peace in the midst of personal trials and distress is so beautifully embodied in the Hebrew concept "shalom," which can be interpreted as a restful state of peace and blessing.

If life is seen as continuing to move ahead and unfold through the experience of fatigue, something of value and significance can be discovered in the process. Although fatigue may persist, suffering may be alleviated. Hence, nothing changes but nothing will ever be the same. Caregivers who are willing to embrace this paradox will provide survivors frequent opportunities to explore their present reality. This can be time-consuming but often yields great results. As cancer survivors describe their fatigue, one soon realizes they are subtly editing their story with each telling. Through this kind of repeated verbal processing, they gain new insight, and through insight, a new sense of direction. The struggle and distress created by fatigue can yield to a sense of rest and blessing as a result of these new insights.

In religious language, the spiritual response to this ongoing struggle might be expressed in the form of the following prayer:

O Lord, I am so tired of this fatigue. I can no longer do the things I need to do, or fulfill my obligations to those who depend on me. It is so hard for me to live like this. I want to be the person I used to be. But if this is what I am called to now, please take the pieces I have left, and rework them into something of value and meaning. Let me find peace and strength in your love, and in the tender care of the others who love me, until my own strength is renewed.   Amen.

References

Bridges, W. (1980). *Transitions: Making sense of life's changes* (pp. 92, 96, 112–113). Reading, MA: Addison-Wesley.

Dean, G., and Ferrell, B. (1995). Impact of fatigue on quality of life in cancer survivors. *Quality of Life– A Nursing Challenge, 4*, 25.

Ferrell, B., Grant, M., Dean, G., Funk, B., and Ly, J. (1996). "Bone tired": The experience of fatigue and its impact on quality of life. *Oncology Nursing Forum, 23*, 1545.

Frankl, V. (1963). *Man's search for meaning.* New York: Pocket Books.

Giblin, P., Wicks R., and Parsons, R. (Eds.) (1993). *Clinical handbook of pastoral counseling* (vol. 2, p. 314). Mahwah, NJ: Paulist Press.

Heathcock, J. E. (1975). Religious language and pastoral care. *Bulletin of the American Protestant Hospital Association*, 120–121, 124.

Lamsa, G. (1957). The Holy Bible from ancient eastern manuscripts: Containing the Old and New Testaments translated from the Peshitta, the authorized bible of the Church of the East. Philadelphia: A. J. Holman.

Leech, K. (1992). *The eye of the storm: Living spiritually in the real world.* New York: HarperCollins.

Leon-Dufour, X. (1973). *Dictionary of biblical theology* (p. 47). 2nd ed. New York: Seabury Press.

Madden, M. (1970). *The power to bless.* (Preface, pp. 1, 15, 117–125, 142, 150–151). Nashville, TN: Broadman Press.

Mays, L. (1981). Cancer management, the clergy, and the human spirit. *Cancer Journal for Clinicians, 31*, 51, 53.

Nightingale, F. (1859). *Notes on nursing.* London: Harrison and Sons. (Reprinted in offset in 1946 by Edward Stern & Co., Philadelphia).

Post-White, J., Ceronsky, C., Kreitzer, M., et al (1996). Hope, spirituality, sense of coherence, and quality of life in patients with cancer. *Oncology Nursing Forum, 23*, 1572, 1578.

Winningham, M. (1996). Fatigue: The missing link to quality of life. *Quality of Life–A Nursing Challenge, 23*, 5.

Prayer for the Fatigued

Turn my weary thoughts to you,
Dear One, who answers prayer;
But hold them—I'm too weak
To raise them unassisted here.

I once could serve and sing and praise
—Those were much stronger, healthier days.
But now my heart is weighted down
By pain and great distress.
And unclear thoughts just fly around
Like birds without a nest.

I long to turn my thoughts to you,
Dear One, who answers prayer.
But thoughts and words don't seem to come
And when I would, my lips are dumb
And fevered restlessness is there.

Dear Father, bring my mind to rest
Your presence is my only cheer.
Hold me, your child, to your breast
And comfort in this helplessness
For you have said you would stay near.

Fatigue From Opposite Ends of the Stethoscope

Theodore P. McDade

One of the hardest things involving fatigue is that many of my family and friends didn't have any clue of what I was experiencing. One of my sisters asked me once if I had been making up the tiredness to get attention. Yeh right!! She said I felt fine last week.

Brenda Heil, 33 years old, 9-year survivor

Background

My interest in the profound fatigue often experienced by cancer patients stems from many experiences. As a physician, I have both compassionate and scientific motivations. My first academic exposure occurred while pursuing graduate studies in biomedical and human factors engineering at MIT's Department of Aeronautics and Astronautics, where I learned about the similarities of fatigue produced by prolonged hospital bed rest and the microgravity of spaceflight. More recently, first as a medical student and now as a surgical resident, I have witnessed the influence of fatigue on cancer patients struggling with the effects of both their disease and its treatment. Clinically, it is often the issues of life and limb that receive priority attention. Yet, fatigue is something that not only contributes greatly to the difficulty of these patients' lives, but also possibly even endangers them. In a sense, it is the very existence of a fatigued body and spirit that provides the setting in which a struggle can occur at all. It is a struggle I understand intimately. Prior to medical school, I was diagnosed with acute myelogenous leukemia (AML), and following induction chemotherapy, underwent allogeneic bone marrow transplantation (BMT) while in first remission. Those months as a patient on Proger 6 North at New England Medical Center taught me a lot about fatigue. As hard as those lessons were to learn, harder still has been seeing a loved one suffer in his own battle with cancer. Perhaps that is the strongest contributor of all to my commitment to such issues. Before a review of the literature from a surgical perspective are a few of my reflections on life as a cancer patient. These are of very private struggles that occur with profound fatigue, yet are not often talked about. If the words at times are brutally honest, and even a bit unpalatable, it is only in an attempt to provide at least a hint of what such experiences can be like. With that spirit in mind, it is hoped that the reader may temporarily enter what was my world, as a young man in late August and early September of 1989.

The Patient's Perspective

Apparently satisfied that my status had not perilously changed overnight, the small group of doctors briskly exited single file from my room, having completed their usual routine of questions, poking, and prodding. Prior to the diagnosis with leukemia, I'd had plans of going to medical school; hence, I enjoyed "morning rounds" and always tried to be alert and sitting up for them. But that was becoming more difficult with each day. The chemotherapy and total body irradiation that had led to my recent BMT were beginning to take their toll. I'd felt quite strong for a while, but things were rapidly changing. Even waiting in a wheelchair, to be transferred back upstairs from my last radiation treatment, had been like a form of torture with my lack of normal postural muscle endurance.

After the door clicked shut, I could see through the glass as the doctors removed masks, gowns, and gloves, and disappeared. Though I looked forward to human contact in my isolation room, I was ready for their departure. Sliding my rear end toward the foot of the bed, I quite literally hurried my head back down to the pillow. I wasn't simply relaxing; there was a *need* to do that. I didn't really feel sleepy. Nor did I lack the physical capacity to remain propped up with my back against the pillow for a bit longer. And I wasn't dopey from narcotics (though at times I experienced that, too). Instead, there was an all-over heaviness, most pronounced in my head, driving me to seek out a horizontal posture. It was a heaviness so deep, it was almost an ache. And yet, I didn't have a headache. I was simply worn out, fatigued in a way I'd never known before.

My search for comfort, however, was soon interrupted. I opened my eyes to the hollow sound of the room intercom clicking on, followed by a pleasant voice greeting me. It was not long after the change of shift for the nurses, and my day nurse was smiling through the window in the door. After a friendly "Good morning!" she suggested that we begin our morning routine, if I was feeling up to it. Though it was nice of her to provide a choice, I knew that at best I could only delay things. As part of the BMT protocol, to limit potential germs while my immune system was so weakened, I was supposed to shower daily with

About the Contributor

Ted McDade's insights, from the patient's perspective, the engineer's perspective, the researcher's perspective, and the physician's perspective, make him uniquely qualified to write this chapter. Prior to his medical studies, Ted received a bachelor of science degree in electrical engineering from Clarkson University (1985) and a Master of Science degree in biomedical/human factors engineering from the Department of Aeronautics and Astronautics, Massachusetts Institute of Technology (MIT), Cambridge (1989). He had experience with the National Aeronautics and Space Administration centers at the Jet Propulsion Laboratories (Pasadena), with the Johnson Space Center (Houston), and with the Man-Vehicle Laboratory at MIT, and has a research background studying digitized bioelectrical data on muscle fatigue assessment. More recently, his research focus has been on cancer.

Hibiclens (chlorhexidine), a strong antimicrobial cleansing solution. Because I usually had at least three intravenous (IV) lines running simultaneously, all with separate IV pumps on wheels, just getting to the shower was an awkward two- or three-person task. What had started out as a refreshing way to start the day had more recently become a somewhat dreaded test of endurance. Figuring I might as well get it over with, I agreed to go ahead with everything. My nurse said she'd be back in 10 or 15 minutes.

Ever since awakening, I'd wanted to get rid of some of the IV fluids finding their way into my bladder and was glad I'd have time to do so while I still had some privacy. Unfortunately, I also had been having diarrhea, another side effect of my treatments, and now felt pressure building there again as well. Damn! I dreaded what that would mean for me. It was more than the burning and cramping. That part of it was bad enough. It was also the effort that it required. I'd had to get up twice during the night, and both times had postponed things as long as possible. However, a spasm deep in my gut told me not to try to delay this time.

Sitting up, I swung my feet over the edge of the bed. The act of "going to the bathroom" wasn't quite so simple as I'd always known it to be while healthy. First of all, I wasn't going anywhere. Because of the diarrhea, my weakness, and all of the IV lines connected to me, I now had a bedside commode. Hence the importance of timing for privacy. In addition, everything had to be measured and analyzed. So urine had to be collected separately from the diarrhea. For that, I had to use a plastic urinal jug. I would take care of that first. Though it seemed almost impossible to use one of those damned things in bed without making a mess, I had learned to conserve energy whenever possible. Standing would be a foolish waste of strength I would soon need. It could also be dangerous; I had already previously "grayed" out and struck my head on the floor while trying to urinate. A repeat of such a fall could be deadly with my low platelet count. The last thing I needed at this point was an intracranial bleed. Sliding up the bed a bit, just out of view from the door, I positioned myself right on the edge of the mattress, thereby providing clearance for the urinal jug to be held upright. Grasping my hospital gown, I pulled it up and sideways to uncover myself. Damn it! I was sitting on the lower part of the gown. A combination of twisting,

After receiving a bone marrow transplant for leukemia, he went on to medical school at Jefferson Medical College in Philadelphia, where he graduated in 1996. He is currently a surgical resident at Massachusetts General Medical Center in Boston. In Chapter 22, Ted presents a poignant contrast between his experience with fatigue as a bone marrow transplant patient and the risks it presents to patients from a surgeon's viewpoint.

His current greatest personal challenge is in learning to be a father. He and his wife are the proud parents of a new baby!

leaning, and tugging succeeded in freeing the gown, but not without a price. I could feel my heart beating rapidly in my chest. Picking up the urinal jug with a quivering hand, I moved it into position. Still leaning on the mattress with my other hand, I would need to use it too. Sitting up straight, I hurriedly parted the fly opening of the hospital pajama-style pants and attempted to begin the task at hand. But starting a stream without simultaneously opening the floodgates of the diarrhea was not easy. It was taking time for my body to find the proper balance of relaxation and control. Yet, in this position, time was not a luxury I could afford. Christ! In my current condition, the performance of a simple bodily function, usually requiring virtually no thought at all, had become a complicated production. As the fluid level finally began to rise in the urinal, so too did my need to lay down as soon as possible. Counting the seconds, it was all I could do to wait for the last droplets. After carefully setting down the urinal jug, I collapsed back onto the pillow.

Within moments, another spasm prompted me to sit up again. Slipping my feet into moccasins at the bedside, I stood up slowly, moving my feet farther apart for added stability. A quick survey of my IV lines confirmed that a counterclockwise spin would be necessary to avoid becoming entangled. After two steps forward, I did so, turning my back in the direction of the commode. Grasping each side of the long hospital gown, I drew it up in front of me, collecting it into a bundle above waist level. Cradling it with my left hand, I peered over it and untied the drawstring pants using my right hand. Pausing, much like a weight lifter before attempting a challenging effort, I mustered all of my strength in preparation for the next few moments. With one last glance I confirmed the location of the toilet seat. My left hand pressing the crumpled gown to my belly, I simultaneously bent at the knees and waist as I lowered my pants with the other hand. When they had reached my knees, I was in what felt like a low squat, but my rear end had yet to find its target. In reality, I was bent over far more at the waist than at the knees. The quadriceps muscles of my legs simply couldn't lower me with control to that level. As they had reached their limits, I unconsciously had compensated by bending more at the waist, thereby shifting my center of mass forward. I strained as if bearing a great weight, but it was only that of my own body. Continued effort failed to produce contact with the commode, and I was quickly losing energy. To avoid falling, I either needed to abort the attempt completely or else quickly grab onto something. Not wanting to lose any hard-earned progress, I opted for the latter. Pulling my knees apart against the pants allowed me to let go of them without tangling up my feet, and permitted me to step around to the right while still in my awkward squat. With my right hand on the toilet seat, my triceps could now assist with the lowering process, my backside finally perching on the edge of the seat. Centering myself, I allowed the diarrhea to escape, and doubled over with forearms flat across knees and my face pressed onto my arms. It was as close as I could get to laying down under the circumstances. Once finished, I raised myself up onto my elbows. But I still had to face the part I dreaded the most. Healthy individuals do many personal things in the course of a day with hardly a thought.

By this point in my therapy, however, that was no longer true for me. I had to break down even the most routine processes into individual steps that I could accomplish. I'd never realized the highly complex interaction of multiple muscle groups in the arms, legs, abdomen, chest, and back that allows one to perform the bending, twisting, and leaning required to simply use toilet paper effectively without falling. It was troubling and embarrassing that this private task, mastered in early childhood, could now be so problematic. No modification in technique seemed to diminish the struggle. Out of necessity, I'd learned to simply share the effort among multiple postures, thereby allowing greater endurance. While still seated, I starting the cleaning process from behind, but quickly became exhausted, quivering violently like an underprepared marathon runner about to collapse before reaching the finish line. With abdominal and back muscles simply unable to continue the twisting and leaning, I switched to awkward attempts from the front. Finally, after doubling over again to rest, I struggled to my feet, hurriedly completing things while standing.

Crawling back into bed, I lay staring at the ceiling. With heart racing, and an uncomfortable sensation of perspiration, I tried to shake my overwhelming feeling of weakness. In a minute or two, I heard a noise at the door. Entering the room was my nurse, accompanied by a transplant nurse in training, both suited up with mask, gown, and gloves. It was time for my real challenge of the day. We talked and joked as they got things ready. While the trainee began moving IV bags from ceiling hooks, grouping them with those on wheeled IV pumps, and untangling tubing, my nurse addressed the sites where the IV lines entered my skin. First, she needed to examine the triple-lumen Hickman-type catheters penetrating both sides of my chest. This long-term variety of the so-called central line is threaded through veins nearly to the heart. These can provide IV access for months because they are tunneled through the chest wall and have a cuff that theoretically limits travel of bacteria up the tunnel and to the vein. Nevertheless, they must be carefully managed to avoid infections, and clear plastic occlusive dressings are used to keep their entry sites clean and dry. The nurse and I unsnapped the hospital gown at the shoulder so the dressings could be double-checked prior to my shower. Next, the more standard peripheral IV line in my right arm needed dressing modifications. Despite the availability of multiple ports for each catheter in my chest, sometimes even more IV lines were temporarily needed. To waterproof the IV site in my arm, the nurses would cut the fingers off of latex gloves and pull the remaining hand and wrist sections over the IV, taping it securely. With these preparations complete, it was time for me to get out of bed. Unfortunately, I already felt worn out.

Pushing off of the mattress with my hands, I stood up among the array of four IV pumps on wheels. Each nurse handled two of these.

"Are you okay on your feet?"

I quite frankly felt pretty shaky, but as a 26-year-old man being assisted by two young women, I responded with perhaps predictable false bravado.

"Sure. No problem."

Now that I was standing, it was truly a race against the clock. My endurance would be limited. I had barely managed to stay on my feet the day before. I wanted to quickly get into the bathroom adjoining my room, but the IV pumps were like four ball-and-chains, attached to me by a tangle of IV tubing. I entered the cramped quarters first, standing close to the shower stall. The toilet and sink filled most of the remaining space. One at a time, the IV pumps were maneuvered over the doorway baseboard. By leaning slightly into the shower, I allowed space for the last IV pump to be squeezed into the bathroom. Reaching around the IV pumps, the nurses helped me off with the hospital gown and asked if I was all set. I had a reputation for being a bit shy, so they were basically making sure I could remove the pajama-type pants and get into the shower without assistance. Once I answered yes, they assured me that they would be right outside the door if I needed them, and then closed it, leaving me alone.

One of the rules of the transplant room was that I was to treat anything below knee level as dirty, and therefore a potential hazard given my reduced ability to fight infections. So, upon untying the drawstring waist of the pants, I let them fall down my legs, but retained one side of the cord in my fingers. Alternately lifting my feet out of the crumpled pile, I pulled the pants away with the drawstring, carefully stepping back onto my shoes to

You Think You Have It Licked

You know, after treatment you think you have it licked. But now you're wearing down, so each day becomes a matter of dull, gray endurance. You talk to the doctor. "Well, what do you expect?" he says, "You had cancer." So a few months go by. It doesn't get any better. Maybe it's worse because you're comparing it with what you used to do, with what your friends are doing. You go back to your doctor. "Well, what do you expect?" he says, "You're getting older." (How can you age 30 years in one year?) So a few more months go by.

You go to your doctor again and tell him you're barely making it. "Well," he says, "What do you expect? You're overweight. You need to lose weight." So in the next few months, I try to diet. But now I add weakness to the fatigue. A few months go by and I go back to the doctor. "What do you expect?" he says, "You're out of shape. You need to exercise." So I join an aerobics class. I thought I was going to die. I was more tired afterward than before. There was no way I could keep up with that! With the little energy I had left after the classes, I hated the aerobics instructor (all of 21 years old), with her lithe little figure and her trim little tush. Just wait until life has jumped on you, sweetheart, I hissed under my breath, as I crawled out the door for the last time. But the energy was poorly spent. I sat in the car, in the parking lot, for over an hour, trying to pull myself together enough to drive home. So I went back to the doctor. "What do you expect?" he said, "You're depressed. I'm writing you a prescription for this new miracle antidepressant. That should do it." So I felt a little better, spent a lot of money, but didn't have any more energy.

About that time, I got on the Internet. At least it was a social activity that didn't require jumping around, dieting, getting dressed up, going out, and acting cheerful. Someone wrote and asked me, "Did you go through menopause as a result of your treatment, too? I found the book The New Ourselves Growing

avoid touching the floor. After waiting for the water to warm up, which seemed like forever, I began my shower. The water felt wonderful, but the need to lay down again was rapidly becoming stronger. As quickly as possible, I covered my body with the strong pink cleansing agent, but before I could even begin to rinse off, my knees began to shake. There was no way I could make it back to my bed fast enough. I began to panic. I was going to fall, and I simply didn't have the energy to will myself to keep standing. Though I should have called for help, my shyness was compounded manyfold by embarrassment at the loss of body hair. As my legs buckled beneath me, I went down onto my hands and knees in a semi-controlled fall. Once stabilized, I rolled to a seated position and slouched against the shower stall, leaning my forearms on upraised knees. The ice cold of the shower tiles against my bare buttocks reminded me that I wasn't supposed to be touching the floor, but it was too late. Hopefully it was pretty clean. Hanging my bald head with exhaustion, I stared blankly as sudsy water ran down my abdomen and thighs, the three streams briefly joining over the smooth hairless skin at my groin, spilling off of each hip and between my legs before circling the drain and disappearing. Where was the strong young man who mountain climbed, scuba dived, and bicycled 80 miles on hilly roads as his favorite distance? His energy had so quickly faded.

Older *by the Boston Women's Health Cooperative helped me." So I got the book and it explained many of the changes in my body. So if I didn't feel more energetic, at least I understood some of the changes my body was still going through and I felt a minuscule improvement in my self-confidence.*

Then someone wrote about cancer-related fatigue. And I thought, WOW, this thing is real! I'm not going crazy, I'm not losing my mind! Other people have this, too. And then someone wrote about "pacing" to help save energy. She explained how her husband bought her an inexpensive pedometer so she could pace how far she could go by certain times of the day so she didn't collapse before the end of each day. She said after six months of keeping a record, she didn't even need the pedometer anymore and offered to send it to me. Then someone told me how to start a little, short, kind, love-your-body exercise program. I started at three minutes a day, three days a week. But do you know what? It didn't make me feel worse! In fact, within two weeks (six minutes a day, three days a week), I was starting to feel better. It took me six months to work up to doing a 30-minute walk, five days a week. Between that and pacing, I started to come alive again.

Sure, I still have big-time limitations. I'll never be the same. But at least I don't feel confused and victimized all the time. I still see my oncologist for my six-month checkups, but I haven't seen my other doctor for a long time. Why didn't someone tell me about all this earlier? Better yet, why didn't someone tell him *about all this earlier? It would have saved me a lot of time, money, grief, and aggravation! And to tell the truth, I now have enough energy to strangle him!*

60-year-old survivor of stage III breast cancer

Not wanting to upset the nurses with my situation, I struggled back onto my feet after a brief rest. Quickly recleansing the body parts I'd allowed to touch the floor, I shut off the water and pulled open the shower curtain. Staring back at me from the mirror above the sink was a bald young man wavering on shaky legs. I hardly recognized myself. A towel and a clean hospital gown with pants had been left for me, draped over one of the IV pumps. I dried off only as much as necessary and slipped on the hospital gown. The pajama-style pants would have to wait; I simply didn't think I could keep from falling if I tried to lift my legs high enough to put them on. Calling to my nurse, I was relieved to see her open the door almost immediately.

"How did everything go?" she asked with a cheery smile.

"Pretty well," I responded, avoiding mention of any difficulties. "But I'm really going to have to sit or lay down soon," I added with a bit of urgency.

With this she began the process of extricating me from the crowded bathroom, eventually working all four IV pumps through the door. Her assistant had just completed changing the bedding, so she came over to help out. Instead of the confident stride of a young man, I covered the dozen or so feet to the bed with the cautiously placed steps of an elderly person. While her assistant now took responsibility for three of the four IV pumps, my nurse held onto me with her one free arm. By the time our odd little caravan had crossed the room, she was supporting much of my body weight. Sitting heavily onto the bed, I laid down immediately. Like a weight being lifted off of my shoulders, gradually things became better again. No longer struggling, I could once again chat and laugh with the nurses who had long since become my friends. My marathon for the day was over.

Of course, I'd still have many other seemingly little things to do that day, none of which would be easy. At some point soon, I'd have to think about getting started with cleaning my teeth. Who would have ever imagined that could seem like such a daunting task? And later, after more rest, I'd want to try to sit up for a while during my family's visit. That was always my biggest priority. My challenge then would be to hide my fatigue. Why subject my parents and sister to such visible reminders of the difficulty of my current existence? Besides, those visits were moments to cherish, without distractions. So for now, I would simply rest. At times I felt like a hibernating bear, but it seemed to be what my body needed. That, along with modifying the ways I usually did things, was all I could do to manage my fatigue, trying to have faith that if my treatments worked, eventually I would feel normal again someday.

I'm one of the lucky ones: I survived. Eventually I regained a feeling of normalcy. Interestingly, fatigue had been my only symptom prior to diagnosis, but I had dismissed it as natural, given my busy graduate student lifestyle. As its level had steadily increased with advanced disease and treatment effects, feeling any other way had become more and more of an abstraction. And yet now, the opposite is true. Since recovering from my illness, I have married, run a ten-kilometer road race, returned to bicycling and skiing, led multipitch rock climbs, been scuba diving to over 80-foot depths, entered and graduated from medical school, and pursued surgical training, to name but a few happy activities. Not only have I been able to get back to a full-time job, but as a surgical intern, I have worked an average of 110 hours each week for 12 months, taking care of patients every third night while on call, in addition to the typical 15 hours each day. But those things didn't happen right away.

On leaving the transplant unit, I was too weak to walk up a single flight of stairs. Getting across a room to get to the bathroom was about the limit of my endurance, and often I needed to rest in a chair halfway along. I couldn't read even a magazine article, because both the attentional and physical energy that that demanded was simply too much. Nevertheless, I became impressed with the rejuvenating powers of the human body. Soon I was walking a bit farther within my family's home. Within a couple of weeks, I was able to walk in the yard completely around the house. Next, I purposely began to attempt small numbers of stairs. In perhaps three months or so, I was finally feeling like I could do nonstrenuous daily activities without undue worry or exhaustion.

Taking walks amidst the fall foliage around my parent's New Hampshire home, I increased distances gradually up to a couple of miles along the quiet country road. I even went cross-country skiing within those first few months, although admittedly the pace was very slow. By six months, I was very active again, returning to Boston to resume taking premed classes, and whatever of my former activities once again presented themselves as opportunities. I probably was a bit too ambitious, having to briefly enter the hospital a couple of times for fevers and other complications. Nevertheless, I was getting a taste of normalcy again, and since then, I've pretty much lived life at full speed.

The Surgeon's Perspective

As a physician, I currently see things from the other side of the hospital bed. From a surgical oncology perspective, cancer fatigue and its intimate association with activities of daily living (ADLs) relate to both quality of life issues and potential risks of morbidity and mortality.

Quality of life should be maximized for patients whenever possible. Nevertheless, when necessary, the human capacity to endure even extensive periods of great hardship can be quite remarkable. This capacity, however, can be limited without hope for a positive change. The ability to offer nothing more than palliative care to patients with widely metastatic disease is, unfortunately, still a relatively common clinical situation. It is perhaps for this group of patients that quality of life issues, and therefore the effects of fatigue on performance of ADLs, may be most critical. Even if for no other reason, fatigue cannot be considered a minor side effect of cancer and its therapy. Limiting patient morbidity and mortality is a part of surgical philosophy that is reinforced from the earliest days of a surgeon's career until its end, through strictly scheduled (usually weekly) "M and M conferences" (morbidity and mortality conferences) designed to provide lessons from recent complications. It is thus natural for surgeons to view cancer fatigue from that perspective.

What are the identifiable potential risks to the cancer patient that may be associated with fatigue? Further complications or even death may stem from three broad categories of risk that fatigued oncology patients commonly face. These may be categorized as (1) injuries secondary to falls, (2) pathology relating to diminished mobility, and (3) conditions associated with metabolic stresses and release of inflammatory mediators.

Falls sustained by patients while attempting to accomplish ADLs either while hospitalized or once at home are of concern for reasons of both hemorrhage and fracture. While there appears to be little in the literature specifically investigating the incidence and impact of such events in cancer patients, their occurrence in more general terms is well understood. Fortunately, most falls of patients on a surgical service do not result in serious injury (Gomella and Lefor, 1996).

With respect to falls, cancer patients are a unique subgroup. *Spontaneous bleeding* is common, either due to the tumor itself or from associated coagulopathy, with low platelet count secondary to marrow invasion, splenomegaly, and/or treatment side effects being most common (LeMarbre and Boyarsky, 1992). Platelet counts below 10,000 to 20,000 cells per cubic millimeter (mm^3) (10–20×10^9 per liter) are associated with spontaneous bleeding, and thrombocytopenia in this range is considered reason for prophylactic transfusion of platelets. When a patient has been challenged with trauma, however, there is a significant risk of bleeding when platelet counts are up to 30,000 cells per mm^3. The transfusion threshold increases to 50,000 cells per mm^3 in the presence of known active bleeding (Shadduck and Crowley, 1992; Bick, Strauss, and Frenkel, 1996). Hemorrhage in a patient after a low-force traumatic mechanism (<15-foot fall) can occur anywhere, but is less likely to involve classic large deceleration injuries (e.g., thoracic aortic disruption) and more likely to involve bleeding from small vessels (Hoyle, 1994).

A search for potential sites of blood loss should address both the abdomen and the head. Intracranial bleeding is one of the most catastrophic potential sequelae of such injuries. The incidence of intracranial hematoma secondary to falls, in the general population, has been reported to be 39.8%, with emergent neurosurgical intervention being necessary 32.3% of the time (Zwimpfer et al, 1997). Though these percentages may be lowered if they are controlled for height of fall (e.g., falls from bed or chair only), this is balanced at least somewhat by the expected increased risk associated with a thrombocytopenic group.

Falls sustained by patients can also result in *fractures*. These can include fractures of the maxillofacial bones, upper extremity, rib, spine, pelvis, and lower extremity. Fractures of the femoral head and neck (hip fractures) are responsible for a high degree of morbidity. In the infirmed patient, such injury may produce a cascade of such troubles as pneumonia, blood clots, systemic infection, and multiple-organ system failure, and ultimately often leads to death. What is the risk of hip fracture related to falls? In a Swiss study of hospitalized or institutionalized individuals 65 years or older, major falls occurred 1.6 times per patient-year on average, resulting in fractures 5% of the time, with hip fractures accounting for 20% of these (Staubli, 1996). Other studies determined associated risk factors, such as advanced age, female gender, osteoporosis, decreased quadriceps strength, decreased endurance with prolonged recovery phase, low body mass index (less padding), presence of chronic comorbidities, cognitive impairment (e.g., related to narcotics), balance or gait impairment, and the presence of hazards in the living environment (Kannus et al, 1996; Nguyen et al, 1996; Schwendner et al, 1997; Tideiksaar, 1996; Tinetti et al, 1995). Many of these parameters are often applicable to cancer patients.

Early ambulation remains a mainstay of postoperative care because of the extremely dangerous situation that diminished mobility produces for the patient. The profound fatigue of cancer patients may prolong a period of total bed rest, thereby increasing the likelihood of a number of serious complications. These include pneumonia, blood clots, pressure sores, and loss of muscle mass (producing yet further risk). One of the most dreaded complications is a massive pulmonary embolism, often rapidly leading to death despite immediate appropriate actions taken by hospital personnel.

Pulmonary embolism occurs when blood clots form in deep veins, usually of the lower extremities, become free floating, and are swept through the right side of the heart to lodge in branches of the great artery that leads to the lungs. Any subsequent flow of blood or nutrients to the affected lung segments is thus blocked. In 1856, Virchow described a triad of causative factors for *deep venous thrombosis* (DVT): stasis, hypercoagulable state, and endothelial damage to veins (Knudson, 1998). The fatigued cancer patient may be at risk from all three of these. Venous pooling in the lower extremities is increased with immobility. Paraneoplastic syndromes of hypercoagulability are commonly associated with cancer. And direct venous wall injuries can occur with placement of large-bore catheters and have been associated with thrombosis (Knudson, 1998). What are the risks of DVTs? Approximately 20% of all asymptomatic (undiagnosed or untreated) calf DVTs eventually embolize (Greenfield and Proctor, 1998), and one out of every three to six of these will cause death (Zelenock, 1998). Even DVTs uncomplicated by pulmonary embolism have a high likelihood of producing lifelong venous insufficiency, with its associated pain and stasis ulceration of the legs. When assessed for DVT risk factors, surgical oncology patients are likely to have many, including malignancy, immobilization, surgery with general anesthesia, any surgery lasting longer than 30 minutes (even under local anesthesia), placement of central venous catheters, and prior history of DVT (Greenfield and Proctor, 1998; Knudson, 1998). Appropriate DVT prophylaxis may include pharmacological anticoagulation and use of compression stockings and/or mechanical intermittent lower-limb compressive devices. If DVT occurs despite such precautions, anticoagulation must be initiated unless contraindicated (5%–10% of all patients; higher percentage with cancer therapy), in which case, a Greenfield filter should be surgically placed in the inferior vena cava to prevent pulmonary embolism (Zelenock, 1998).

Early vigorous ambulation is also the gold standard for avoidance of pulmonary infectious complications (pneumonia). Doing so increases carbon dioxide production, ventilatory drive, and frequency of deep-sigh breaths and coughing, and redistributes pulmonary blood flow, thereby normalizing lung physiology and limiting atelectasis (alveolar collapse) (Maier, 1998). Daily ambulation is more likely with active encouragement, proper pain control, optimized nutrition, and early removal of unnecessary IV lines, drains, and bladder catheters.

Finally, metabolic stresses and release of inflammatory mediators may be associated with other life-threatening risks to the profoundly fatigued cancer patient, such as sepsis or acute myocardial infarction (MI). Sepsis is a significant risk to any critically ill patient. Fatigue leading to immobility sets the stage for infections secondary to atelectasis and long-term bladder catheters, which can subsequently become systemic. In addition, fatigue can impair nutritional intake (Grindel, 1994), which in turn has been associated with increased risk of sepsis (Cangiano et al, 1996). MI is also a concern. Vital exhaustion, as measured by a subjective questionnaire score, has a positive predictive value for risk of MI (Appels, 1997a), with changes in the hypothalamic-pituitary-adrenal axis believed to be involved (Appels, 1997b). Chemotherapy and surgery may increase such risks. For example, cyclophosphamide is associated with 1% to 5% risk of cardiac toxicity, with case reports of MI (Bearman et al, 1988; Goldberg et al, 1986; Wang et al, 1996).

Noncardiac surgery has a well-described perioperative cardiac risk, resulting from patient-specific, anesthesia-specific, and surgery-specific factors, the first of which has the greatest impact (Wirthlin and Cambria, 1998). These patient-specific factors, such as the comorbid conditions of infirm, fatigued patients and preexisting coronary artery disease, should be assessed prior to any surgery. Intermediate- to high-risk patients benefit from further work-up, such as perfusion scanning, and appropriate perioperative minimization of cardiac load via adequate pain control and, if necessary, β-blockade (Eagle, 1997; Gojer and Williams, 1995; Palda and Detsky, 1997).

Such changes in immune function and metabolic demand on the heart can result from what is collectively known as the *surgical stress response*, a constellation of biomolecular disturbances that have been correlated with the occurrence of postoperative fatigue (Christensen and Kehlet, 1993). In this phenomenon, surgical trauma induces endocrine hormonal changes, as well as release of numerous cytokines, arachidonic acid metabolites, complement, free oxygen radicals, and nitric oxide (Kehlet, 1997). Changes in serum levels of the trace elements copper and zinc also occur, for as many as 45 days (Cordova and Escanero, 1992). Both subjective fatigue symptoms and functional deficits are observed for up to three months, though they are most pronounced over a 30-day period, with peak levels at one week (Hill, Douglas, and Schroeder, 1993). Examinations of percutaneous muscle biopsy specimens following elective cholecystectomy have shown decreases in protein synthesis for a similar duration of somewhat longer than one month (Petersson et al, 1990). Interestingly, an important predictor of prolonged postoperative fatigue is the presence of significant preoperative fatigue, most common with oncology patients, the elderly, and those with low total body protein (Schroeder and Hill, 1993). Current means of reducing the surgical stress response include limiting the duration of procedures, minimizing blood loss, maintenance of normal core body temperature, optimization of fluid resuscitation, adequate analgesia, and increased nutritional intake (Christensen and Kehlet, 1993; Wirthlin and Cambria, 1998). Future modalities may well involve manipulation of cytokine cell signaling pathways.

Common Themes From Both Perspectives

Once serious illness has been viewed from both sides of the hospital bed, it is essentially impossible to separate the influences of each perspective on one's thoughts. Though initially quite distinct, they tend to draw each other to a common whole. Thus, the essence of profound fatigue, as often experienced by cancer patients, seems identical to me regardless of which perspective I choose. Both have led me to the same primary themes. Cancer fatigue can be a potential obstacle to a successful course of therapy. As a patient, I worried many times that I simply might not make it through my treatments. As a physician, I now see things more concretely as potential sources of morbidity and mortality. It sounds more scientific, but essentially it still boils down to worries about the patient. Cancer fatigue is also a very significant hardship, the burden of which should be lightened whenever possible. I felt this with every part of my being as a leukemia patient. In the role of a physician, it has been hard to witness the similar difficulties of others as patients. And as a son, it has broken my heart to share some of the struggles of daily living more intimately once again, while caring for my father at home during his last days of life. Although his bravely fought private struggle with cancer is not my story to tell, part of why I tell my own story of life as a cancer patient is for him. Dad was a surgeon and a tremendous and natural teacher, and there is still much that can be taught about what happens each day to cancer patients. Indeed, it is the daily and seemingly mundane events that are so important in the lives of fatigued cancer patients.

> *It is the daily and seemingly mundane events that are so important in the lives of fatigued cancer patients.*

Where Do We Go From Here?

If there is just one message that I can impart to physicians, nurses, and other caregivers about cancer fatigue, it is that what one sees in these roles is generally just the tip of the proverbial iceberg. Physicians assess, make decisions, and by necessity, disappear again. Nurses have a much closer association with patients, owing to their increased time of contact and multiplicity of roles. Certainly many of my nurses assisted me through innumerable hardships. After holding a container of my bloody vomit in one hand, while helping support my exhausted upper body with the other, surely my nurse on that evening knew a bit about my life at that time. Even while busily giving medications or hanging blood products, my nurses could share a lot with me. And yet no one, not even family, could be with me for every minute of the day. Only a fly on the wall could know what happens between caregiver tasks or visits from family and friends. I would recommend to doctors and nurses that they attempt to see with the eyes of such a fly. What could be causing the greatest distress to the patient, trying hard not to cry during a solitary struggle in the dark of night? What might be left unsaid because it's rather embarrassing? And what is so routine to healthy individuals that it would never be imagined to be a problem? These are potential opportunities to make a real difference in the life of a cancer patient.

Possibilities for Research

There are many possibilities for future research in cancer fatigue. The true incidence and impact of the various potential morbidities previously described have not yet been studied specifically among cancer patients. A retrospective review could be quite informative. With the modern trend toward managed care and ever-shortening hospital stays, what are the differences between the hospital and home environments? Are these important? In terms of fall-associated morbidity, an interesting question is what activities of daily living are most commonly involved. Are there device modifications or unique approaches to burdensome or dangerous tasks that might make them easier or safer? What are the indications for and appropriate use of physical and occupational therapy and rehabilitative medicine specifically for cancer-related fatigue? These are opportunities for truly improving cancer patient care.

Recommendations for Personal Survival

For the patient and the family, I have no easy answers, but rather perhaps a few philosophical recommendations:

- Struggle neither too little nor too much.
- Learn when to struggle, for there are times you should.
- Try to relax between the battles: This requires an ability to find an inner peace.
- When it is permissible, grit your teeth and get out of bed occasionally but feel no guilt for "excess sleep." It is nature's magic.
- Use every trick you can think of to do things for yourself, as safely as you can.
- Ask for help when needed and do not judge yourself harshly for needing it.
- If your struggles involve highly personal issues, question carefully your hesitations to ask for assistance. Are they rooted in anything relevant to your current situation?
- Take things one day at a time.
- The beauty of the human spirit is that despite great hardships, something positive can still be found with another day. Look for it.
- At times it is hard to believe life can ever be good again. With faith, hope, and good fortune, hardships can become distant memories.

References

Appels, A. (1997a). Exhausted subjects, exhausted systems. *Acta Physiologica Scandinavica Supplementum, 640,* 153–154.

Appels, A. (1997b). Why do imminent victims of a cardiac event feel so tired? *International Journal of Clinical Practice, 51,* 447–450.

Bearman, S., Appelbaum, F., Buckner, P., et al. (1988). Regimen-related toxicity in patients undergoing bone marrow transplantation. *Journal of Clinical Oncology, 6,* 1562–1568.

Bick, R. L., Strauss, J. F., and Frenkel, E. P. (1996). Thrombosis and hemorrhage in oncology patients. *Hematology/Oncology Clinics of North America, 10,* 875–907.

Cangiano, C., Laviano, A., Muscaritoli, M., et al. (1996). Cancer anorexia: New pathogenic and therapeutic insights. *Nutrition, 12*(1 suppl.), S48–S51.

Christensen, T., and Kehlet, H. (1993). Postoperative fatigue. *World Journal of Surgery, 17,* 220–225.

Cordova, M. A., and Escanero, M. J. (1992). Changes in serum trace elements after surgery: Value of copper and zinc in predicting post-operative fatigue. *Journal of International Medical Research, 20,* 12–19.

Eagle, K. (1997). Surgical patients with heart disease: Summary of the ACC/AHA guidelines. *American Family Physician, 56,* 811–818.

Gojer, B., and Williams, K. (1995). The role of scintigraphic perfusion imaging for predicting ischemic cardiac events in noncardiac surgery. *American Journal of Cardiac Imaging, 9,* 213–225.

Goldberg, M., Antin, J., Guinan, E., and Rappaport, J. (1986). Cyclophosphamide cardiotoxicity: An analysis of dosing as a risk factor. *Blood, 68,* 1114–1118.

Gomella, L. G., and Lefor, A. T. (Eds.) (1996). On-call problems: Fall from bed. In *Surgery on call* (pp. 106–108). Stamford, CT: Appleton & Lange.

Greenfield, L. J., and Proctor, M. C. (1998). Pulmonary thromboembolism. In J. L. Cameron (Ed.), *Current surgical therapy* (pp. 891–894). St. Louis: Mosby.

Grindel, C. (1994). Fatigue and nutrition. *Medsurg Nursing, 3,* 475–481.

Hill, G., Douglas, R., and Schroeder, D. (1993). Metabolic basis for the management of patients undergoing major surgery. *World Journal of Surgery, 17,* 146–153.

Hoyle, R. M. (1994). Mechanisms of injury. In M. A. Lopez-Viego (Ed.), *The Parkland trauma handbook* (pp. 15–18). St. Louis: Mosby Year Book.

Kannus, P., Parkkari, J., Sievanen, H., et al (1996). Epidemiology of hip fractures. *Bone, 18*(1 suppl.), 57S–63S.

Kehlet, H. (1997). Multimodal approach to control postoperative pathophysiology and rehabilitation. *British Journal of Anaesthesia, 78,* 606–617.

Knudson, M. M. (1998). Prevention of venous thromboembolism in surgical patients. In J. L. Cameron (Ed.), *Current surgical therapy* (pp. 899–903). St. Louis: Mosby.

LeMarbre, P. J., and Boyarsky, S. M. B. (1992). Complications of cancer and cancer treatment. In J. F. O'Donnell, C. T. Coughlin, and P. J. LeMarbre (Eds.), *Oncology for the house officer* (pp. 164–166). Baltimore: Williams & Wilkins.

Maier, R. V. (1998). Postoperative respiratory failure. In J. L. Cameron (Ed.), *Current surgical therapy* (pp. 1103–1108). St. Louis: Mosby.

Nguyen, T., Eisman, J., Kelly, P., and Sambrook, P. (1996). Risk factors for osteoporotic fractures in elderly men. *American Journal of Epidemiology, 144*, 255–263.

Palda, V., and Detsky, A. (1997). Perioperative assessment and management of risk from coronary artery disease. *Annals of Internal Medicine, 127*, 313–328.

Petersson, B., Wernerman, J., Waller, S., et al. (1990). Elective abdominal surgery depresses muscle protein synthesis and increases subjective fatigue: Effects lasting more than 30 days. *British Journal of Surgery, 77*, 796–800.

Schroeder, D., and Hill, G. (1993). Predicting postoperative fatigue: Importance of preoperative factors. *World Journal of Surgery, 17*, 226–231.

Schwendner, K., Mikesky, A., Holt, W., et al. (1997). Differences in muscle endurance and recovery between fallers and nonfallers, and between young and older women. *Journals of Gerontology. Series A, Biological Sciences and Medical Sciences, 52*(3), M155–M160.

Shadduck, P. P., and Crowley, N. J. (1992). The hematologic system: Thrombocytopathies. In H. K. Lyerly and J. W. Gaynor (Eds.), *The handbook of surgical intensive care* (pp. 594–597). St. Louis: Mosby Year Book.

Staubli, M. (1996). Iatrogenic falls. *Schweizerische Medizinische Wochenschrift/Journal Suisse de Medecine, 126*(14), 576–583.

Tideiksaar, R. (1996). Preventing falls: How to identify risk factors, reduce complications. *Geriatrics, 51*(2), 43–55.

Tinetti, M., Doucette, J., Claus, E., and Marottoli, R. (1995). Risk factors for serious injury during falls by older persons in the community. *Journal of the American Geriatrics Society, 43*, 1214–1221.

Wang, B., Cao, L., Liu, H., et al. (1996). Myocardial infarction following allogeneic bone marrow transplantation. *Bone Marrow Transplantation, 18*, 479–486.

Wirthlin, D., and Cambria, R. (1998). Surgery-specific considerations in the cardiac patient undergoing noncardiac surgery. *Progress in Cardiovascular Diseases, 40*, 453–468.

Zelenock, G. B. (1998). Inferior vena caval interruption. In J. L. Cameron (Ed.), *Current surgical therapy* (pp. 895–898). St. Louis: Mosby.

Zwimpfer, T., Brown, J., Sullivan, I., and Moulton, R. (1997). Head injuries due to falls caused by seizures: A group at high risk for traumatic intracranial hematomas. *Journal of Neurosurgery, 86*, 433–437.

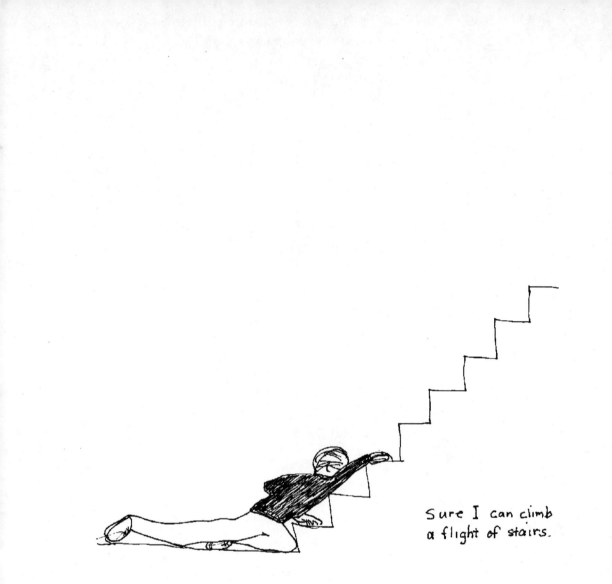

Sure I can climb
a flight of stairs.

Issues in Fatigue and Cognition: Quality of Life in a Survivor

Tricia C. Corbett
As interviewed by Maryl L. Winningham

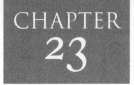

I'm hungry, but I'm too tired to eat right now.
Brenda Heil

Nobody realizes that some people expend tremendous energy merely to be normal.
Albert Camus

Dr. Winningham: How was your tumor diagnosed and how long ago was that?

Ms. Corbett: It's been ten years this month since it was discovered. I had been having problems for at least two years with short-term memory. I was experiencing aphasia (object-noun words)—finding words, especially simple object nouns like *table* or *door*—and a general feeling of fatigue that increased over time. No amount of rest seemed to help. This fatigue was quite different from anything I had experienced before. I also began to notice that I had difficulty sequencing—performing simple tasks that required multiple steps, like fixing breakfast in the morning.

During this time, I had gone to three different physicians—my GP (general practitioner) and two neurologists. The fact that I had had two babies in two years, the youngest being only a few months old, greatly complicated getting a diagnosis because "of course I was tired," and "of course I was having memory problems." It was written off as a simple matter of postpartum depression or "maternal amnesia." Maternal amnesia? One of them actually sold me his newly published book on how difficult neurological diagnoses were, with stories of some of the diagnoses he had missed.

About four months before my diagnosis, I began to lose hearing in my right ear and had periods of dizziness—I called them the "whirlies"—especially in the dark. If I couldn't see, I couldn't stay upright. I was told I had Meniere's disease. I went to see a friend who was an ear, nose, and throat specialist. He tested my hearing, found a sensory loss, and sent me for an MRI (magnetic resonance imaging) study. The tumor in my right frontal lobe lit up like a light bulb. I sent a copy of my diagnosis to my neurologist-author with a note saying, "You missed this one, too." He apologized.

In all fairness, frontal lobe tumors are very difficult to diagnose; indeed, they are often called the "silent tumor." People then really did not know what the frontal lobe did—we still don't know that much—so identifying what it was *not* doing was very difficult. Manifestations also seem to differ from person to person. To make matters worse, I had a slow-growing, diffuse tumor called a *glioma,* actually a mixed glioma called an *oligoastrocytoma,* which did not displace architecture and was insidious. I never had a headache or seizures. This was a shotgun shell-sized tumor down the midline, which unfortunately extended into the corpus callosum so they couldn't remove it all.

Dr. Winningham: You mentioned loss of memory, hearing, and balance, and they suggested you were depressed. Were you depressed? What made them think so?

Ms. Corbett: I want to clarify one thing that is very important to me. I was not depressed then and I am not depressed now. I think one of the main problems is that many symptoms, not only of frontal tumors, but also of fatigue in general, have superficial manifestations of depression. For that reason, and since depression is such a common "wastebasket" term, these conditions are misperceived and misdiagnosed. We need to find a much better way to differentiate depression and such symptoms as fatigue, flatness, or apathy which can result from other pathologies as well. I was not depressed, but the health care system does not seem to have a very large arsenal of names with which to distinguish a wide range of conditions that appear similar. So the fault is one of insensitivity and lack of specificity by health care providers in making the diagnosis.

After surgery and radiation, I had about a 1½-year memory loss. Looking back, it was like a blank. I don't know what it was from, but I was taking phenytoin. When I stopped taking it, my memory immediately started getting better. I had problems with the CT (computed tomography) scans. I am allergic to iodine. They told me the amount of iodine they use in the isotope for the scan was so small I wouldn't react—but I did. And it even

About the Contributor

Tricia C. Corbett, with a master of science in public health from the University of Washington, is an interesting woman. As a ten-year survivor of brain cancer that was treated by surgery and radiation, she is statistically unusual. But her character, her creativity, and what she has accomplished make her even more remarkable. Shortly after the beginning of an interview in which I sought to learn more about cognitive deficits and fatigue, as well as the potential for rehabilitation, I recognized that this was not just a patient interview as part of another chapter. What she had to say warranted its own chapter: There is much for us to learn here.

happened more than once! It is so frustrating not to be believed, especially when you are struggling with the enormity of brain surgery and you're so tired of arguing. If they would just listen. I'm afraid I wasn't a very docile patient. I was also very tired during the seven weeks of radiation and it seemed like a couple of months afterward.

Dr. Winningham: It took you a while to recover. In the meanwhile, you were a mother with small children. What did you do?

Ms. Corbett: I was fortunate to have a nanny! After all, I had a baby and a two-year-old, and commotion absolutely shut me down. The nanny was a "get well gift" from my father, and I don't know what I would have done without her.

Dr. Winningham: So you are now a ten-year survivor! It is still relatively rare to see people with that kind of tumor who have survived that long. How has life been since then? What kind of residual effects have you had? I hear from others that there is little follow-up and information available. It seems to be every person for themselves.

Ms. Corbett: Well, within a year after my surgery, I was back to being a very high-functioning professional. I was fine except for some mild aphasia and a few short-term memory problems having mostly to do with schedules. I was compulsive about my calendar and keeping lists to compensate. During this time, I served for six years, and eventually was president of, a national educational accreditation council for one of the health professions. We accredited professional schools and departments in medical schools that provided graduate education in this area. This involved rigorous two- to four-day visits on site, with the requirement that a draft of our findings be finished before we left. I chaired nearly 20 of these visits in an eight-year period and still occasionally do visits. My first trip was absolutely exhausting, and I realized I would have to be very prepared and highly organized to reduce the stress of these trips. As a result, I became a good chair. I would tell my team ahead of time that if I tired, I tended to have trouble finding words and wouldn't mind at all if they helped me out. I did fine—I did not seem to have any trouble with work-related, academic activities.

Tricia Corbett is a keen observer, applying scientific problem-solving techniques with strategic self-advocacy to articulate issues others feel but have difficulty communicating. Questionnaires and investigative techniques developed by "healthy" professionals who work in the field of cognitive alterations, fatigue, and head injury often do not seem to reflect a comprehension of the nature or degree of their patients' distress. As a result of her scientific training, Tricia is a perfect bridge between the strange and sometimes bewildering world of experience and the objective world of science. Those who wish to understand some of the uncommon characteristics of cognitive impairments and cancer-related fatigue could profit from absorbing the experience shared here. We are grateful for her candor.

Interestingly, I did have trouble with the simple day-to-day activities of daily living. That was a puzzle. It seemed like the more routine the task, the more trouble I had getting it done. I had difficulty with such things as getting the kids off to school, getting meals prepared (and I love to cook), laundry, and housekeeping chores. The biggest problem with meals was the sequencing problem–and having everything ready all at once. My husband irritably suggested that I cut back on my professional work and pay attention to getting things done at home. The ability to function in my professional life but not at home made little sense to me. Then it occurred to me that perhaps day-to-day routine did not engage my brain at the same level as my professional work. Maybe different chemical systems of the brain were being engaged for the different roles. If this was a deficit problem, why would it affect one area of cognitive function and not the other?

Dr. Winningham: Has your status continued at that level?

Ms. Corbett: No. About three years ago, I began to notice several changes. I first noticed that I was beginning to lose a significant amount of hair in the area of my head that was irradiated. I began to have trouble with my vision. My eyes took a great deal of scatter radiation. I know the effects of radiation damage can be delayed in many ways. Then I began having what I called "dead brain days" when I literally struggled to do anything. I would know, when I got up in the morning and couldn't wake up, that I was going to have a bad day. I felt jet-lagged. The odd thing was that these days did not happen with any regularity. I tried to find a pattern–something that triggered it–anything, but I couldn't. It was a malaise that I had never experienced before.

Besides this mental fatigue there were other ways my cognition was affected, most of them intermittent. I began having trouble "gestalting" things–putting together the whole picture. My inductive logic was impaired. It's like I can see every single cell in a film clip of a story, but I can't put them together to make a story. Let me give you an example:

A friend was coming over to pick up some papers. I had errands to run, so I told her I would leave the material in an obvious place in the garage. I went out and placed the papers on the bike rack behind the van and put a can of paint on them so the dog or the wind wouldn't scatter them about. I went into the house, got my keys, and left on my errands. A few hours later, I returned and noticed a lot of loose papers littering our neighborhood road. I pulled into the garage, went into the house, and called my friend to make sure she had gotten the material. No, she couldn't find it. I went out and discovered the litter was the material I left for her. The damn dog had scattered the material–but how did he get the paint can off? I went back to look for the can and couldn't find it. Very odd. I called my friend to say the dog had gotten the materials off the van and scattered them about. "But the van wasn't there when I came," she said. The car was there, but not the van. Normally, I would have figured this out immediately. As it was, the whole sequence of events had no continuity, no meaning. It never even occurred to me to ask: "What's wrong with this picture?" I have more stories like this than I care to admit.

Difficulty "gestalting" is one of several problems I call temporal problems. These relate to a feeling I often have of somehow living outside of time. Like being in parallel worlds—one foot here, one foot with the spirits. Oddly enough, these times seem to enhance my creativity. They are often peaceful times with great clarity; I usually write my best poetry during these times. The poem at the front of the book, "Las Phantasmas de Tiral," is what it's like to be there.

I began to notice I was having trouble holding more than one thing in my head at a time. Sometimes it's a struggle to hold even one thing in my head—to concentrate long enough to get one simple, little thing done. I started to have trouble remembering appointments and things I was to do. I would write it in my calendar, but I would forget to look. It wasn't just simple forgetting; it's like the need to look *now* and to do something *now* did not connect. People just don't understand. This is not lack of responsibility. You are working harder at living than ever before, but you seem to have those gaps, those disconnections.

I just couldn't process too many stimuli at once. Background noise or interruption would bother me a lot. I started becoming confused, befuddled, easily. This wasn't like me at all. I wasn't working full-time anymore. I was just on the clinical faculty because I wanted to spend more time with my boys. I was spending more time at home, but was still traveling for on-site visits. Then, I noticed on one visit in particular, that I had trouble concentrating. Even with all that I could do to focus . . . I was scared. I was still interested, but very tired. Each time, it took me longer to recover after I returned home.

Like I said, I had trouble doing more than one thing at a time. I started having difficulty following recipes at home, at getting timing down to make a meal, to coordinating what had to be ready and when. I also began struggling with monitoring my behavior and emotions. Part of it was not recognizing how I was coming across to people—I wasn't connecting. It's like I didn't act the way I felt, but I was unaware of the incongruity. People thought I was angry or irritated with them when I wasn't. My feedback loop was messed up. Other times I reacted so fast—before I could think and choose an appropriate response. I was losing control of my emotions and my ability to behave accordingly. My responses, good and bad, were more intense than called for.

I was also becoming increasingly agitated and irritable. I could not seem to filter incoming stimuli. I became confused more easily. Commotion, background noise, and interruptions drove me to distraction and tears. I found myself emotionally labile, popping off at my husband for very little reason and yelling at my kids. I noticed my mind tired easily, even on good days. I took naps not because my body was tired, but because my mind was, or I was, emotionally drained. I couldn't seem to regulate my energy levels—conserve energy. It seemed to be all or nothing, and I had little control over it. I couldn't keep up with extended family interactions as I became increasingly tired. I just couldn't function and cope with that.

It took me a while to recognize what was going on and be able to articulate what I was doing and how I was feeling. I was sure most of it was related to long-term radiation damage. I was having follow-up brain scans every four months and for three consecutive sessions, I ticked off my list of problems to my neurosurgeon. He said none of the other long-term survivors as far out as me had complained of any problems. He said it sounded like menopause to him. I knew it wasn't menopause. No one seemed to understand what was going on.

I don't know how much others noticed, but it was obvious and overwhelming to me. Things continued to deteriorate and I became increasingly frustrated, angry, anxious, miserable, and guilty for what I was putting my family through. I withdrew, increasingly, from social activities. I cried at the drop of a hat and no longer trusted myself around people. My emotional and behavioral volatility made me worried about conducting site visits. I explained the problems I was having with our executive director. She, of course, had not noticed anything, but I asked to be excused from visits until I could get a handle on what was going on.

Everything came to a head two years ago at our annual Corbett family summer gathering on the Oregon coast. I was nervous about my ability to cope with the commotion and demands of keeping 12 of us going for the week. When we arrived, I told the family that I was having some problems and what they were, that I would try hard to keep up my end of things and to please cut me some slack. They listened but I knew it would be hard for them to understand. I also knew they did not want to hear that I was having problems, much less see them. They wanted me to be okay, to be the old Tricia. My brother-in-law, in particular, indicated I was just making excuses to shirk my responsibilities and not do my share. He not only cut me no slack, he took even the smallest opportunities to confront and chastise me. It was a disaster. I was so overwhelmed and feeling so cutoff that I could not think of one place to turn. For the first time, I actually thought of killing myself as the only way out. That really scared me. I woke my husband in the middle of the night, told him I could no longer cope, that I was ruining everyone's vacation and wanted to go home. I was in a state of total despair.

When we returned home, I immediately went to my neurosurgeon. Before I even had a chance to describe my horrible experience, he asked me to tell him again what things had been bothering me in the last year. This time he listened. He said he had three other patients in the last two months come in with the same complaints. And you know what? They were all males. They weren't in menopause! He was puzzled too and admitted that he was not sure how to proceed.

Now here is a problem. As far as I know, there are no significant databases on the effects of cancer treatments on long-term survivors, especially brain tumor patients. There are not very many of us around, so the "n" available for studies is very small and not likely to be statistically significant. Very few follow-up studies have been done. You are either here at five or seven or ten years or you're not. Little attention has been paid to your quality of life–how you live–how you function–that far out. I told him something needed to be done about this. He agreed. I also told him that as far as I was concerned, I had a radiation-induced brain injury. About this time, the scans started showing my problem as a recurrent tumor, but it was difficult to differentiate tumor from radiation injury. Only in the past two or three years have new techniques evolved.

In addition to scans, neuropsychological testing such as is used in traumatic brain injury rehabilitation centers and with accident victims may pick up on some of this. But here, again, was a problem. I am fully aware, as bright as I am, I may not look very bad. On good days you may not notice; on bad days I may not be able to do anything. Most of those tests require a drop of at least one standard deviation for anything to be considered significant. I thought it was worth trying to document what was happening to me. In addition, I thought I might at least learn some techniques that would help me with functioning.

I asked if there was someone at the university medical center who dealt with brain injury problems. Yes, there was. I had a brain injury because I had had a brain tumor. I thought maybe some of the rehabilitation techniques would transfer from traumatic brain injury to tumor brain injury. So I got a referral to the brain injury clinic in the rehabilitation center.

Dr. Winningham: That was very creative, considering none of the experts had thought of it.

Ms. Corbett: I went in and sat down with these rehabilitation people. I told them I wanted to consult with them, that I could give them more information than most people and most professionals could. I wanted them to help me quantify and deal with my deficits, and I thought I could help them because I had watched the development of my deficits and felt I could articulate this fairly accurately. I wanted to identify the effects of the radiation on the full range of my functioning. They provided a complete work-up of physical and neurological functioning, psychometric testing, and behavioral and emotional measures. Of course, that just happened to be a "good day." Of course, I aced everything but a motor test (thumb clicks), and I had a little trouble with sequencing. The only thing I couldn't do even when I had a tumor was shut my eyes and stand up without falling over!

Dr. Winningham: I have a hypothesis about why that happened, but we can discuss that later. What did the rehabilitation staff do for you?

Ms. Corbett: First, they wanted to take the view, "You're a professional, you did well on your tests, you are a very bright woman. We do not see any cognitive deficits. We don't need to bring your family in for an 'official briefing' like we do for others." No deficits compared to what?

Dr. Winningham: So their professional conclusion was, "very bright woman, so far out on parameters, no obvious mental deficits." That was obviously a good day. Did they ever see you on a "dead brain day"? That seems to be one of the problems.

Ms. Corbett: Oh, no! On bad days, I could barely get out of bed, so of course, they only saw the good days. You see, from a medical perspective, the experts really don't understand what is going on, they don't know what it means, and they really don't know what is standard functioning or normal for you. They do their tests and they come up with nothing.

Dr. Winningham: This really seems to be a problem of sensitivity versus specificity, isn't it? Are the measures specific to picking up on that kind of problem (if it exists), and are they sensitive to picking up how much of a problem it is? It seems our tools, our instruments, are currently very dull, being neither specific nor sensitive.

Ms. Corbett: That certainly sounds so. Although the deficits didn't show up, I was having trouble with work for the first time. It was not so much having difficulty thinking, but having the energy to think. I could still get through site visits, but I was exhausted at the end, and it took weeks to recover.

I became frightened I would be caught in a situation I couldn't pull off. I was having all kinds of problems with everyday activities, but the tests didn't look at that. I don't think anyone was aware of that. I finally asked to back off from my responsibilities until I could figure all this out. None of the tests were of any help with this.

There were two problems. First, we didn't have a baseline of how I functioned in the past, either prior to or after the surgery. So how are we to determine the extent of any deficits related to the radiation? We can't! Second, I am fully aware that because I am fairly bright and on the extreme end of the statistical bell-shaped curve, what is a significant drop in functioning to me may not look that bad to them. Most of these tests seem to require a drop of at least a standard deviation for the results to be even considered significant. We talked about this, and the differences we might see depending on whether I was tested on a good day or a "dead brain" day.

What I have been most confused about and would most like to understand is, if there is enough damage that you can see it on the scan, it seems that you should have a consistent deficit. How is it that it is so unpredictable, manifesting itself so profoundly on some days but not on others? It's difficult to explain and it's one of those questions that cannot typically be answered by rehabilitation and neuropsychological evaluations.

Dr. Winningham: Now that is a problem with people and statistics, but that's how the tests are derived. Means and standard deviations don't say anything about a single human being, do they? All the computer programs and actuarial projections by an insurance company don't mean anything with respect to an individual. They are merely group data to give a general picture and help in management. In fact, it is unethical, if not immoral, to demand that a single human being with a health-related problem fit into a pile of computer printouts. That's the problem we're having today in health care.

Ms. Corbett: It's also–it's especially–a problem of communication, like we talked about earlier.

Dr. Winningham: I got us off the track. Back to rehabilitation.

Ms. Corbett: About communication . . . here is a key: Avoid trying to figure out how to explain to them how you feel. Rather, think in terms of things they will understand, in terms of their vocabulary, the vocabulary in which they have been taught to communicate.

Dr. Winningham: That's sad. The patient, who is struggling with so much, has to struggle to communicate distress that the professional cannot or will not understand!

Ms. Corbett: It is similar to statistics (data/numbers) versus interpretation (what the data mean/significance). If you keep going to a physician and say, "Doctor, I'm always tired," you are going to get zip for a response. They are not used to dealing with this. They have not been trained in this. This is not anemia or thyroid. And of course it's not menopause. But it's hard to figure all this out when you can barely crawl around. You can think to do things, but you can't get yourself moving. How do you explain that?

Dr. Winningham: And then you come into the clinic and do well on all their tests!

Ms. Corbett: I told the rehabilitation staff, on the contrary, just talk to and about me as a patient. We reviewed the results and talked about them. They did hear my complaints: The psychological/emotional and social work interviews did identify problems. So in regard to these problems they were very helpful.

Pharmacologically, we tried a serotonin booster (fluoxetine [Prozac], 10 milligrams daily) and in little over a week I saw dramatic improvements in my irritability, agitation, and emotional lability. I was calmer and able to think more clearly. Instead of being totally overwhelmed, I could see what was bothering me and make environmental adjustments to control it. This was akin to a miracle for me and my family!

The family feedback session with the rehab staff was also very helpful. It validated that I indeed had deficits that interfered with my abilities to function at home. We dealt mostly with memory, emotive volatility, and my difficulty performing household tasks. It gave my husband and boys an opportunity to provide feedback on my behavior at home, vent their frustrations, and ask questions. The hardest thing for them to understand was why I am okay some days and not others. It also gave us an understanding that we were all in this together and could take steps that would help. We were also offered family counseling if needed. We haven't needed it yet, but it's reassuring knowing the option is there. I think the session was a great relief to all of us–instead of having constant family disruptions and tension, we are all helping mom function better and are focusing on the good times.

Dr. Winningham: Can you give an example of things that helped with your family functioning?

Ms. Corbett: I have worked hard to identify those things I either have difficulty doing or do not feel comfortable doing. If they are important, I look for an alternative way to do them, or to change the circumstances so that I can deal with them more effectively. It's really not that I can't do them; it's more the prices I pay in mental energy and stress that make them difficult. I have also identified the things I can still do well and am concentrating on them. For instance, I have to be able to keep my family going. I have to. I look for ways to reduce the amount of mental energy needed for everyday tasks. Most of the problem is simply remembering that I have to do them. It takes a tremendous amount of energy to keep things in my head, like my daily schedule; that I might forget also causes anxiety.

I have become a faithful "to-do" list maker. I write down what I need to do for the next day with appropriate cues and phone numbers, if required, and I organize and prioritize my itinerary. I try to anticipate anything that may distract me (like not having a phone number I need) and take care of that ahead of time. I try to organize myself in a way that if I am sitting down to make a series of phone calls, I will not have to get up for anything!

Dr. Winningham: I have had people tell me, "I make lists, I have a planner, but then I forget to use them. It sounds like such a lame excuse, but it's true, and it's very embarrassing." Do you have a problem with that?

Ms. Corbett: Well, I did. I would completely forget to refer to it. It's like a temporal discontinuity. Somewhere in my mind I was aware I should be doing something. Another place in my mind, there was an awareness of a list. But I couldn't bring the two together–that the list would show me what to do. It is a strange feeling.

Dr. Winningham: It sounds like you learned techniques to deal with that. What were they? I'll bet a lot of other people could benefit from applying similar techniques.

Ms. Corbett: Sometimes I would have trouble remembering to look at my calendar for the things I needed to do that day that take me out of the house. I now cue myself to check the calendar and list by placing a small red flag in the hallway to the kitchen and in my car. I see the flag; I know to look and do so immediately. I have practiced that so it is almost reflexive.

Dr. Winningham: Some people tell me they habituate to cues like that. After a while, they become numbed to the cue and it loses its effect. Did that ever happen to you?

Ms. Corbett: I never habituated to these but if I did, I would simply change them.

Dr. Winningham: Back to your family functioning. What was one thing that was affected by your family rehabilitation counseling?

Ms. Corbett: Again, making a list was one. For example, along the same line with what I said about multitasking, sequencing, and my trouble being cued to do things: My husband or one of my sons would say, "Remember to get this done today" or "Could you do that for me?" Before, I was likely to forget, and they would be frustrated or disappointed. As we learned to adapt, they said, "Remember . . ." and I would say, "Put it on the list." Now everyone knows to put it on the list so I can access the information in a consistent manner.

Dr. Winningham: What other techniques did the rehabilitation team share with you that you found helpful?

Ms. Corbett: The staff also gave me ways to exercise my cognitive functions such as working crossword puzzles, playing Scrabble and Jeopardy and thinking games, and memorizing lists. I have found that these activities really help, especially if I am having trouble focusing or concentrating.

The rehabilitation experience didn't accomplish everything I hoped it would, specifically the verification of my cognitive deficits, but what we were able to accomplish made it an unqualified success as far as I'm concerned. I know they are there if I need them.

Dr. Winningham: So what do we call this fatigue thing? It has been suggested that what healthy people think of as fatigue is not what we are talking about in cancer.

Ms. Corbett: Well, I think that depends on the source, the etiology of the fatigue. Some people with cancer may experience fatigue due to treatment-induced anemia, thyroid problems, clinical depression, and other commonly recognized causes. I think cancer patients and survivors as a group, or even as individuals, experience a broad range of fatigues with varying etiologies, some of which are well understood and others of which are not. I believe the fatigue we are referring to is neurologically based.

The fatigue I am describing, and have heard others attempt to describe, is much more akin to profound apathy, flat affect, or perhaps even despair, than to physical exhaustion. Physical exhaustion is clearly different. And let me emphatically say that depression and despair are not the same thing. Maybe some people have a sense of what mental or emotional fatigue is like, but it is the profound and random nature of this fatigue that is so difficult to fathom if you have never experienced it.

We must be cautious not to dump all fatigues into one clinical basket. Just as cancer is a number of different illnesses with differing etiologies, pathologies, and courses, so, I believe, is fatigue. I think we know very little about the fatigue we are talking about, the "cyclopsia" (my word), and even less about effective interventions for it.

Dr. Winningham: In Chapter 4 of this book, Hockenberry-Eaton and Hinds tell about some of the metaphors children use to talk about fatigue. Pictures the children have drawn are really very expressive. Perhaps in the end, it is art that is most effective in bridging the communication gap.

Ms. Corbett: Yes, I believe that's true. Art may be very useful. Metaphors may help communicate experiences where words are inadequate.

Dr. Winningham: Susan Kesler, a nurse in Salt Lake City who has worked with impaired elderly, refers to this as "Swiss cheese memory"–unpredictable holes in memory and cognition.

Ms. Corbett: Swiss cheese memory—that's good! A healthy person may think they understand it, but they have no real clue as to the nature and extent of it. I not only knew something was wrong, I knew what was wrong. I am fairly scientific and objective and I still had trouble getting anyone to understand. This kind of fatigue is very hard to communicate. This is not anemia, or thyroid, or depression, and it certainly isn't menopause. I believe it is neurologically based. But figuring out a way to communicate this is very difficult when you can barely function . . .

Dr. Winningham: . . . and when your attention span is limited.

Ms. Corbett: Sometimes you simply do not have the word to describe how you are feeling. You either dance around the problem in muddled explanations, or you use words like *fatigue,* which are sort of close, but not close enough. Here the miscommunication starts. People think they know what the word *fatigue* means and don't really listen to what you are trying to say.

What I Learned From Joe

One day, Dr. M., one of our oncologists, asked me to talk with Joe and his wife, Grace, about some concerns Joe had. He said Joe had colon cancer with limited lymph node involvement and was on a chemotherapy pump; his Karnofsky score was 90 (90 out of 100 being high functioning). "He's doing fine," I was assured. "He can do anything he wants. His prognosis is actually very good if he stays on the chemotherapy."

After I introduced myself, Joe said, "Look at this" (he "made a muscle" with his left arm and pointed to it). "I've lost 50 pounds of muscle because of the cancer and the chemotherapy that guy has me on. What's he trying to do to me? I outta sue the SOB." He sounded very macho. Grace proudly explained that Joe was an "important businessman with lots of clout" in the community before his retirement two years ago and that he "had made plenty of money in contracting." I asked Joe what he was doing since he retired, how active he had been, what his activity patterns looked like. He said he was working with his son in his business and still helped out a day every week. He wanted to do more, but he said the cancer and treatments were "killing him." I promised to call him at home the following afternoon and follow up on our conversation.

The next afternoon:

"Hello," I said, "Can I speak with Joe?"

"He's in bed," said Grace gravely, almost secretively.

"Why is he in bed?" I asked.

"He's sick," said Grace.

"Really?" I asked (thinking he looked pretty good yesterday in the clinic). "Why? What's he got?" (I was thinking maybe he had caught a cold or flu.)

Dr. Winningham: That is a major problem in assessing any symptoms. I used to tell students to get the patients to use their own words. We tend to use labels (our preconceived notions) and the patients adopt them because they figure we'll understand. A good example is with cardiac patients. They may come in complaining of an aching in their left arm and pressure-type pain in their chest. The great health care professional says, "Your angina. . . ." The next time patients come in, they say, "My angina. . . ." We may lose a lot in the translation. In fact, what patients are experiencing this time may be very different. That difference may be clinically significant. It makes no difference. We've obscured that significance with a vague word. No wonder we have become so dependent on lab tests! Now we get fatigue, where there is no definitive meaning, let alone lab test, and we're stuck! Even worse, the patient is stuck!

Ms. Corbett: Well, I made up my own word–"cyclopsia." "I am suffering from cyclopsia." You can look it up. It's not in the dictionary. So if you want to know what it means, you have to ask. It is my word for my unremitting, unrelenting, overwhelming inability to func-

---

"He has cancer," intoned Grace.

"Oh," I said. "When is he getting up?" (I thought he was taking a nap.)

"He's not," countered Grace firmly. "He's in bed."

I was dumbfounded. Maybe I had not understood something obvious. I could see no reason he would be in bed.

"Why," I blankly asked, "Is he sick?"

"Well, of course he's sick," Grace said a little more loudly. "He's got CANCER."

"Oh," I said, trying to figure out my next move. I was surprised by the finality of her statement. "Well, can you have him call me when he gets up for supper?"

"He's not getting up," said Grace in an irritated tone of voice. "But if you insist, I can take a note when I take him his supper."

"Why do you have to take him supper in bed?" I asked, dumbfounded.

"Because," said Grace, "He's sick! HE'S GOT CANCER!"

And then I understood why Joe lost 50 pounds of muscle. It had little to do with cancer or chemotherapy. Over the next years I would meet many people who thought a diagnosis of cancer meant giving up, going to bed, and dying. They would get "pumped up" for the clinic visit or some other event during the week, exhaust themselves, go to bed the rest of the time, and gradually slip downhill. They believed bed rest was some kind of cure. They saw the exhaustion as evidence of sickness, and they believed going to bed was somehow curative. They weren't dying from cancer, they were dying from expectation and bed rest.

Maryl L. Winningham

tion, the befuddlement that frequently overtakes me. This is my acute jet lag of the brain. If they have to ask, they listen.

Dr. Winningham: By cyclopsia, do you mean how you feel when you have this exhaustion, or the ignorance of health care providers who have no idea of what this is like?

Ms. Corbett: Well, it's more, and it's different from exhaustion. It's more that I simply cannot function. There's a difference. But, the answer to your question is both, in a sense. I chose the term *cyclopsia* because of the Greek legend in Homer's *Ulysses*. The cyclops had only one eye and limited vision (eventually he had no eye). That's how I feel sometimes. Most people have not had the experience, the vision, to understand the particular fatigue this word defines. I also chose this word because for most people it is seemingly familiar, so it catches their attention.

Dr. Winningham: This sounds like the term *pneumonia,* which is incorrect without defining the kind of organism or condition that caused it. If the cause is not known, it should be called *pneumonitis.* So it is the etiology that defines it.

Ms. Corbett: Yes. Now *fatigue* is such a wastebasket term. It's now becoming very popular. But we have to learn to recognize the sequelae unique to each particular kind of fatigue and try to associate them with etiologies and mechanisms of pathology. We must learn to identify the precise cause of the fatigue in order to treat it.

I want to repeat that: We need specific research that addresses and differentiates causes of fatigue and cognitive impairment. Then we need research to design interventions. It is truly a multidimensional problem.

Another problem is that of communication. Patients often don't know how to communicate what is happening to them or what is different. They don't have the words that plug into the professional vocabulary. That's where art may be useful. Metaphors may help communicate experiences.

Dr. Winningham: Like "Swiss cheese memory"?

Ms. Corbett: Exactly. It helps communicate a dimension that is not verbal. Don't forget, with extreme fatigue, whether related to specific head injury or not, your mind is not functioning at its best. How do you bridge that gap? The professionals don't comprehend (and some even doubt), and the patients can't explain. In the end, the patients are frustrated and little is done to change the situation and find solutions that work. That's where I was different; I found ways to get help in adjusting to this. No, it wasn't 100%, but it helped me cope better in terms of everyday living. And it was something that could be done. My scientific background has been very helpful to me. I know how to design scientific studies, how to analyze for flaws. I look upon this as a scientific study with an "n=1." So now I look at me. One of the problems is, again, that the experts who make up tests and interventions don't truly understand. They haven't experienced it; they can't put themselves in the "Swiss cheese" frame of mind. They don't know how to test for it, how to identify it, and they certainly don't understand how it affects everyday life. If they see you on a good day, they can't imagine that you have bad days when you can barely function, so they only see a very biased piece of the story. That is not objective observation, which is supposed to be the basis of good medicine, and it certainly is not good science.

Dr. Winningham: Do you have anything you would like to pass along to those who are struggling with experiences similar to yours? Things you have learned that have helped you?

Ms. Corbett: By far the most helpful thing for me was our family discussion with the rehabilitation staff. It verified that I indeed had deficits that were disruptive to the family. Like I said, it gave my husband and the boys the chance to ventilate their frustrations and ask questions. It gave us a chance to troubleshoot in a way that had positive and constructive outcomes. This is a family problem, not just an individual problem. It affects every member.

Dr. Winningham: How are you doing now?

Ms. Corbett: I think I am doing quite well. I still have occasional problems with memory and aphasia. I use "whatchamacallit" and "thingamajig" a lot and describe an object when I can't find the word for it. I let people know I have these difficulties. I still have my "dead brain days" now and then, but they are fewer and farther between. I need my naps and my family agrees that I should do whatever I require to function better. They take my down days in stride. I am continuing to look for ways of overcoming my problems, like ways to conserve my mental energy and to reduce commotion and stress. I actually see it as rather a fun challenge. My main concern now is whether the damage and impairments from the radiation will plateau or continue on a downhill course. Nobody seems to know the answer to this—it's a wait-and-see proposition. We carefully study my scans for any changes, but I am aware that there was quite a significant time lag between when I noticed problems and when the scans actually showed the damage. I just had my semiannual MRI. There didn't seem to be anything new.

Dr. Winningham: How would you summarize your attempts to adapt to your limitations?

Ms. Corbett: Well, first, I got help. I got it. It was my idea to go to the brain injury clinic. It still amazes me that a referral for rehabilitation of some kind was not offered, especially when you consider the potential benefits resulting from it. I also try to avoid situations that are stressful or physically tiring. If I cannot, I take steps to control the stress. This includes preparing for the situation so that it will take the least amount of energy. I have also learned to say no! I'm learning to take care of myself graciously, but firmly, and without guilt.

Dr. Winningham: From your experience as well as your studies, are there any insights or curiosities you would like to share with other professionals that may stimulate creative problem solving about this problem?

Ms. Corbett: Yes, I have a mixture of observation and intuition. Some of it is simplistic; some is not. My deficits were due to radiation damage. I have tried to be a keen and objective observer not only of the difficulties I have been experiencing, but also of the effect of various interventions we have used. I have noticed a few things, but I do not fully understand the possible significance or the mechanisms underlying them.

The most dramatic improvement that I have had is due to treatment with a daily 30-milligram dose of fluoxetine. My emotional, behavioral, and some cognitive deficits markedly improved. As I understand it, fluoxetine is a serotonin booster. Serotonin is a neurotransmitter. It made me wonder how much of the deficits might be due to problems with the excitability and the electrical-chemical conductivity of the neural membranes. I don't know if this might have anything to do with the death of neurons or selective damage to the neural membranes. Maybe it reflects a problem with the production or storage of the neurotransmitters. I recently read a study where the use of the dopamine booster methylphenidate had markedly improved cognition, apathy, and initiation-related impairments in cancer patients and survivors. I would be interested in finding out if studies have been done on other neurotransmitters such as norepinephrine, acetylcholine, or glycine.

Dr. Winningham: Just as there are probably many etiologies for fatigue, there are likely many corresponding treatments. By the way, the reference about methylphenidate was from a study on brain tumor patients. I would like to caution readers against making assumptions about off-label uses of drugs when there have been no clinical trials to test for efficacy and safety.

Right in line with your speculations on neurotransmitters, I have a hypothesis I'd like to share with you and see what your thoughts are. Remember how you said the physicians wouldn't believe you when you tried to explain your problems? You also talked about how well you did on your neurological tests, and your good-day, bad-day roller coaster. There is a phenomenon regarding the role of excitement and epinephrine on behavior. Tell me, in emergencies or during a period of excitement, can you rise to the occasion and do whatever is necessary to get through?

Ms. Corbett: Yes, I can carry on in an emergency and do what must be done. I get an adrenaline rush. So in that respect, I can carry on. My actions and decisions are sound.

Dr. Winningham: Even on a "dead brain day"?

Ms. Corbett: Yes.

Dr. Winningham: Like the day you went in for rehabilitation testing! Now, tell me, how do you feel afterward?

Ms. Corbett: Afterward, I get prolonged, persistent exhaustion that may last for several days. I have to do what I can on good days to compensate for my bad days when I may be able to do very little.

Dr. Winningham: Are you aware that Florence Nightingale made that observation? She said ill people can do a great deal when they are excited, that they may look quite well. It is afterward that they "crash," and even have trouble sleeping. She said the "afterward" effect was the real indicator of the true state, not the performance. As you probably know, Nightingale was a great observer of illness behavior as well as a public health statistician. We've filled this book with some of her quotes. Unfortunately, 140 years later, we still haven't fully appreciated what she had to say.

Ms. Corbett: I remember reading about her contributions to public health. I didn't know about her excitement observation, but it's true! There is a tremendous cost to excitement. Most people only see you during the "rise to the occasion" time and assume that's how you are. They don't know that may be the exception rather than the rule. And it contributes to erroneous clinical conclusions about functioning.

Dr. Winningham: We talk about "white coat hypertension" among patients who develop high blood pressure when they come into their physician's office. I would like to propose we call this "white coat artifact." I think we have greatly underestimated its effect on our observations of patient functioning. It reminds me of the story of the old lady carrying her piano out of the burning house. I have also observed patients get some kind of temporary amnesia when the physician walks into the room.

   The scenario goes like this:

   Physician: "How are you today, Joe?"

   Joe: "Great, doc. I'm doing fine."

Right before this, Joe had been giving you a 30-minute litany about his aches, pains, and how miserable he is. He was not lying. At that moment, when the physician was with him, he truly felt great. Afterward, he dragged himself out and didn't understand why he felt so deenergized and rotten for the next few days.

Ms. Corbett: You know, that's true. That's a real possibility. Clinics are stressful places at best.

   There are several things I've noticed, intuitive things, but I don't understand the mechanisms behind them. They deal with receptors, I think–maybe they will give some researcher insight for research and treatment. About serotonin receptors: The first thing we tried was fluoxetine; this produced a miracle for me, with respect to cognition. I am not suggesting this may work with someone else. What a difference for me! But–and this is important–it still did not help with physical fatigue or initiative. I still have cognitive problems that are exacerbated by physical fatigue. I think physicians must be open to working with patients on an individual basis to see what works best until we have definitive data based on clinical trials.

   I wonder if the dopamine receptors are associated with this and how. I don't know anything about the brain biochemistry, I'm just guessing.

Dr. Winningham: What would you like to say to the health care providers and experts who read this chapter?

Ms. Corbett: There are several things I would like to respectfully tell them: Patients or survivors experiencing this fatigue syndrome need help. You need to listen carefully to what they are trying to tell you. You need to encourage them to use alternative forms of communication if they cannot find the words; for example, "Can you describe an image in your mind?" "Can you draw it?" "Can you free associate?" Please do not assume that you know and understand what patients are trying to say. Even if you do, it helps them to express it. If you don't have time to listen, send them to someone who does. These people can be helped. We do survivors a great disservice if we do not provide the full range of services needed for functioning and quality of life. We should strive to have integrated oncology and rehabilitation programs of service from the time of diagnosis and treatment, to quality survivorship.

We need to mount a concerted research effort to identify and understand the effects of the various cancer treatments on the human body over time. I know it is a very complex and multidimensional problem, but it is made from our own successes in treating cancer. Mean survival rates are increasing. So, also, is the number of those who now need a focus on the status of their survival. We need to address specific research to differentiate causes of fatigue and cognitive impairment; then we need to address research to effective interventions. Its multidimensionality requires a team approach.

Dr. Winningham: What would you like to say to patients and their families who are experiencing this?

Ms. Corbett: Some people waste a lot of energy—and much of their lives—trying to figure out what happened to them and why. They are angry and frustrated. They keep thinking back to how it was before and wishing they were there. Get over it. You can't change anything; you can't change the past. You have to accept what has happened, establish where you are, and go from there.

I have found that it is helpful to explain difficulties you might have, or that you are struggling with. People won't understand why you sometimes act the way you do. They will try to explain it in terms of their own experience. You have to tell people, to explain to them: I have this deficit, I forget, I get irritable. I don't mean it, but it happens. And do you know what? Now and then someone will cut you some slack. Most of them still won't understand; you have to know it won't change how they react to you. You have to accept that. It's difficult because you are trying to be helpful. You must accept that or you'll always be frustrated and angry.

For much of my life, I was impatient with people who couldn't keep up, who weren't achievers. Now I am the one who can't keep up anymore. As I have learned to be more patient with myself, I have learned to be more patient with others. I have also become much happier.

Be kind to yourself. Do the things you need to do to improve your ability to function. If you need naps, take naps. Do things that make you feel good about yourself. Think of something to enjoy before you get out of bed in the morning. Find the things that comfort you. There will be bad days, and these special comforts can get you through. Maybe it is a favorite song. I have an old prayer, a Navaho prayer called "The Night Way," that gives me comfort and courage when I need it most. It helps me see my way clear and gives me hope. I would like to share it with you:

The Night Way

In beauty may I walk.
All day long may I walk.
Through returning seasons may I walk.

Beautifully will I possess again.
Beautiful birds . . .
Beautifully joyful birds.

On the trail marked with pollen may I walk.
With grasshoppers around my feet may I walk.
With dew about my feet may I walk.
With beauty may I walk.

With beauty before me may I walk.
With beauty behind me may I walk.
With beauty above me may I walk.
With beauty all around me may I walk.

In old age wandering on a trail of beauty,
lively, may I walk.
In old age wandering on a trail of beauty,
living again, may I walk.
Until all is finished
In beauty.

(This prayer is available on greeting cards through the South West Indian Foundation, P. O. Box 307, Gallop, NM 87305.)

PART

V

New Beginnings

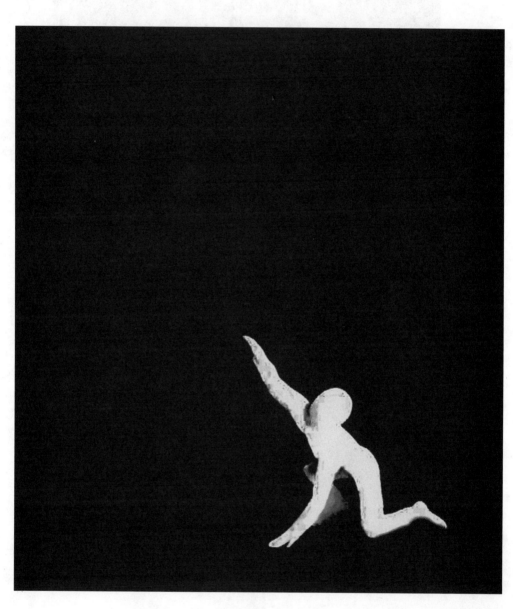

Coming Back

Toward a New
Understanding of Fatigue

Maryl L. Winningham
Margaret Barton-Burke

With our readers, we would like to share this challenge:

Confidence in the Future

I have not lost courage. The misery I have seen gives me strength, and faith in my fellow men supports my confidence in the future. I do hope that I shall find a sufficient number of people who, because they themselves have been saved from physical suffering, will respond to requests on behalf of those who are in similar need. . . . I do hope that among the doctors of the world there will soon be several beside myself who will [share] "the Fellowship of those who bear the Mark of Pain."

Albert Schweitzer, *On the Edge of the Primeval Forest*
and *The Forest Hospital at Lambarene*

One of the great advantages of editing a book like this is that we were the first to read it. We are honored by the insights shared with us by all who contributed to this book. It is fair to assume that anyone reading this book will be challenged by new ways of viewing that amorphous thing called the cancer-related fatigue syndrome (CRFS). One thing is certain: This CRFS phenomenon is *real*, it is *devastating*, it demands *recognition*, and it requires a *response* from all involved in cancer care.

Why did it take so long for oncology professionals to recognize this problem? Although several have been presented, perhaps the most significant reason is that we could not see "the forest for the trees." The CRFS is such a global phenomenon, it affects the most intimate corners of all aspects of life. Perhaps we forgot that for those with cancer, life is about living, not just about tumors, or medical procedures, or blood tests. In oncology, we have been used to looking at discrete measurements such as blood values, x-ray films, tumor size, toxicity scales, cell receptor status, genes, and treatment dosing. We see people for a few moments in time and forget about all the other times. As health care professionals, we have been so consumed with so many detailed things for so long that we rarely take time to stop and see how big the forest really is. These continual breakthroughs and quantifications of the disease called cancer are the trees. To take this metaphor to its logical conclusion, the forest becomes the person or persons with the CRFS. This book is about the many parts of the forest. Treating cancer is not only about finding ways to help people live longer, but also about finding ways to help people live.

Some salient ideas stand out from the chapters and are worth some reflection:

- The entire health care system is physically as well as emotionally exhausting, perhaps even destructive, to people with cancer. Many of the things we do to patients and their families (or ask them to do) are thoughtless and insensitive; they serve to promote anxiety, physical exhaustion, sleep deprivation, physiological insult, and emotional stress. Children with cancer, in particular, seem to be more observant and articulate about this than adults. It is amazing that patients survive at all, despite all the things we do to them!

- As health care providers, we seem to be remarkably unaware of what patients' lives are like. We have little knowledge of how they have to physically adapt and emotionally cope with the effects of the CRFS. Hopefully, this book will help everyone understand a little more of the struggle people encounter as they try to maintain normal lives in the face of the CRFS and other overwhelming symptoms. It is also hoped that we sharpen our assessment skills to see beyond the "epinephrine rush" where people perk up in the hospital or clinic, to the reality of their lives outside.

- There is a great deal of ignorance among health care disciplines regarding the expertise that each of the other team members can bring to identifying and solving the problem of the CRFS creatively. Through multidisciplinary research and practice, multiple solutions can be theorized, and tested, and specific scientifically based interventions can be refined. Tumor boards, rounds, and case conferences would be more useful as we start bringing this material to the table. This book should help each of us understand what other oncology professionals do, or what their perspectives are.

- The experiences and expertise shared in this book should profoundly challenge how we conceptualize the CRFS and motivate us to search for innovative solutions. We are still in the infancy of CRFS research. The implications are enormous. Fatigue is also a major component of the misery associated with most other chronic illnesses. Many things we learn about the CRFS may also be applicable to patients with congestive heart failure, rheumatoid arthritis, acquired immunodeficiency syndrome (AIDS), diabetes, chronic obstructive pulmonary disease, postpolio syndrome, multiple sclerosis, myasthenia gravis, and a host of other illnesses.

- There are literally hundreds of ideas in this book that provide insight into better ways of measuring the many dimensions of the CRFS. Experts from several disciplines have offered a broad variety of viewpoints and information on numerous issues related to the CRFS. By examining the CRFS from this broader perspective, by sharing with investigators from multiple disciplines, it is hoped that revolutionary changes in the field of CRFS regarding measurement, research, and practice will move both our knowledge and our understanding beyond the current state into a new realm.

- We have seen obvious irrationality, permitting patients to become so debilitated as a result of therapy, allowing them to suffer from unnecessary deficits in oxygenation (anemia) and nutrition (cellular deprivation or starvation) at a time when their bodies need the benefit of anabolic metabolism to counter the stress of disease, treatment, and a host of psychosocial and economic threats. This is the hallmark of antiquated medicine! Maintaining nutritional and oxygenation status should be viewed from a broader perspective—as a primary goal for medicine and an integral part of rehabilitation. An enlightened, forward-thinking, prophylactic approach is needed with a view to keeping patients as healthy, as active, and as involved in life as possible during as well as after treatment.

- One of the most remarkable and consistent findings in discussing the contents of this book with its many contributors, as well as those with cancer and their families, was frequent mention of the overwhelming and even long-lasting cognitive effects of the CRFS. Although this has been examined in select studies, it is clear that we have not begun to understand the magnitude of this problem in everyday life.

- It is also clear that the disability and health care systems have been unable to comprehend how the CRFS, a symptom with few or no visible characteristics, relates to disability and impairment. Patients and families need to have the CRFS recognized by the medicolegal system so they can get the help traditionally available to other patient populations. Recent work by Cella and colleagues (1998) features suggested ICD-10 criteria and a brief, structured interview to confirm diagnosis. This is a significant start because it may provide a unified basis for identifying individuals with special intervention needs.

- There are few provisions for rehabilitation of fatigue and cognitive impairment. We need to vigorously pursue rehabilitation efforts and train professionals who are qualified to evaluate and develop appropriate interventions. Beyond this, we need to develop consistent protocols—formats to clarify the nature of the CRFS for employers and disability services–and to provide patient advocacy services for vocational rehabilitation and appropriate employment.

A conclusion usually means the end of something, usually a text, a paper, or a speech. That is not the case with this book, and it certainly is not the case for the topic of the CRFS. With each new and additional chapter in this book, the concept of the CRFS evolved and changed to encompass areas of knowledge and expertise that were not necessarily broached in earlier clinical or research arenas. Tens of thousands of individuals are desperate for help. Someday we may be one of them. No single discipline will be able to find solutions. It will be essential to work together, to share insights and research findings with one another, and above all, to listen to cancer survivors. After all, they are the truest experts on fatigue that we know.

Reference

Cella, D., Peterman, A., Passik, S., Jacobsen, P., and Breitbart, W. (1998). Progress toward guidelines for the management of fatigue. *Oncology, 12,* 369–377.

Index